"*Civic Medicine* offers a striking and pathbreaking perspective on medical knowledge in early modern Europe. Transcending influential approaches in which physicians and patients are viewed as caught up in the networks of the medical marketplace or else of modernising territorial states, Mendelsohn and his team focus instead on the role and activities of physicians in civic office across the continent. This provides a stimulating, holistic vision of the early modern physician and his world, now grounded in an enriched sense of community rather than the market or the state."
 – *Colin Jones, co-author of* The Medical World of Early Modern France

"At last we are beginning to understand early modern physicians as full-fledged members of their urban polities, holding offices, taking oaths, and entering into the world of the experts who knew how to employ paper technologies. According to the authors of this volume, even the attentiveness of physicians to carefully written descriptions of medical cases arose more from civic humanism than from medicalization, medical police, professionalization, the new science, or even commerce. In revisiting the history of city physicians, these studies offer new insights into medicine's civic past."
 – *Harold J. Cook, author of* Matters of Exchange: Commerce, Medicine, and Science in the Dutch Golden Age

W0113644

Civic Medicine

Communities great and small across Europe for eight centuries have contracted with doctors. Physicians provided citizen care, helped govern, and often led in public life. *Civic Medicine* stakes out this timely subject by focusing on its golden age, when cities rivaled territorial states in local and global Europe and when civic doctors were central to the rise of shared, organized written information about the human and natural world. This opens the prospect of a long history of knowledge and action shaped more by community and responsibility than market or state, exchange or power.

J. Andrew Mendelsohn is Reader in History of Science and Medicine in the School of History at Queen Mary, University of London, having previously taught at Imperial College London.

Annemarie Kinzelbach has published extensively on medicine, health, and society in early modern Germany.

Ruth Schilling trained in early modern urban history and is Junior Professor for the History of Science at the University of Bremen and scientific coordinator of exhibitions and research at the German Maritime Museum.

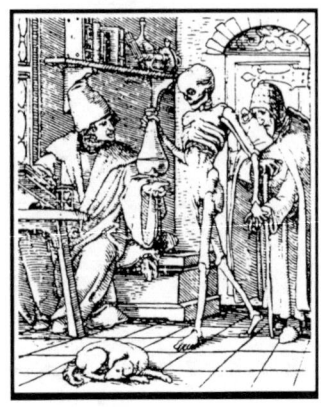

The History of Medicine in Context

Series Editors: Andrew Cunningham (Department of History and Philosophy of Science, University of Cambridge) and Ole Peter Grell (Department of History, Open University)

Titles in the series include

Pathology in Practice
Diseases and Dissections in Early Modern Europe
Edited by Silvia De Renzi, Marco Bresadola and Maria Conforti

"It All Depends on the Dose"
Poisons and Medicines in European History
Edited by Ole Peter Grell, Andrew Cunningham and Jon Arrizabalaga

Health and Welfare in St. Petersburg, 1900–1941
Protecting the Collective
Christopher Williams

The Afterlife of the Leiden Anatomical Collections
Hands On, Hands Off
Hieke Huistra

Civic Medicine
Physician, Polity, and Pen in Early Modern Europe
Edited by J. Andrew Mendelsohn, Annemarie Kinzelbach, and Ruth Schilling

For more information about this series, please visit: www.routledge.com/The-History-of-Medicine-in-Context/book-series/HMC

Civic Medicine

Physician, Polity, and Pen in Early Modern Europe

Edited by J. Andrew Mendelsohn, Annemarie Kinzelbach, and Ruth Schilling

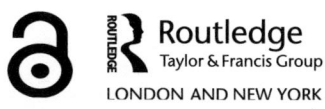

Routledge
Taylor & Francis Group

LONDON AND NEW YORK

First published 2020
by Routledge
2 Park Square, Milton Park, Abingdon, Oxon OX14 4RN

and by Routledge
605 Third Avenue, New York, NY 10017

First issued in paperback 2021

Routledge is an imprint of the Taylor & Francis Group, an informa business

British Library Cataloguing-in-Publication Data
A catalogue record for this book is available from the British Library

Library of Congress Cataloging-in-Publication Data
A catalog record has been requested for this book

ISBN 13: 978-1-03-209058-0 (pbk)
ISBN 13: 978-1-4724-5358-7 (hbk)

DOI: 10.4324/9781315554693

Typeset in Sabon
by Integra Software Services Pvt. Ltd.

Contents

Figures and Table

Figures

Cover: Frontispiece of 1,300-page encyclopedia or "Treasury of All Medical and Natural Things," with vignettes of knowledge and practice surrounding a physician writing at a desk beneath rays of sunlight behind a crowned eagle with sword and scepter, symbolizing enlightened government. Johann Jacob Woyt, *Gazophylacium medico–physicum, oder Schatz–Kammer medicinisch– und natürlicher Dinge* (Leipzig: Lankisch, 1761). Courtesy of Charité, Medical Humanities: Bibliothek für Geschichte der Medizin und Ethik in der Medizin, 14195 Berlin, Thielallee 71

Table

Contributors

Laura Di Giammatteo studied history of philosophy at Chieti and Pisa and completed her doctorate at the Istituto Nazionale di Studi sul Rinascimento, Florence, on *Magia e medicina a Helmstedt: l'insegnamento di Aristotele, Melantone e Bruno nell'Academia Iulia* (2013). She has held scholarships at the Warburg Institute, the Herzog August Bibliothek, and the Forschungszentrum Gotha and was a member of the ERC-funded project Ways of Writing: How Physicians Know, 1550–1950. Her most recent publication is "Liddel's *Ars Medica* (1607): The Effective Method as Foundation of Medical Knowledge and of Ethics," in Pietro Daniel Omodeo and Karin Friedrich (eds), *Duncan Liddel (1561–1613): Networks of Polymathy and the Northern European Renaissance* (2016).

Fritz Dross studied history and information science at the Heinrich-Heine-University in Düsseldorf and is Assistant Professor at the Institute for the History of Medicine and Medical Ethics at the Friedrich-Alexander-University Erlangen-Nürnberg. He has authored many articles on early modern and modern medicine and *Krankenhaus und lokale Politik um 1800: Das Beispiel Düsseldorf, 1770–1850* (2002). He works mainly on medicine in urban environments, history of leprosy and of epidemics, and the history of hospitals. His recent publications include two co-edited volumes of the annual journal *Historia Hospitalium* (2016 and 2017) and "'Man Does Not Live by Bread Alone': Feeding Confraternity in Early Modern Nuremberg Leprosaria," *Food & History*, 14 (2016).

Annemarie Kinzelbach has published extensively on medicine, health, and society in early modern Germany. She has been affiliated with the universities of Ulm, Berlin, Erlangen-Nürnberg, and Heidelberg and was a member of the ERC-funded project Ways of Writing: How Physicians Know, 1550–1950. Her recent publications include *Chirurgen und Chirurgie-Praktiken: Wundärzte als Reichsstadtbürger 16. bis 18. Jahrhundert* (2016) and "Medicine in Practice: Knowledge, Diagnosis and Therapy," with Stephanie Neuner and Karen Nolte, in Martin Dinges et al. (eds), *Medical Practice, 1600–1900: Physicians and Their Patients* (2016).

Elaine Leong recently joined the Department of History at University College London, having led the Minerva Research Group on Reading and Writing Nature in Early Modern Europe at the Max Planck Institute for the History of Science, Berlin. She has held Wellcome Trust and Leverhulme Trust Fellowships and has published widely on early modern science and medicine. She co-edited *Secrets and Knowledge in Medicine and Science, 1500–1800* (2011) and is the author of *Recipes and Everyday Knowledge: Medicine, Science, and the Household in Early Modern England* (2018).

J. Andrew Mendelsohn is Reader in History of Science and Medicine in the School of History at Queen Mary, University of London, having previously taught at Imperial College London and held visiting professorships at the Ecole des Hautes Etudes en Sciences Sociales (Paris), Université Pierre et Marie Curie Paris VI, and Tel Aviv University. He has published on knowledge and society, from the sixteenth to the twentieth century, in German, French, British, and U.S. history and co-led the ERC-funded project Ways of Writing: How Physicians Know, 1550–1950. His recent publications include "Common Knowledge: Bodies, Evidence and Expertise in Early Modern Germany," with Annemarie Kinzelbach, *Isis*, 108 (2017) and "Empiricism in the Library: Medicine's Case Histories" in Lorraine Daston (ed.), *Science in the Archives: Pasts, Presents, Futures* (2017). His current project is on the European *longue durée* of physicians in governance and the methods of empirical inquiry and judgment this generated.

Gianna Pomata is Professor of the History of Medicine at Johns Hopkins University. Her research interests include the social and cultural history of European medicine in the early modern period, women's and gender history, and the history of historiography. Her publications include *Contracting a Cure: Patients, Healers, and the Law in Early Modern Bologna* (1998); *The Faces of Nature in Enlightenment Europe*, co-edited with Lorraine Daston (2003); *Historia: Empiricism and Erudition in Early Modern Europe*, co-edited with Nancy Siraisi (2005); and an edition and translation of Oliva Sabuco, *The True Medicine* (2010). She has worked on the history of epistemic categories, genres, and practices in early modern European medicine, with particular attention to medical empiricism and its role in the history of scientific observation. Her current work takes a cross-cultural approach to the history of medical genres and epistemologies, and she is writing a cross-cultural history of the medical case narrative. In 2016–2017 she was a Fellow of the Wissenschaftskolleg zu Berlin.

Valentina Pugliano is Research Associate and Lecturer in History and STS at the Massachusetts Institute of Technology, having previously been a Wellcome Trust Fellow in the Department of History and Philosophy of Science, University of Cambridge, and a Junior Research Fellow of Christ's College, Cambridge. Her research interests encompass the social and cultural history of medicine, craft technology, and science in southern Europe and the

Mediterranean world in the early modern period. She is currently completing two books: the first, based on her doctorate completed at Oxford University, on the role of Italian Renaissance pharmacy and its artisans in the development of early modern natural history; the second on the network of diplomatic medicine and public health established by the Venetian Republic in the eastern Mediterranean and the Mamluk and Ottoman Levant, ca. 1400–1730. Her recent publications include "Pharmacy, Testing and the Language of Truth in Renaissance Italy" in the *Bulletin for the History of Medicine*, which received the Jerry Stannard Memorial Award 2017, and "Natural History in the Apothecary's Shop," in E.C. Spary et al. (eds), *Worlds of Natural History* (Cambridge University Press, 2018).

Marion Maria Ruisinger trained in medicine and medical history and is Director of the German Museum of the History of Medicine in Ingolstadt as well as adjunct professor at the Institute for the History of Medicine and Medical Ethics at the Friedrich-Alexander-University Erlangen-Nürnberg. She has authored many articles on early modern medicine and *Patientenwege: Die Konsiliarkorrespondenz Lorenz Heisters (1683–1758) in der Trew-Sammlung Erlangen* (2012). Her fields of research include medical museology, history of surgery, history of patients, and healthcare in modern Greece.

Ruth Schilling trained in early modern urban history and is Junior Professor for the History of Science at the University of Bremen and scientific coordinator of exhibitions and research at the German Maritime Museum and Leibniz Institute for German Maritime History. She was a member of the ERC-funded project Ways of Writing: How Physicians Know, 1550–1950. Her publications include *Stadtrepublik und Selbstbehauptung: Venedig, Bremen, Hamburg und Lübeck im 16. und 17. Jahrhundert* (2012), and a biographical study of a town physician, *Johann Friedrich Glaser (1707–1789): Scharfrichtersohn und Stadtphysikus in Suhl* (2015).

Sabine Schlegelmilch is Assistant Professor at the Institute for History of Medicine, University of Würzburg. She trained in classics and German literature in Würzburg and London. Her interdisciplinary doctoral thesis in classics, archeology, and Egyptology was published in 2008. Most recently, she is the author of *Ärtzliche Praxis und sozialer Raum im 17. Jahrhundert: Johannes Magirus (1615–1697)* (2018), focusing on a town physician, and co-edited *Medical Practice, 1600–1900: Physicians and Their Patients* (2016). In addition to medical theory and practice in the sixteenth and seventeenth centuries, her research interests include medicine in film and television.

Michael Stolberg holds the chair in history of medicine at the University of Würzburg. He is the author of many articles and books on early modern medicine, including *Experiencing Illness and the Sick Body in Early Modern Europe* (2011) and *Uroscopy in Early Modern Europe, 1500–1800* (2015), and recently co-edited *Medical Practice, 1600–1900: Physicians and Their Patients* (2016). He coordinates a long-term database project on early modern physicians' letters (www.aerztebriefe.de) and is currently working on a book on the world of learned medicine in sixteenth-century Europe, drawing especially on physicians' personal notebooks, practice journals, and correspondences.

Acknowledgments

This book is the product of the first of three working groups convened as part of the research project Ways of Writing: How Physicians Know, 1550–1950, led by Volker Hess (Charité University Medicine Berlin) and Andrew Mendelsohn (Queen Mary, University of London) and funded by the European Research Council (AG 295712).

The authors met three times in 2013–2014 for intensive discussion of initially very rough ideas and drafts and continued to collaborate in writing and revising in 2014–2016. The third meeting was a collaborative workshop of the ERC project at the Charité Berlin Institute for the History of Medicine and the Minerva Research Group Reading and Writing Nature in Early Modern Europe led by Elaine Leong at the Max Planck Institute for the History of Science.

We are grateful to Stefanie Voth and the staff of both institutions for helping make these meetings possible. Colleagues at both institutions and from other universities generously contributed as commentators and discussants. For this our hearty thanks go to Lars Behrisch (Utrecht), Dominique Brancher (Basel), Tricia Close-König (Strasbourg), Oliver Falk (Charité Berlin), Silvia de Renzi (Open University), Alexa Geisthövel (Charité Berlin), Kaspar von Greyerz (Basel), Alexander Kästner (Dresden), Ursula Klein (MPIWG Berlin), Harun Küçük (UPenn), Sebastian Kühn (FU Berlin), Marion Mücke (Berlin-Brandenburg Academy of Sciences), Roberto Poma (Université Paris-Est), Christelle Rabier (EHESS Marseille), Thomas Schnalke (Berlin Museum of Medical History), Claudia Stein (Warwick), Mary Terrall (UCLA), Klara Vanek (Munich), and Alfred Stefan Weiss (Salzburg). We are grateful to series editors Andrew Cunningham and Ole Grell, former Ashgate editor Emily Yates, and Routledge editor Max Novick for enthusiasm for the book and editorial support.

Chapters were completed in 2015. The manuscript was reviewed in 2016. Revision or editing of chapters was completed in 2017. References after 2015 in the notes are confined to updating details on previously forthcoming publications.

Introduction
Civic Medicine

J. Andrew Mendelsohn

Communities great and small across Europe for eight centuries have bound doctors by oath of office and contract for public service. Physicians provided citizen care, helped govern, and often led in public life. *Civic Medicine* stakes out this timely subject by focusing on its golden age, when cities rivaled territorial states in local and global Europe and when civic doctors were central to the rise of shared, organized written information about the human and natural world. This opens the prospect of a long history of knowledge and action shaped more by community and responsibility than by the market or the state, exchange or power.

Two narratives animate how we understand medicine and society in past and present. One starts from above, from doctors. It runs from academic learning through patronage and corporation to expertise and the state, professionalization, scientization, medicalization, biopolitics. The other starts from below, from patients. It runs from the body and illness through recipes and regimens to the plurality of healers and remedies, demand for and production of drugs, whether materia medica or modern pharma, the medical marketplace, healthcare in consumer society. The first story is about control. The second story is about choice, or culture. *Civic Medicine* proposes a third narrative. It is about community. It starts "from between," from communication. It runs from the city—polity as *polis, civitas* more than *urbs*—through civic medical office, healthcare for all, written interaction and administration for the "common good," the medical republic of letters within and not aloof from *res publica*, the medical public sphere. This volume outlines and situates this story through case studies, surveys, and historiography. Civic community and responsibility for health promise as rich a history of knowledge, values, norms, and practice as those traced by power, in all its theorized and historied forms, and by economic and cultural exchange. These narratives are ultimately all one; written information and interaction are central to all three; and this volume explores their interweaving. Yet each tells something different about what medicine, knowledge, and society have been and can be.

This volume began from the idea that studying physicians in civic office would be a good way to get at knowledge and polity in history. There

DOI: 10.4324/9781315554693-1

were several reasons to expect this. Medicine meant both natural and social knowledge. It meant practical and liberal arts as well as sciences. Physicians comprised by far the largest group of occupational knowers of the human and natural world until the nineteenth or perhaps the twentieth century. Most medical public office has been civic. This meant it has been local yet—doctors being doctors, cities being cities—highly networked, even global. And this meant civic medicine has been very widespread and long lived. Governance was a key area alongside natural history and philosophy, humanist scholarship and information management, translation and publishing, and organized science, in which physicians acted, and often led, beyond their practice as healers. Our hypothesis is that these activities were all related. They were related not so much by ideas and ideologies—of the body and body politic—as via practices that became common to the life of learning, both with and beyond books, and the life of community. Since late medieval times, these shared practices have increasingly been practices of writing. More specifically, they have been practices of written information and interaction and indeed written-down oral interaction. This hypothesis promised, finally, to relate local polity and public service to empirical renewals of medicine and natural inquiry throughout these centuries and especially in the sixteenth and seventeenth. For recent work had pointed to civic doctors or official "town physicians" as creators of new genres of observation and masses of it.[1] Somewhat unexpectedly, along the way of this collective inquiry, a new picture of the early modern physician and his world began to emerge: a picture of community of wellbeing more than "medical market" or "medical police," in which physicians stand out from the many other healers as writer-communicators at the core of their polities.

Polities, historians have recently shown, are made as much of interactions as of institutions. These interactions tend to be rich in information and productive of it. Digging behind discourses and theories, seeing in the archives not only sources but the media of past society, historians here and there since the 1980s and everywhere since the late 1990s, have unearthed communicative practices of governance and everyday local political interaction. Historians have also learned to see practices of scholarly information and communication; of reading and writing, both learned and vernacular; of scientific observation and matters of fact; of print and publics; and of expertise in society and polity. These have been pursued mainly as separate histories. To study civic doctors would be to study their confluence. And it would be to try to understand knowledge and polity without starting from big concepts, each with the specificities and limitations of having been developed around sources from one or another of these domains and one or another period much shorter than the many centuries traversed by political communities and their physicians.

We soon found we would have to work on foundations. For virtually no systematic attention has been paid to physicians' civic activity.[2] It appears mainly in older local histories and biographical studies and in more recent histories of urban medical systems.[3] The only historical survey of the "town and state physician" is now nearly 40 years old (1981). It is organized by national context, with chapters on Italy, France, Germany, and so on.[4] This gives a static picture if taken as more than the important groundwork it was. The present volume offers instead primarily an analytical and subject-defining study without pretense to coverage of time and place, yet also the beginnings of a dynamic map of physicians' civic activity—of communities, knowledge, and practice in motion, in Europe and beyond. Instead of a chapter on Germany, there are three. Two are set in one metropolis of commerce, the arts, humanism, printing and the book trade—Nuremberg—yet in nearly opposite guises: on the one hand, as a city-state that bound *all* resident doctors to the commonwealth by oath of office (Chapter 4 by Dross); on the other hand, as a crossroads of global information and an epicenter of civic doctors' unofficial public and publishing action (Chapter 11 by Kinzelbach and Ruisinger). Warsaw in the early eighteenth century became the capital of a newly constituted kingdom and thus a case for studying what happens when a royal physician becomes involved not in court culture or diplomacy, but in the public life and published construction of a capital city (Chapter 9 by Schilling). Instead of touring Italy in a few pages, the reader will visit two very different places in detail: grand Milan and humble Mesagne. Unusual among Italian health boards, Milan's had physician members with executive powers as well as duties of counsel and reporting. This makes Milan not one case study but a window on the relations between executive administrative function, being a learned physician, acting for a community's health, and making natural knowledge—and how all this happened in and around work on paper (Chapter 5 by Di Giammatteo and Mendelsohn). Mesagne in Apulia, at the opposite end of Italy, was a typical town with its *medico condotto*. Not every such place and its civic doctor generated knowledge or novel information, but Mesagne shows what kind of knowledge could be generated when this did happen—namely, civil and natural history, ethnography, *observationes*—and with what effect on knowing disease (Chapter 8 by Pomata). Nördlingen was a free Imperial city in the Holy Roman Empire: like Mesagne, a town with its doctor in office, but offering, in this case, through its unusually well-preserved city archive, a study in the practice and politics of the most common form of evaluative activity: certification (Chapter 6 by Kinzelbach). The chapter on Prague is less about Prague in particular than about the learned physician in general making—literally writing—his way in communal rather than academic or court life (Chapter 2 by Stolberg). Venice, the trading empire, invites writing about somewhere else, which its *medici condotti* did when they were elsewhere. The Venice chapter is about Damascus, its Venetian *condotto*, and his doctor's diary, and hence two polities in one (Chapter 7 by Pugliano). A host of towns and cities appear in Chapter 3 by Schlegelmilch, a survey of communication between physicians and local authorities seeking services for their communities.

This book includes no chapter on an academic medical center like Padua, Paris, Leiden, or Edinburgh. Medical culture in these places tended to be more scholastic than civic, or divided between court and faculty, as it acrimoniously was in Paris.[5] Or was that in fact generally so? Further study may tell. Meanwhile, academic medicine is not missing from the story. Appropriately, it appears in translation and translocation—from Latin to vernacular, from Montpellier university lecture halls to English households via London as political and printing center of a public as much as domestic medicine (Chapter 10 by Leong).

This puts England on a map from which it has been largely missing.[6] The still standard survey on the town and state physician lacks a chapter on England, where few such offices existed or lasted long. That was far from the case in Spain and the Low Countries, though they too are missing from the 1981 volume and appear here only in Chapter 1 by Mendelsohn, leaving major opportunities for research. France did appear in the 1981 volume on the town and state physician. This is no less intriguing than England's absence, for early modern France had virtually no permanent town physician offices like those elsewhere in continental Europe and the chapter instead mainly concerns occasional royal distribution of free medical supplies in the provinces. Absence of offices like *medico condotto* or *Stadtarzt* or *protomedico* or *stadsgeneesheer* or *archiatro* need not mean absence of any version of the history suggested here. No place in Europe escaped the public sphere of medical print.[7] Moreover, as the present volume shows, the story of civic medicine is not only of official functions, but also of the unofficial public life of communities.

The approach was to mobilize available historical expertise on mostly little-known archival and published material to address a series of simple questions—simple but with wide implications. These structure the volume as follows. First, entrée. How did physicians enter at all into community life? Often outsiders, how did they belong, so as to be able to take action? The answer appears to be: less distinctively as healers (here they were part of the greater plurality of practice around health, illness, and well-being, from astrology to bone-setting to dietetics and provision of remedies) than as scholar-communicators. To be good at this was to keep journals and notebooks of local information (Chapters 2 and 7). To keep account was not only to run the business of one's medical practice, but to be accountable. Second, office and service. What brought and bound together physicians and the communities they served? What were the shared values, expectations, agreements, and forms of communication? Exploring the archives reveals an evolving apparatus of oaths, contracts, and instructions and a remarkably vibrant and competitive world of candidacy for office, with acquisition and evaluation of credentials and know-how (Chapters 3 and 4). There was a lot more going on here than patronage or perfunctory officeholding. What sorts of knowledge and capacity were valued, and why, become important questions. Third, knowing and intervening. What did physicians do in and around office as scholar-communicators? In what ways did they serve? And how did this relate to knowledge-making, health care and the healing art, political community and public affairs? Evaluating and reporting (Chapters 5 and 6), documenting and locating or localizing (Chapters 7–9), translating and translocating or perhaps universalizing (Chapters 10 and 11): these three preliminary answers emerged by synthetic overview (Chapter 1) of the case studies comprising this volume and of wider published and archival sources, as well as several mainly unconnected historiographies. Chapter 8 delves more deeply into the most specific question at hand: in what ways did being physician to a community affect how physicians understood disease and wrote it down? Fourth, scope and interface. These questions run throughout the volume. Was the civic in fact local? In what ways and with what implications does civic medical office show generality and portability of values and practices beyond the local? How transportable were civic-doctor functions among polities and cultures? Did civic medicine have a wider geography that could revise our primarily diplomatic, colonial, and imperial interpretations of European medicine abroad (Chapter 7)? What interfaces were there with the royal court (Chapter 9), household and university (Chapter 10), republic of letters and commercial enterprise (Chapter 11), and wider sphere of vernacular print (Chapter 10)? The approach and conclusions of this volume can be tested on places not covered here by taking seriously multifaceted physicians' full biographies, looking beyond medical practice, and focusing on what the everyday written word did.

Notes

1 Gianna Pomata, "Sharing Cases: The *Observationes* in Early Modern Medicine," *Early Science and Medicine*, 15 (2010): 193–236. Notes in this introduction have been kept to a bare minimum; for historiography, see Mendelsohn, "Public Practice," Chapter 1 of this volume.
2 Two members of our group had begun working in this direction: Ruth Schilling, Sabine Schlegelmilch, and Susan Splinter, "Stadtarzt oder Arzt in der Stadt? Drei Ärzte der Frühen Neuzeit und ihr Verständnis des städtischen Amtes," *Medizinhistorisches Journal*, 46 (2011): 99–133.
3 Another member of our group had pioneered in this research: Annemarie Kinzelbach, *Gesundbleiben, Krankwerden, Armsein in der frühneuzeitlichen Gesellschaft: Gesunde und Kranke in den Reichsstädten Überlingen und Ulm, 1500–1700* (Stuttgart, 1995); a large and recent example is Elisa Andretta, *Roma medica: anatomie d'un système médical au XVIe siècle* (Rome, 2011).
4 Andrew W. Russell (ed.), *The Town and State Physician in Europe from the Middle Ages to the Enlightenment*, Wolfenbütteler Forschungen, 17 (Wolfenbüttel, 1981).

5 Colin Jones, "The Médecins du Roi at the End of the Ancien Régime and in the French Revolution," in Vivian Nutton (ed.), *Medicine at the Courts of Europe, 1500–1837* (London, 1990): 214–67.
6 But see Steve Sturdy (ed.), *Medicine, Health, and the Public Sphere in Britain, 1600–2000* (London, 2002).
7 On the language of public good in early modern English medical publishing, see Mary Fissell, "The Marketplace of Print," in Mark Jenner and Patrick Wallis (eds), *Medicine and the Market in England and Its Colonies c. 1450 – c. 1850* (New York, 2007): 108–32.

1 Public Practice

The European *Longue Durée* of Knowing for Health and Polity

J. Andrew Mendelsohn

Since around 1980, medical history has innovated by refocusing from physicians to patients and disease. Patient-centered historiography revitalized the history of medicine and opened vistas of social and cultural study: of health and the variety of healers, of the body, of the medical market, consumer, and household. But this came at a cost. It turned the physician into a doctor. He was more.

Four times he was appointed Bürgermeister of Chemnitz in Saxony: Georg Agricola (1494–1555), physician. Every new student of the history of science and technology encounters Agricola as the author of the great humanist technical work *De re metallica*. Few remember that he was a physician by training and practice as well as civic doctor or medical officer (*Stadtarzt*, often translated as "town physician") and a head of government. Through his scholarship and correspondence, he moved in a world of knowledge as wide as global Europe, yet he was also doubly bound to the civic community in which he practiced medicine: by the oath of mayor and by that of medical officer, which made him an administrator of poor relief among other duties. He was also inspector of schools. Agricola's public activity extended beyond the civic sphere: he served as official Saxon historiographer and as a diplomat between city and court.[1] Though unusually prominent, Agricola is nonetheless exemplary of the public function of physicians in early modern Europe and of the centrality of written communication to that multifaceted activity, which are twin themes of this volume. A later example from a very different part of Europe is Epifanio Ferdinando the Elder (1569–1638). A life-long town physician (*medico condotto*) in the southern Italian region of Apulia, the mayor of his town and its leading historian, Ferdinando also advised regional rulers and wrote a health regimen for the Pope. He authored an important collection of medical cases and pioneered the ethnography of illness and healing ritual: his classic description of tarantism (from Taranto, the main city of Apulia) is still read by anthropologists today.[2] From the sixteenth through the eighteenth centuries and indeed before and beyond, physicians across Europe—north and south, Catholic and Protestant (and pre-Reformation), agrarian and protoindustrial—fulfilled a range of public functions while

DOI: 10.4324/9781315554693-2

practicing medicine and contributing to knowledge. Many doctors' working lives were more civic than academic or corporative or commercial. And
contrary to modern concepts and realities of "civil society" as opposed to
"the state," physicians' civic activity comprised both.[3] Even individually
paid—or what we call "private"—medical practice belonged, in many communities, to public duty for the common good.[4] This frame invites repicturing the early modern physician and his world. That world stretches
back, in many ways and places, to the thirteenth or fourteenth century and
up to the twentieth.

There is a wider point to this. Our understanding of natural knowledge
in the age of Renaissance and Scientific Revolution (and down to the present) has come to be profoundly economic. Knowing emerges from and for
making, and therefore also exchanging, and in some narratives dominating.
Values and practices of producing and consuming, of prospecting, collecting, trading, possessing things and information about them and how to use
or make them, comprised much of natural history as well as the chemical
and mechanical arts and sciences, including materia medica. Yet this may
be only half the picture and thus a distorting view to boot. Physicians
figure in it, but even more centrally in the missing half: natural knowledge
emerging from and for political community (rather than commerce or the
fiscal-military state); from and for the political and juridical activity of
living together amid disagreement, inequality, and uncertainty (rather than
from and for making and exchanging, or taxing and making war). Can
a profound relationship be demonstrated between natural knowledge and
polity—in addition to the market, the workshop, the colonial or trading
empire, and the territorial state, yet perhaps also affecting how we see
them?[5] We could do worse than begin by keeping "polity" historically and
theoretically vague and examining those with civic doctors.

To go back to looking at doctors would be retrograde. Instead, we can look
through their lives at the practices and values that intersected in their activities, especially those of physicians active in office and public life. I mean this
as a one-sentence program of research.[6] It is based on two observations. First,
even in functionally less differentiated societies, like those of early modern
Europe, physicians stand out as major figures of intersection. Second, the
practices that intersected in physicians' lives were mainly of communicating
rather than—as with many other knower groups—of making, or of measuring, counting, and calculating.[7] This communicating was not primarily rhetoric, the usually recognized distinctive contribution of Renaissance men of
letters to public life. It was descriptive, evidentiary, evaluative, and often
explanatory about observable events, materials, and conditions in the human
and natural world. These points comprise the specificity and generality of
studying knowledge and society by studying physicians. In so far as apothecaries, barber-surgeons, and midwives were figures of intersection and fulfilled public functions, which in many places they did, they too come into this
story.[8]

Thus, there is a second wider point to repicturing the world of the early modern physician. His multifunctionality highlights differences of domain against the background assumption (made influential through the sociology of Talcott Parsons and more recently Niklas Luhmann) that what makes premodern societies premodern is that they are less differentiated into functional systems—politics, religion, economy, science, law, art, medicine, sport, and so on—than are modern societies. Therefore, the assumption continues, for understanding societies and their historical development, it is important to study the processes of differentiation or, to cite a similar concept from history and sociology of science, boundary work.[9] Medical history has long done something similar by studying professionalization, corporatism, and medicalization.[10] Instead, the multifaceted physician invites us to discover empirical rational practices that cut across areas of social life, corporative groups, institutions, and occupations—practices, moreover, that did not wane amid the differentiations of modernity, but grew over a *longue durée*.[11]

At the core of this chapter is an attempt, especially in Section III, to work out what some of those communicative cross-cutting empirical rational practices were. Moreover, this attempt should show that these activities created information yet did more than inform; that they made knowledge without being *for* making knowledge; and that they progressed—became ever more refined, elaborated, comprehensive ... these will be observations in search of a language—without being progressive. And, finally, it should show that they were practices more of the common good than goods exchange; and of polity in the root sense of *polis* rather than *state*. Serving the common good, let it be clear from the outset, is not to be confused with altruism. Public office was a burden that physicians sought. It brought income and could help them climb socially and professionally. However, physician officeholding is not to be confused with disguised self-interest. That physicians could gain from it does not reduce the whole to this for that, patrons and clients, and the pursuit of status.

This brings us to a third and indeed unavoidable wider purpose in repicturing the world of the early modern physician: to work out a new model of knowers acting for the common good. Civic medicine does not fit existing models. Nor does it share their problems and limitations. Three major ones emerged in this same period: Renaissance civic humanism and its Christian variant (Erasmus, Vives); the social policy side of the Reformation (and its Counter- and Radical variants); and the rise of university graduates in public administration, perhaps also "cultures of expertise" in public life.[12] These three modes of knowers acting for the common good might be called classical, Christian, and expert. Education and poor relief feature in all three. Therefore, because education usually involved physicians as teachers or writers and poor relief was arguably the "major context" of early modern health care provision,[13] physicians can be found at work in all three yet altogether fit none. The model suggested by looking at physicians in public life will not apply everywhere but has the instructive benefit of being less subject to what Natalie Davis in 1968 called the "debate on the *engagement* of humanists in civic affairs," a debate that became an impasse to this day.[14] Preoccupation with sincerity and motive has obscured the deeper question of the historical forces and forms through which learned knowers acted in civic affairs and with what effect.

To set up these arguments (Sections I–II) requires introducing into the history of science and medicine what can be regarded as a recent revolution in how we understand past politics and government. It also requires setting aside categories like state and civil society. The civic doctor pertained to both. I use polity—from *polis* in the sense of political community—to encompass both, making distinctions as needed. Implications follow for history and theory of knowledge and society and prospects for research (Section IV). Finally, Section V looks beyond 1800 toward the present. Throughout, the notes provide extensive though far from comprehensive historiography based on several mostly separate research literatures.

From Meaning and Culture to Knowledge and Polity

If asked about medicine and society in early modern Europe, a historian would have to decide which of several mostly separate stories to tell, or hope the listener would be all ears and happy with miscellany. There are histories of plagues and public health or "medical police," of charity and poor relief, of hospitals in all their variety. There are histories of practitioners and patients, households and the medical market and patients as consumers, of corporative organization (guilds and colleges of physicians, surgeons, apothecaries) and unlicensed practices around it. There are histories of universities and medical education, of anatomy, surgery, materia medica, learned medical theory and practice, relations among the four main healthcare groups, and their growing regulation by government, not to mention wider histories of healthy living and cultural meanings of health and disease. All of these stories are important, yet the increasing evidence is that each is not a patch in a quilt but an artificial slice out of an interactive whole, in which, moreover, the interaction was crucial to the creation and development of the activities themselves.[15] Moreover, what was shared was not only meaning—cultural history's main focus—but knowing. And as only some of the stories in the collection have ostensibly been about knowing, historiography has until recently tended to foreclose asking how people knew (including knowing what to do and how) and prevented opening this question from epistemology of learned medicine to all of the stories in the collection.[16] To be sure, historiography since the 1980s has yielded useful organizing concepts: the medical market, medical pluralism, and corporative medicine, or putting it all together: "corporative medical community + medical penumbra = medical world." Yet even these capacious organizing concepts are themselves *about* plurality (of healers and healthcare) and, moreover, leave the rest to encyclopedic overview.[17]

That which we thought we were done with, the doctor's perspective, offers a way out. The point of departure is the physician in civic action, often through public office but also beyond its duties. There is a justification for this. If we look at doctors in the history of health and healing before 1850, they get a relatively small chapter, and women turn out to be the main providers.[18] If we look at doctors in the history of polity and community, we find them central. This is especially true of what I shall call plural Europe, the decentralized Italian, German, Dutch, and Swiss political spheres in which cities and towns were either sovereign or more or less self-governing. This perspective puts the centralized monarchies of France and England, traditionally dominant in historiography of science and medicine after the early 1600s, in a new light. It may also help situate medical Spain.[19] The centrality of physicians to civic life is especially true of the period roughly 1500 to 1800. This period began when permanent municipal health offices were established or, where they already existed, were newly filled by university-educated physicians instead of practitioners trained by apprenticeship. Where medical office had been limited mainly to a contract for healthcare, as with the medieval Italian town physicians or *medici condotti*, in the sixteenth century it expanded in public functions.[20] This is therefore the period that began when communities *made* doctors integral to local governance and civic life—in ways that touched the lives of many and perhaps most inhabitants. The contrast could not be greater with the early modern physicians likely to be most familiar to Anglo-American readers and to appear in a course in history of medicine: namely, the College of Physicians of London with their distinguished representative William Harvey and their modern descendants denying the very communicability of the medical art. In their "detachment from active political life, ... isolation from civic responsibilities," and "studied avoidance of the public realm," the English metropolitan medical elite was not only atypical of medical Europe, it was the tiny polar opposite of a whole continent of civic medicine.[21]

No historical survey of early modern doctors in public life has been attempted in the nearly 40 years since the proceedings of a conference on the town and state physician held at the Herzog August Bibliothek in Wolfenbüttel appeared in 1981.[22] To build now toward a synthesis is, first, to move from surveying the offices to studying the practices of their holders in depth; second, to recognize and explore doctors' multifaceted public activity beyond civic office or even, in England and France, in its relative absence;[23] and third, to take the civic doctor less as a topic in itself than as a key to open up study of knowledge and society around political communities and public good rather than market, court, and state. For these reasons, though town and court have largely separate historiographies, physicians at court also belong in the picture.[24] They too were multifaceted, and some of their activity was similarly public.[25] Moreover, physicians with court appointments often also had civic ones at some point in their lives or even at the same time; and in some cities where the court resided, royal physicians fulfilled the functions of town physician, as they did in Hanoverian Celle until 1671.[26] Finally, barber-surgeons, apothecaries, and midwives belong in the picture. Their practice, too, was in many ways public.[27] And they, too, had public functions beyond medical practice, some in common with those of town physicians, such as certifying, reporting, and testifying.[28]

Why study physicians at all in order to learn about things public? The old intertwined answers are, in chronological order: professionalization, state-building, and some version of social disciplining or rationalization. From as early as the thirteenth century, physicians' corporative activity exemplified or even led the emergence of the professions and their role and power in society.[29] From the sixteenth and seventeenth centuries, as guilds and other corporative bodies "became agents of central government," corporative medicine "was skilfully woven into the fabric of the modern state," and physicians in office served, alongside jurists and pastors, as administrators in state-building and among its rank and file on the ground.[30] And from the eighteenth century, they contributed knowledge, norms, and practices to the creation of "modern" disciplined, productive individuals and populations, a process so closely related to health that it is often regarded, following Michel Foucault, as medicalization or biopolitics.[31]

None of these grand medical narratives of modernity has been rejected at the macro-historical level of a "before and after" contrast. But their underpinnings in social and political history are under major revision. All see too much in terms of the state or control, however subtly these are conceived. All overestimate power and regularity, whether from above or in pervasive human technologies, especially in cities but even on the land. All ignore the sheer volume, vigor, and reciprocity of political communication between authorities and citizens or subjects at all levels of society, communication that was important enough to be written (or put from speech into writing) and archived by government. A few historians studying medicine and government in the archives saw this, and took a critical turn before much of social and political history did, but medical history was headed elsewhere and their work was not followed up.[32] Meanwhile, in the 1990s, increasing numbers of historians moved from studying political discourse and constitutional, administrative, and legal history to the history of governing practice and political interaction in localities. What they found was not rule from above, which turned out to be far weaker than it had once appeared in the minutely regulating ordinances of the "well-ordered police state," in draconian pre-Enlightenment penal codes and punishments, in the theory and symbolic practices of absolutism, in cameralist treatises and machine metaphors of government, and in later imagery of the state and how it "sees."[33] They found enormous participation in governance, initiative from below, and less obedience and domination (as in Max Weber's three forms of legitimate rule or *Herrschaft*) than constantly negotiated consensus.[34] Thus an urban polity—and there were several kinds, from the independent sovereign city-state to the federated one to the capitals and administrative centers of territorial states—in the vast swathe of Europe that still appears in state-of-the-art history of medicine and science as the home of "Enlightened Despotism" and "authoritarian, reactionary states"[35] was often something more like an Aristotelian *polis*, a republican political community governed by an elected council. There was inequality of wealth, standing, and political influence (as there is in modern liberal democracies), but also vigorous political communication—petitions, elections, supplications, grievances, accusations, denunciations, outright revolt, tactical avoidance—and constant negotiation of consensus. Even the politics and governance of a Habsburg territory in the age of "absolutism" defies analysis and description in standard oppositional terms of discipline and disturbance, obedience and resistance, rule and cooperative association, "above" and "below." And an in-depth study of a city whose economic elite was unusually able to prevent political participation reveals not smooth control and production of subjects, but centuries of conflict.[36] Across the spectrum, interaction itself—oral, written, performed—constituted the polity among social and political unequals. None could escape, though each could try to use, the ideals and values of good government, *bonne police, gute Policey*, peace, justice, and the "common good," which can be understood as the community-based opposite to the more familiar "reason of state" in early modern politics.[37] Moreover, as histories of state-building "from below" have got longer and wider, histories of the public sphere or informed public opinion and communication as a political force, in dialog with the ideas of Jürgen Habermas, have stretched back from the eighteenth century to the Middle Ages.[38]

Something similar is happening in history of knowledge. Studies are showing how descriptive and explanatory knowledge were generated and not only transmitted in oral and written communication.[39] Participation in the making of natural knowledge is now found to have been far wider than once assumed: "from below," but also horizontally from outside the usual learned groups and institutions.[40] Thus by *communication* in this chapter, I mean not language, representation, discourse, meaning, or culture, but interaction and more specifically *interaction with a surplus*—of information generated or transferred or tested or used in some other documented way.

The method proposed here is therefore to concentrate (1) on the places where physicians most held office and participated in public life and where the unit of government was also a political community, that is, cities and towns rather than territorial states; and (2) less on the canon and discourses of medicine, science, and politics than on acts and practices of communication, with a surplus. These included both talk and ink rather than manifesting transition from oral to written and print culture.[41] The new political history lends far-reaching meaning to the occasional remark found in medical historiography that the doctor's perceived capacity to "give counsel" made him "the indispensible interlocutor of other *experti et probi viri* [i.e., experienced and virtuous men]—judges, urban officials, priests [or pastors], inquisitors—who consulted him to deliberate with competence and rectitude in complex situations requiring multiple approaches."[42] The social history of medicine may have run its innovative course. Its operative terms seem redundant ("social" or "cultural"), or placeholders for an uncertain object of study ("medicine," or is it health and wellbeing, healing, the body, disease and culture, or, following the logic of medicalization or biopolitics or the health consumer and *souci de soi*, what is it not?).[43] A new political history of knowledge, or rather a knowledge history of polity, with physicians at its core, beckons. This would be not a history of medicalization or biopower, or prescriptive analogy between body and body politic, medicine and government.[44] Nor more generally would it be a history of knowledge shaped by political interests, nor of co-production of natural and social order or of "science" and the "state" and its subjects (since neither was necessarily being produced).[45] It would be a history of ways of knowing and ways of living together. Both were abuzz with communication. Knowing was less dominated by learned elites than we think. And living together ranged from more to less equal yet was usually constrained above as well as below by powerful norms, because the powerful depended on negotiated consensus. This would be less a knowledge history from below than a knowledge history "from between" and "on the ground," where physicians found themselves with everyone else.

From Standing in Society to Acting on and for It

If the doctor's perspective is going to tell us anything new about knowledge and society, then the way to begin is not with the learned physician in the learned world, the scholar among scholars (we have a rich and growing history of this), but with the scholar at large.

But where in society and wherefore? Social mobility and self-fashioning, patronage and privilege, rank and distinction, status and habitus—these form an important first stop in this inquiry.[46] It must not become the last stop. Moreover, looking at doctors in the polity, rather than among their own, alerts us to the fact that there are two relevant stories of social place and its behaviors rather than one. Both are deeply shaped by Pierre Bourdieu's concepts of social practice and the forms of capital. They bear differently on what writing did for physicians and what physicians did with writing. On the one hand, book-ensconced in their portraits, often pen or paper in hand, physicians' self-fashioning partook of scholarly habitus.[47] On the other hand, from ruffed collars in the sixteenth century to powdered wigs in the eighteenth, physicians adopted civil and courtly dress, manner, speech, and hand. In the last of these, however, they could turn to advantage what they had, and elites of council and princely court did not: years of training in the written liberal arts and humanities. And they could address a slightly different audience, or even the same one, for purposes of acting on as well as standing in the polity. The gold-headed cane was good for positioning in aristocratic and patrician life; the well-wielded plume, for positioning in the *civitas* and carrying out its responsibilities. A few physicians accumulated wealth; many accumulated notes—hundreds or indeed thousands of pages of excerpts and observations, hundreds or thousands of often information-rich letters, not to mention objects of art and nature.[48] A learned physician's mastery of the arts of writing (and reading and listening) and the information in his often voluminous notebooks were capital not only for standing alongside governing elites—or just behind them, in processions and ceremonies—but also for acting alongside them in governance. Like many a doctor, Ferdinand Jakob Baier, a town physician or "Physicus" of Nuremberg from 1730 to 1773, as well as a counselor and first physician ("Consiliar. & Archiater") to the Margrave of Brandenburg, inherited his father's working archive of notes and cases, just as a son might inherit wealth. When, as was equally typical, the son published some of this capital—30 precious forensic cases (which the father Johann Jacob had made his own though they were signed by the medical faculty of which he had been dean)—he displayed his academic family's accumulated medico-political savoir-faire, and indeed son like father was elected president of central Europe's most important learned scientific society, the Academia Naturae Curiosorum, or "Leopoldina."[49] Yet by publishing, he also made this knowledge capital available as guidance to other physicians and collegia on *how to* in public affairs.

How to *be* with words is one chapter in the story of physicians and their political communities; how to *do* with words is a whole series of chapters. The former is a story of distinction (Bourdieu), of being learned; the latter, of interaction, of learning—and continuing to learn. Understood as an historical anthropology of how societies learn through the intersection of writing and political life, Jack Goody's work is a more relevant guide than Bourdieu's.[50] If learned practices distinguished physicians from most others around them, they were equally a means by which physicians acted in the world and learned from it.[51] The physician was a man of letters yet, as so many doctors' full biographies show, this was letters often in the service of things public. Agricola used his erudition and learned practices to make himself useful in novel ways to the polity—evaluating systems and problems of weights and measures, analyzing and synthesizing information about natural resources and practical arts and industry to improve them. Doctors who published nothing important did the same, just less usefully. Writing in classical forms of verse and letters integrated Agricola's younger contemporary, the Bohemian physician Georg Handsch, into the civic sphere of Prague. Scholarly methods of note-taking and commonplacing (*loci communes*) used in the library also got him out of the library and made the learned doctor a learner at large, who paid close attention to what townsfolk knew about health and who accumulated this knowledge for use.[52] This was not only scholarly practice at work. It was scholarly impetus.

Scholar in town, scholar in office: the second way to begin is with the fundamental fact that starting around 1500, and earlier in the Italian and Iberian peninsulas, the learned physician was hired as such by society, that is, by communities and governments, which had previously been happy to hire barber-surgeons as town medical officers.[53] Physicians' academic training was valued less for its content than for its form: advanced oral and written communication.[54] We might expect this meant the arts of rhetoric and oratory that were revived in the Renaissance and marked the entry of scholars into political life. That appears not to be the case. Communities were not looking to hire a medical Cicero. What they valued was the ability to take up forms of written communication with which the writer had little or no previous experience (and in which there was no formal schooling) and adapt those forms for various purposes. Physicians demonstrated this particular ability to write—not literacy as such but political literacy—by performing it in the application for public office. Such applications were modeled on a more general form of everyday political writing, the supplication, which—along with the petition, the grievance, the accusation, the notification, and formal ways of responding to all of these, as well as the certificate and the written counsel (*consilium, Gutachten*) and generally all manner of official reporting, inquiry, and correspondence—were the written ways in which political communities perpetuated themselves through continual rounds of conflict, uncertainty, disagreement, inquiry and information-gathering, negotiation, decision, and the pursuit of interests.[55] Thus communities sought competence in something broader than the healing art, yet which medicine exemplified in the scope of its interaction with social groups and strata: being adept at learning how to carry out increasingly paper-based forms of living together. In short, medicine was *this*, too—as much public as "private" practice. Or it was becoming so in this period.

Applying for office involved the physician in formal modes of political community. Assuming office did the same, for this was done by swearing an oath or signing a contract or both. Oaths of office were both written down in record books and performed orally, and indeed renewed annually in ceremony at the town hall.[56] This made civic doctors just like any other officeholder or corporation whose integration into the polity and specific functions were expressed in the most binding way known to premodern societies.[57]

Office could mean primarily a contract for medical services to the people of a community, as in the medieval post of *medico condotto*.[58] Office could also mean a range of public duties including but also extending far beyond the provision of care. This was true of the *Stadtarzt* position in German, Swiss, and Dutch towns and cities (sometimes classicized by its holders as *poliater*, from *polis* and *iatros*, physician, later replaced by the term *Physicus*) and that of *Archiater*, chief physician, in large cities or city-states. It became increasingly true of the *condotto* post in Italian towns in the later fifteenth and sixteenth centuries, though already in medieval times these included duties of reporting on wounds and deaths.[59] Office, finally, could mean public functions alone, to the exclusion of attending patients, as in the Spanish, Italian, and Austrian post of *protomedico*: whether as head of a medical collegium or as presider over a health "tribunal" (the Spanish model), or as a single appointment by a city council, sometimes, as in Milan, an appointment to a health board alongside jurists and a presiding senator.[60] In the larger Italian cities, the *condotti* system was replaced altogether by a new surplus of doctors. Doctors' public functions expanded enormously in the fifteenth and sixteenth centuries through the creating of medical colleges with regulatory and administrative functions, and new posts such as *protomedico, provvisatoria alla sanità*, and health officer for plagues. Their functions also expanded through the creation of lay health boards to which physicians gave counsel or, in some places, belonged. By the sixteenth century in Italy, "every Collegiate physician was, in a real sense, a state doctor," which in practice meant primarily local governance.[61] In northern Europe in the seventeenth and eighteenth centuries, territorial governments appropriated and expanded the town physician model into that of the *Physicus* or medical officer responsible for an urban or rural district.[62]

Historiography hitherto has aimed to work out this institutional variety as well as influences across Europe and change over time. Yet despite this complexity, the duties of civic doctors can be relatively easily listed: provision of health care to those unable to pay for it; examining wounded or dead bodies for purposes of justice; examining the sick poor for allocation to hospitals; providing reports and written counsel on a wide range of publicly relevant cases or on more general questions of the health, environment, and resources of a community; serving on health boards or adjunct to them; inspecting pharmacies and developing pharmacopoeia; overseeing medical services (barber-surgeons, apothecaries, midwives) and medical education or even providing public instruction; working with authorities to enforce laws against unlicensed practice; organizing response to epidemic disease and indeed remaining in town to do this; and administrating poor relief. By the eighteenth century, *Physici* were being required to catalog local plants and other naturalia, investigate their properties and utility, and research and compose medical geographies.[63]

Physicians' public activity, moreover, reached far beyond even this expansive job spec.[64] Various kinds of polity invited various wider modes of physician involvement and initiative in public life. These ranged from the physician as mayor (Agricola in sixteenth-century Chemnitz) to the chief health officer serving on administrative boards with jurists and senators (Alessandro Tadino in seventeenth-century Milan), to the royal physician active beyond the court in a capital city (Christian Heinrich Erndtel in eighteenth-century Warsaw), to the physician hired by one city to work in another city altogether—on public payroll for taking care of envoys and citizens abroad and for diplomatic reporting alongside (Cornelio Bianchi acting medically for Venetian trade and political presence in sixteenth-century Damascus). Public writing was another mode of involvement and initiative in community life, ranging from the doctor as local historian and curator of a community's ongoing construction of itself through historical memory (many examples in polities great and small, from Venice to Epifanio Ferdinando's Apulian town) to the physician as a creator of everyday public information and an organizer in ink of shared cumulative and predictive experience by putting out an annual almanac (Johannes Magirus in seventeenth-century Anhalt) or by editing and publishing a learned news and review weekly (the Nuremberg medical collegium in the eighteenth century). Still another mode was to be involved in creating and sustaining civic institutions of useful knowledge, such as the city botanic garden for training doctors and apothecaries founded in Bologna in the sixteenth century while the scholar-naturalist Ulisse Aldrovandi was *protomedico* and a senator, his home, too, an internationally networked civic institution, as a constantly growing, frequently visited encyclopedic museum and archive of the natural world. And finally there was the physician as civic teacher: from the public lecturer in anatomy, such as Frederick Ruysch and Nicolaes Tulp in Amsterdam, to the city instructor and examiner in everything from midwifery to natural philosophy, such as the celebrated humanist scholar and naturalist Conrad Gesner, *Stadtarzt* of Zurich, to the seven civic doctors who in unbroken succession from 1589 to 1660 taught *Physik* in the north German county seat of Schleusingen at the regional Gymnasium, an activity the Leopoldina recognized in its rosters, for any teaching role from the doctoral to the municipal, as "Prof. Publ."[65]

From many examples like these, three concentric spheres of activity and responsibility can be discerned: that of public office, non-medical as well as medical; that of the civic beyond official duties; and that of still wider communication—from learned societies to the republic of letters to vernacular medical publishing to the diplomatic and news networks of Europe, the Mediterranean, and beyond.[66] These spheres and wider networks differed from one another. Yet much of this activity beyond office belonged to sustaining and bettering polity.

It is easy to miss what is remarkable here. The physician did not have to be an altruist to do all this. Nor did he have to be a reformer. And though everything in this whole constellation of public activity was shot through with goals and values of the common good, these belonged to no particular moral and intellectual tradition of what the good is and how to achieve it, either classical or Christian. Unlike, say, poor relief by redistribution of wealth, poor relief by civic medicine excited little dispute. That makes it exciting for us, because it takes us, in Braudel's metaphor, below the storms and even the great swells of political history into its oceanic currents and *mentalités*. Civic medicine was not mainly what eloquent learned men, whether Ciceronian or Erasmian or Lutheran, exhorted communities to do.[67] It was what communities legislated and contracted for themselves—from learned men.[68] Major problems and limitations in the existing models of learned knowers acting for the common good fall away. Such models are dogged by doubts about sincerity and motive, about the usefulness of higher learning for real politics, about political and religious divides and disagreeing traditions and reformations that prevent or scuttle action for the common good. Here, in contrast, the claim is, first of all, not about motivation. It is about the forms that knowing and doing took, and on this there can be no doubt (if also much more research to do). Second, civic doctors had civic real jobs, with a list of routine duties. Of course, the "common good" was rhetoric. Yet in oath, contract, and performance of duties detailed therein, it was grimy reality, too. Civic doctors were, in our terms, permanently on call— not just in a hospital but in a whole town, or at least one of its districts. They shared this burden with barber-surgeons and midwives, yet had overall responsibility as well as weekly duties on the ground, if not, as physicians, always hands-on. On Tuesday mornings in Zurich around 1560, the world's greatest bibliographer and one of Europe's most well-connected scholars oversaw examination of the sick poor for allocation among the city's several hospitals.[69] Third, civic responsibility conferred status and drew clientele. It could have been a mere stepping-stone or, if we take seriously complaints about the burdens of office, a millstone around the neck. It was both and neither. *Physicians* hung onto civic office. Felix Platter achieved wealth, status, fame—and stayed in office.[70] Gesner threatened to die from overwork —and stayed in office.[71] Christoph Friedrich Pichler, an obscure eighteenth-century *Physicus*, struggled in uncooperative local situations and fought for his salary and inspection fees for 25 years—and stayed in office.[72] In success and in plight we see the same pattern. Does it matter—can the historian ever really know—whether this was because the status of office was too good to give up (especially to someone else to whom one would then have to answer) or because it gave doctors a way to do good, to be civic? Perhaps precisely the truth of both made the system work. For some 400 or more years, depending on where you look, physicians in plural Europe competed for burdensome, (sometimes badly) remunerated civic responsibility. That could help explain the remarkable *longue durée* growth and functioning of physician-led early modern urban health and welfare systems. It also helps make sense of the anomaly that the intellectual cream of western medicine, in plural Europe, was unusually prone to die of plague, despite the Hippo-cratic injunction to flee. Only where civic medicine's political and legal foundations were far weaker, as in England, or where Calvinism under-mined them, as in the Netherlands, was there a way out (literally of town) —via the argument that a physician's real duty was not to stay with the sick, but to preserve his future utility to the commonwealth by flight.[73] The untimely plague deaths of civic doctors are monuments not to heroic altruism or to some implausibly virtuous sincerity of medical civic human-ism, but to the sheer convergent force of its forms, at once legal, moral, social, political, intellectual, and economic. Forces and values that could keep entire medical city-states going in this way could easily power civic medical intellectual production. This brings us back to knowledge and the pen. The humanist's chief practice for the common good was rhetoric. On this, the whole controverted historiography agrees.[74] But following the civic doctors takes us into very different, no less communicative ways of writing for the public good.

Values Across Spheres, Values in Practice

What can we learn from studying the intersection of myriad domains in the working lives of civic doctors? The long list of those domains includes poor relief, book publishing, editing periodicals, public administration, hospitals, curative medicine, natural history, civil history, geography, local recordkeeping, public health, administration of justice, *police* and *Policey*, counsel to magistrates or governing councils, diplomacy, learned corres-pondence, regulation of trades, municipal teaching, literary and oral cul-ture, botanizing excursions, collecting, and household production and consumption. Logically the gain must lie in the discovery of a relationship among what intersects.

Toward that end, it would be possible to parse civic doctors' multifa-ceted activity into written forms and practices of communication, informa-tion, and knowledge.[75] Take the studies in this volume. Parsing the activity of Dr. Handsch in Prague this way would show us poetry, letters, com-monplace books; Dr. Bianchi in Damascus, a diary; Dr. Ferdinando, a town chronicle, case histories, and mayoral paperwork. The Milan study would reduce to a table of bureaucratic forms, one of which, certificates, would be the subject of the chapter on a German Imperial town where such documents have survived in large numbers. Other chapters would be about genres such as the supplication, the oath, and news in the early peri-odical; and the chapter on Warsaw would contribute to "history of the book" as would the chapter on London. There is not much mileage in this exercise.

Taking the physician's perspective(s) will not yield some new history of communication and its media, information and its management, print and reading, scholarly or humanist method, paper practices from note-taking to tabularization. Nor will it contribute much to the history of rhetoric and literary form as the main mode of learned contribution to public affairs. But it will allow us to identify cross-cutting activities of community and polity—of judgment and decision-making, membership and account-ability, negotiation and control, material and political sustainability—that do things with words about things for communal ends rather than mainly persuade communities by eloquence. And taking physicians as the lens helps sort this activity into some basic forms.

Evaluating/Reporting

Was this man poisoned? Did that woman abort her pregnancy? Can this person be excluded from town because his bodily condition endangers others? Should that person be admitted to charitable community care? Can this marriage be annulled because of impotence? Or that one because of a concealed family history of melancholy? Is this plant product what the merchant claims it to be? Is that a recipe for a recognized drug? What are the qualities of this mineral spring? These are the sorts of question put increasingly to doctors as we move forward in time through late medieval and early modern Europe.[76] All involved evaluating bodies, substances, and environments in situations of uncertainty, disagreement, potential danger, or perceived injustice, or indeed claims to the miraculous. Answering required empirical rational practice—some form of observation or information-gathering, often accompanied by inquiry into causes and an explanation, and reasoning to a recommended decision. Answers came in the form of oral testimony, certificates, *rapports, consilia, responsa*, judgments (*judicia*), *Gutachten*, and so on.

Hitherto only the "forensic" fraction of such activity has received sustained attention from historians.[77] This has been construed as expert testimony in juridical trials since medieval times and, by the seventeenth century, elaboration of legal medicine by figures such as the celebrated Roman physician Paolo Zacchia, *archiatro* of the Papal states and regular medical counsel to the Roman Rota, Catholic Europe's highest court of appeals.[78] The point I wish to make here is threefold. Virtually *all* civic doctors—and sworn surgeons and midwives—dealt with questions like these. They did so at one level or another of proceedings that were, moreover, far more common and diverse than full-blown trials. And the knowledge and practice of doing so was not specialized. A few uniquely placed figures like Zacchia certainly became expert specialists and formulated a "medico-legal" field of expertise, but this was only the cutting edge of the ubiquitous ongoing judging activity of physicians (among others) in and for communities, their individual members, and their governments.

Even early modern drug trials can be seen as part of this wider activity of evaluation for the common good, for resolving disagreement, uncertainty, or possible rule violation, as, for example, in the preparation of medicines. Properties of preparations known or claimed to be materia medica could be evaluated by reading recipes rather than by trying experimentally.[79] And, conversely, evaluating the condition of human bodies could involve various tests in addition to visual and physical examination.[80] Thus procedures as seemingly diverse as determining the nature of a simple or composite substance, the cause of a death, the efficacy or safety of a concoction, the nature of an illness in fact shared practices of observing, testing, reasoning, such that physicians and faculties published collected cases of them under the common rubric of *consilia, responsa*, and so on.[81] In ways only now being explored, physicians' public judgment activity was related to, but not the same as, judging the condition of a patient for prognosis or prescription, the logic and results of which were also written in the form of *consilia*.[82]

Though certificates and *consilia* appear to be as old as spoken testimony, evaluation and judgment increasingly took written and documentary form.[83] So did disagreement over results. And when disagreement overloaded the mechanisms of negotiation, violence ensued on paper. Thus, we find in the south German Imperial city of Nördlingen in the 1590s one medical officeholder tearing apart a certificate issued by another—and yet the torn certificate was reassembled and duly archived in the city hall.[84] The controversy concerned competence to intervene medically yet showed that this had become little distinguished from competence to certify. So paper-bound was competence that, whereas to disagree with another official's judgment was to criticize it in writing, to deny competence to judge altogether was to rip it up. The point holds more broadly. Competence meant being able and allowed to use certain paper-enabled practices that made certain things happen, documented the process, and often justified or explained it. The case of the Milan health board shows how tightly ordered the forms and their authorship were, the further we move into executive powers. In order of ascending exclusivity: Milanese town physicians could write an *avviso* and nothing higher than that in the hierarchy of reporting; the *protophysicus* and the two *conservatori di sanità* could write a *ragguaglio* or a *provvisione*; and only the *conservatori* could write a *grida*.[85] These can be regarded as bureaucratic forms, yet they also comprised a rationality of reporting, of how to judge and intervene on an empirical basis, which therefore was much more elaborated in its method and particulars than the political theory of *prudentia* or whispered counsel to a ruler.[86] Questions of form and structure are more interesting here than those of authority and expert status, though historiography has tended to focus on the latter. Knowledge in the polity sometimes meant power; it always meant constraint—acting only by rules and genre, resolving disagreement only in structured ways. So much was this so that these modes of description, analysis, causal reasoning, evidence, proof and argument flourished in domains as apparently diverse as bureaucracy and family: observed in official proceedings yet also privately archived and handed down from father to son, as we saw from J.J. Baier to his son F.J. Baier, as accumulated knowledge and know-how—worth saving on paper and re-reading, as a basis for acting on and for the polity.

Naturalia as well as human bodies, places as well as cases, came under physicians' evaluative gaze and pen. Physicians in office evaluated vegetable, mineral, and animal substances when they inspected apothecary shops for the public good. They evaluated shipments of such substances when these became the object of commercial controversy.[87] On request or as part of their regulatory duties, doctors inspected, monitored, and judged specific sites of what we would call natural resources, industry, and environment: the qualities and hazards of airs, waters, and places, including places of production such as mines and places of consumption such as mineral springs, rivers, and spas. For these belonged not only to the "Hippocratic" physical geography of a region and its "natural particulars," but also to the geography of its economic and health resources recognized by governments.[88]

All these can be treated as separate topics, as they have been in histories of public health, chemistry, medical practice and consultation, pharmacy, natural history, mining, learned medicine, court medicine, domestic medicine, secrets of art and nature, recipes, legal medicine, and regulation of medical services. Or, looked at synthetically, they can all be seen as instances of evaluation and judgment. This happened according to a set of cross-cutting empirical rational practices. These occurred variously as inquiries, trials, inspections, tests, visitations, and critical reviews of written evidence. Much of this, moreover, belonged to the ubiquitous values and proceedings of social, economic, and environmental regulation known as "good police" (*gute Policey, bonne police*) for the "common good." This was underway for centuries before cameralist writers in the later eighteenth century hived off a specific field of "medical police."[89] And it was the query-by-query, problem-by-problem counterpart to the now better-known activity of evaluating the resources of a whole territory: from the Domesday Book to colonial data-gathering to history of local "natural riches" and cameralist survey. Physicians were deeply involved here, too. When J.J. Baier was not busy with his duties as Nuremberg town physician or, as dean of its nearby medical faculty, judging public cases like those later published by his son as an *Introduction to Forensic Medicine*, he was busy researching the natural history of Nuremberg's territory, especially the value and utility of its minerals, and writing one of the important early local mineralogies.[90] Physicians' natural historical activity has a place in the history of science. To what extent did physicians' case-by-case public judging activity contribute to natural knowledge or to ways of knowing that were useful beyond that activity itself? There is room for further research here. Yet in work that has not received the attention it deserves from historians of medicine, Paula Findlen showed that even "policing the [medical] profession" was part and parcel of scientific culture in early modern Italian urban polities and that civic doctors with public regulatory responsibility were at the core of that scientific culture.[91]

Documenting/Locating

Reports often documented sites and situations as well as evaluating them for decision-making. Thus, much evaluative practice was also documentary practice, and the latter spanned still wider. It is well known that early modern physicians renewed the ancient practice of documenting cases and published these in the form of *observationes*. Civic doctors led this trend,[92] which is now considered central to the renaissance of observation and "empiricism" in the sixteenth and seventeenth centuries.[93] Besides cases, they also began documenting much else: the natural and civil worlds around them, in both present and past; geography and climate; practical arts, their associated natural histories, and whole areas of material production, as Agricola did for mining and metals. On the one hand, such documentation took diverse forms, from manuscript casebooks to published *centuriae* of *observationes* to chronicles of cities or states to a book like a Saxon royal physician's *Warsavia physice illustrata* of 1730, mixing geography, natural and civil history, ethnography, summary of prevailing diseases, cataloging (of plants), and weather tables.[94] On the other hand, the effect of documenting was to *relate* diverse domains through practices of *historia*, commonplacing, taking protocol, or making lists.[95] To dwell on this point would, however, be to see histories of writing, of practices that, though they might take on a life of their own and shape uses and effects, were not carried out for their own sake.[96] Diverse domains were also related through the fact that the documenters were physicians in communities and often to them.

Community meant, first, opportunity and even onus to learn what was locally known, or to learn from what was locally observed, tried, or claimed. Thus, activities as diverse as bioprospecting, data-gathering for natural histories, tapping into folk therapeutic wisdom, conversing with gardeners, sharing recipes, or writing and reading how-to manuals can be seen as different dimensions of listening, especially in communities where listening was likely to bring something new.[97] This could be in a familiar place or an exotic one. And Europe's often fast-growing towns and cities were in a sense both, especially to physicians, who tended to be peripatetic until settling into practice and civic posts with residency requirements, at which point correspondence replaced travel.[98] Integrating himself into Prague in the sixteenth century, Bohemian physician Georg Handsch filled his days with speaking and listening and filled thousands of notebook pages with people's sayings and observations, their medical proverbs and recipes, stories, and so on.[99] Cities and towns were dense with communication, both oral and written. Opportunities abounded to note down what one heard or read. This was a more interactive, continuous, and widely usable method than that of the published call for proverbs issued by the Chancellor of the Faculty of Medicine at Montpellier, Laurent Joubert, to gather the material for volume 2 of his genre-setting book, *Popular Errors* of 1578.[100] Physicians' campaigns against "popular error" documented as much as it disproved, or merely disapproved. Moreover, *both* the documentary impulse and that of critically evaluating assertions of what's what, what causes what, or what works to what effect can be seen as roots of Baconian science. Illustrating Warsaw, the new capital of Poland-Saxony in the 1720s, as an investigable and improvable medico-physical metropolis, royal physician Erndtel compared what he heard people say about the forms and virtues of particular local plants or the sightings of creatures— like the basilisk—with what he could find in the library or archive on these topics.[101] The chronicles penned by the many doctors who wrote their local civil and natural histories depended on written and oral sources and so exemplified second-hand empiricism rather than the first-hand kind by which medicine is usually known for its empirical renaissance: *autopsia*.[102] And second-hand empiricism meant documentary communication and community. Whether in extensive *loci communes* or mere diary jottings to jog memory, physicians learned from their communities and about them, thereby making themselves members and potentially better practitioners.

Community meant, second, being an object of study. This usually meant writing the past or present or both, as a basis for action or prescription or legitimation. Civil history by physicians varied in purpose (from humanist scholarship to official historiography), in scope (from the local to the global), in subject matter (sometimes including health and disease, sometimes not), and in period (from ancient to contemporary, or combining both).[103] Civil and natural history most came together with each other and with knowing, treating, and preventing disease, when civic doctors wrote about their places of observation and action. Even when patronage and personal service to a prince was paramount, as in the case of Baccio Baldini, who signed his biography of Cosimo de Medici as "his protomedico," this position, far from being solely that of a courtier, brought with it the civic sphere of knowledge, responsibility, and action. This included the city's natural and engineered environment, as Baldini made clear in the commentary he published on the Hippocratic *Airs, Waters, Places*. There, he focused especially on the waters of Florence—documenting and evaluating the health qualities and pollutants of its rivers, its water supply and sewerage systems, ducal projects of draining marsh into salubrious and useful land. Writings on place by physicians of Rome focused more on its baths and springs.[104] Writings on place by the leading physician of eighteenth-century Beaune in Burgundy focused on its vineyards and their associated issues of environmental and occupational health. He knew these through the charitable public practice that comprised part of his clientele of 800 patients, and through the regular observations he made of weather, prevailing disease, social behavior in the town, and crops in the fields, "uncovering the inner workings of Beaune's environment and society." All this was documented in case notes accruing to 5,500 pages, which he fittingly bequeathed to Beaune itself rather than a medical son or colleague.[105] And writings on place by the sixteenth-century physician

Tommaso Rangone, better known as a wealthy patron of the arts in Venice, focused more on its climate and "airs," in a regimen he researched and composed for the city. It was the first such work in Italian for the good of a whole urban polity rather than the health of an individual patient.[106]

By the eighteenth century, physicians were writing medical "topographies" of their cities or regions, a task some governments made obligatory for town and provincial medical officers. These were part history part geography, mixing the political and natural.[107] Was genre crucial in all this activity?[108] Yes and no. Commentary, case, chronicle, regimen, topography: physicians wrote in recognizable forms, yet documenting and evaluating flourished athwart genre, just as we have seen them flourish across other sorts of difference.

Community, third and finally, meant membership, responsibility, and accountability. And accountability meant keeping account, another documentary impulse. Even curative medicine for paying patients—private practice—was in a way public by being publicly accountable. Every doctor in Nuremberg swore an oath of office, not only the two *Stadtärzte* who held the most responsibility.[109] From a northern port like Rotterdam to Provençal towns to a capital of Renaissance medical learning like Bologna, written contracts between doctors and patients and tribunals for disagreements governed individually paid medical care. Patient–practitioner agreements and disagreements registered by notaries sometimes detailed expected and actual therapeutic outcomes. Across Europe, paying or refusing to pay were acts of evaluation of medical treatment. And the new legal codes of the sixteenth century made physicians and surgeons liable, in certain situations, for preventable failure to heal.[110] Seventeenth-century court physician Theodore Turquet de Mayerne kept detailed, structured case notes amounting to thousands of pages. Among other purposes, these "were designed to serve as a defense of Mayerne's actions should the case become controversial, as cases involving courtiers were wont to do."[111] Though seemingly worlds apart from medical practice at the French and English courts, a Venetian *medico condotto* in Damascus found himself in an analogous if less exigent situation. Whichever way he turned, Dr. Bianchi was accountable: to his patients, expecting to be cured; to the Venetian state, expecting him to keep merchants and envoys healthy and expecting to be able to interview him on his observations; to the civic sphere of Damascus, in which he had to learn to belong; and to the art of medicine he represented.[112] Moral, monetary, legal accounting for the art encouraged habits of the medical diary or casebook and thus, it seems plausible, fed an emerging culture of taking note of ordinary practice and not only of its extraordinary moments.[113] This was an extension of the growing function of writing for any citizen or subject. The spread of writing in Europe can be said to have begun with accountability: being able to sign one's name meant being able—and required—to account for oneself and one's household in increasingly paper-bound polities.[114]

Public function, public accountability, public record: these have one more dimension worth exploring here, not least because it is unexpected. Corporative or "guild" organization of the medical or any other trade is usually synonymous with secrecy rather than transparency; the privilege of self-governance rather than the responsibility of community governance; special rather than public interest; protected hierarchy and monopoly rather than quality assurance for the common good. Yet both sides are true, and the half-truth of the former, at least in the case of corporative medicine, reflects the fatal defensive turn it took with the rise of a consumer medical market in the seventeenth and eighteenth centuries—only to be resurrected in the "neo-corporatist" form of the modern system of professions and qualifications.[115] Compared to patients choosing freely among all sorts of healers, and compared to individual doctors competing for clientele and patronage, the more corporative the doctors became the more they became representatives of a public rather than private practice. Public here meant (1) exercised collectively by documenting and sharing experience, and (2) accountable and reflected upon by being documented, either publicly in the reporting and archiving activity around evaluation and counsel, or privately, in casebooks, but with publics in mind, both the public of the art and that of the communities served. Even the early modern physicians who most avoided "civic responsibilities" and "the public realm," the fellows of the London College of Physicians, in becoming incorporated, turned themselves from a congeries of elite individuals into an institution of regular and often detailed "semi-public" recordkeeping, mainly for accountability in their censorial activity and examinations of irregular practitioners. Not a record of one's own practice, this was a record of evaluation of practice. Over time, the College moved from Latin to English, the better to show the "truth, honesty, and sincerity" of its proceedings.[116] Florentine physicians, to take the oldest well-studied example of corporative medicine, belonged to a guild—and thereby served the state, the poor, and the commonwealth in other ways, notably by documenting and reporting on communally significant events, dangers, and resources. Here was a guild making the public medical record, an archive of and for empirically based decision-making.[117]

Translating/Translocating—Universalizing?

Doctors not only wrote things down and judged them. They set things in motion—by pen, post, and print. To be a learned practitioner was itself to be fundamentally a mediator: between "learned" Latin knowledge and vernacular conversations with "lay" patients and their kin. In this way, the physician stood out from other healers not only because of something he possessed and they did not—medical "learning," university education, knowledge of the liberal arts and natural philosophy—but also because of something he had to do and they did not: translate. For other healers, practice flowed from apprenticeship without translation, as it could not from libraries, university curricula, and the Latin literature of medicine already so huge and complex as to require canon and compendia to make it usable. Barber-surgeons, midwives, and other healers plied their trades and carried out their duties without having to move back and forth, as the physician did, between languages, both natural and conceptual, between differing structures of knowledge, and between written information, daily conversation, and sensory experience. This was translation in much more than the linguistic sense.[118] It also suggests another way of looking at—and perhaps beyond—the theory/practice problem in premodern medicine.[119]

Historians have recently highlighted the role of intermediaries in the creation and use of practical natural knowledge, especially by governments and trading companies, in Europe and its empires.[120] Physicians stood out in the early modern world of intermediaries because they mediated to make possible their own action and not only that of others. They also stood out because they wrote things down in prodigious volume and detail. Any mediating involved communication, but with physicians, mediating resulted in texts as much as acts (or material products) and often in texts for action, as in health regimens, prescriptions, and written consultations or *consilia*. Physicians were not unique in the indispensability of translation to their profession: jurists, too, could hardly act without mediating and translating between learned Latin legal traditions and the "lay" languages of clientele and everyday government. Analog to civic doctors, the civic jurists employed as so-called *Stadtschreiber* in charge of city administrations created a widely read lay legal literature based on both Latin and vernacular sources. The famous northern humanist Sebastian Brant gave up a law professorship at Basel to become *Stadtschreiber* of Strasbourg. A poet and author of the *Ship of Fools*, not to mention broadsides on monstrous births and the French pox, Brant brought vernacular legal guides to press and lent his name and verse to their dissemination.[121] Nor in their wider translational activity were physicians unique among men of words. All humanist work on nature (much of it by physicians) involved relating ancient texts to exotic contemporary worlds or indeed familiar ones.[122] Beyond medical practice, translational, translocational documenting united physicians' seemingly unrelated mediating activities—as when Agricola mediated between city and duchy via daily dispatch, or when he mediated via note-taking and publishing between mining know-how and natural history, between classical texts and miners, investors, rulers, and informants. Among the informants were not only mining administrators but also physicians who, like Agricola, served as medical officer in Saxon and Bohemian mining towns. *De re metallica* translated all this into humanist Latin for widest European dissemination and was first published, after all, as a dialog based on these conversations.[123]

Under these documentary conditions, to translate was not only to mediate. It was to create or re-create readers and communities of information and knowledge. This happened above all when translation appeared in print. Here, too, doctors stood out. As members of the translocal community of published medicine and of the medical and wider republic of letters, they were highly networked major users of the two key new technologies of rapid post and print. The urban polities that were home to most early modern physicians were also the workshops and hubs of hand-copied and printed communication. Many physicians were involved in the book trade and not only as authors. They translated, compiled, edited. Whereas later seventeenth- and eighteenth-century representatives of the Frankfurt patrician von Uffenbach family appear in histories of science circulating among the scientific societies and collections of Europe,[124] their nearly forgotten forbear Peter Uffenbach (1566–1635), immobilized like any town physician by being contractually bound to the city he served, made himself a center of translation from Latin into European vernaculars, and vice versa, for thousands of pages of natural history and the medical, chemical, and surgical arts. His predecessor in office had done the same.[125] It was apparently something town-bound civic physicians in global communications and printing hubs did.

Translating *into* Latin deserves an additional comment. At times, physicians differentiated their knowledge from that of their patients by shifting from vernacular to Latin writing habits, as they did, for instance, in the Bristol infirmary in the eighteenth century.[126] At other times, especially in earlier centuries, translating vernacular medicine and surgery into Latin enabled translation back out into another vernacular. Latin, that great divider, was also an enabler and accelerator of Europe-wide interactive medical knowledge-making across boundaries of all kinds.

When not thus creating new publics of knowledge from his position at a hub of the European book trade, Frankfurt *Stadtarzt* Uffenbach could be found doing the equivalent for another dimension of physician involvement in public life. In 1620 he was the first Frankfurt physician to sign a forensic report rather than give oral testimony in court. He co-signed with the surgeons. Just as his publishing activity moved vernacular surgery into Latin and Latin surgery and medicine into German for readers of both "high and low standing,"[127] so in his documenting for governance the civic doctor observed and reported together with the city's sworn barber-surgeons.[128] The polity's translational documentary culture grew with each such episode, with each piece of paper written and signed in a collective public or semi-public moment, passed among several or many hands, read by various pairs of eyes, read aloud in council, occasioning further rounds of discussion in talk and ink, archived for reference sooner or later.

Between interaction that yielded an archived documentary and translational surplus (like Uffenbach's forensic report) and printed translation that was meant for regular household and municipal use (like Uffenbach's books) lay a mass of published ephemera, a whole world of everyday action and interaction in and around print and annotation. Most sheets that came off early modern presses were not pages of monographs. They were ephemera like broadsheets, handbills, newspapers, notices, bulletins, pamphlets, and those books in which the user was supposed to make notes yet in which some of the annotating was already done by the author-compiler: almanacs.[129] Much of the information in almanacs was medical (and astrological or meteorological, hence indirectly medical). Physicians made up a large proportion of early modern almanac-makers. A well-studied example is Johannes Magirus, physician in Berlin in the 1640s and then official town doctor of Zerbst, capital of one of the principalities of Anhalt (before moving on to a professorship in Marburg), whose almanac was so successful that he published new annual editions for 26 years.[130] Magirus annotated his almanacs from published *observationes* and other Latin medical literature. The relationship between learned and vernacular here can be understood as "popular enlightenment." Or it can be understood as knowledge-by-translation. Written in like diaries, almanacs can be studied as "ego documents."[131] Yet almanacs also expressed and created shared expectations and experience. They were as much about *we* as *I*. Though publishing almanacs was a good way for doctors to earn on the medical print market, some cities showed just how communal a function this was when they made the town medical officer responsible for preparing and publishing an annual local almanac.[132]

Though necessarily commercial in form, publishing by physicians exhibited and advanced goals and values other than those of capital and trade. It is no coincidence that the world's first Latin weekly was founded by a group of civic doctors, who belonged to the Collegium medicum of Nuremberg and, like all physicians in that city, held public office.[133] They made novel use of commercial structures. Yet they innovated only so far as to serve their goals and no further, that is, not as publishing entrepreneurs. Like these Nuremberg doctors who translated vernacular news and observations into Latin every week, the London practitioners who translated in the opposite direction, from Latin lectures into popular medicine, had income from a product and expenses to produce it.[134] However, whereas trade was life and livelihood for the merchant or the printer, for these physicians the information trade was a means to another end: useful knowledge community, better medicine, the public good. (Personal and professional advance goes without saying—and says little.) In England, in the relative absence of civic medical office and its associated ethos and duties, the London equivalent of the publishing civic practitioner was the publishing radical practitioner. Best known among them was the apothecary Nicholas Culpeper, who teamed with printers to "English" the official Latin pharmacopoeia and generally to destroy any monopoly of learned physicians on medical knowledge. Translation often adapts the products of one culture to another, as when the anthropologist tells the story of Hamlet and hears her listeners "correcting" the story to match their culture.[135] Yet translation also dissolves differences, creating new knowledge by uniting or bridging communities. The community that Culpeper and his publishing associates sought to create was the knowledgeable "commonwealth."[136] Printed and sold, this sort of translation was the public activity of physicians at its most commercial yet potentially most widely communal. In these diverse yet always translational ways, doctors generated in a stream of print a continuum of civic sphere and wider publics. In so far as their readers' medical lives were framed by caring or being cared for in the household, this was also a continuum of medical *polis* and medical *domus* that belied the ancient and modern declared duality of the political and the domestic. Print was sold and bought, yet the cross-cutting epistemically relevant practice here was not economic transaction, or that overworked economism "exchange."[137] It was translation, textual and far more than textual. And by making new communities of knowing, it was learning, in another sense: not what the few had, but what the few and the many could do more or less together.

Why All This Matters

The logic of this chapter ran as follows. Doctors were more than doctors. Their multifaceted activity related several domains of everyday, learned, and public life. In much of Europe, this was accentuated by the fact that many doctors and certainly the influential ones were first and foremost civic doctors, by both official and unofficial purpose and action and often by public self-identification. The life of the polity and the life of the physician shared values, practices, and sworn and contractual obligations of community. With no less-real consequences, this activity happened in talk and ink. Beyond genres, practices, and media of communication, cross-cutting empirical rational activity of a few basic kinds can be discerned, such as evaluating and reporting, documenting and locating, translating and translocating, perhaps universalizing. Implications follow for understanding knowledge and society in past and present. I start with implications within existing categories—medicine, science—and move on to implications that require rethinking the categories and creating new ones.

1 **Medicine, fortress and forum.** The standard picture of the physician in society has been that of learned practitioner: a university man with elite clients and a college of colleagues. He might have a hospital position, a progressive interest in anatomy, a position at court. Yet fundamentally he was a rather defensive *doctor*, the very word for scholar and higher university graduate. He asserted the status, privileges, patronage relations, and knowledge tradition of a learned profession against competing guilds and trades (barber-surgeons, apothecaries, midwives), other learned professions (law, clergy), and empiric "chymical" and

"lay" medicine. Indeed, learned medicine was partly constructed against these. The picture that emerges by taking seriously the full biographies of many early modern doctors and by changing perspective from market to polity could not be more different. Physicians were as much their societies' vital communicators—indeed contracted partly for this— as they were guardians of special knowledge and privilege. In much of Europe, office, oath, and specific duties of public service were at least as important as—and entangled with—profession, patronage, and struggle for a share of the medical market. Medicine was a fortress of learning. Yet it was also a forum of learning, vast and public, among civilization's longest running, all-encompassing forums of knowledge-generating communication, of interaction with a surplus. At times more inclusive, at times less, over the millenium since the first schools of medicine appeared in Europe, medicine is comparable, as we might expect from this timespan, only to law and has had a function no less public.

2   **Civic medicine.** Academic medicine, court medicine, corporative medicine, domestic medicine, private practice: the point has not been to add civic medicine to the patchwork quilt. Like public practice and medical polity, civic medicine is a concept for understanding dimensions of the whole. This is no extrapolation. It happened empirically along the way. Civic doctors were at the center of this story, yet it also quickly filled with medical professors, physicians at court, and practitioners paid by individual patients. All of these were often the same person. From this perspective, what is called the medical marketplace looks more like a medical polity with transactions. Consumer choice was but one aspect. Especially in the communities of plural Europe, transaction for health was governed by values and practices of collective good in at least three ways. First and foremost was regulation: contracts for cure and tribunals to adjudicate dispute; diagnosis and therapy worked out on paper before a notary public; quality and safety control in the form of official pharmacopoeia, pharmacy inspection, and practitioner licensing, training, examination. Second, even among market competitors, such as the apothecaries of a large city, "working collectively to survive and prosper" was more the norm than cut-throat competition. Third, the communities themselves were paying clients for medical services— for the poor or, on the *condotto* model, for all.[138] Likewise, building the big picture of medicine by starting from the polity rather than the academy does not leave out academic medicine but shows it had a whole dimension beyond doctrine, a public function beyond pedogogy. Across Europe, medical faculties were consulted for expert judgment. Thus could physicians reasonably and meaningfully serve in both political and professorial capacities.

What holds for town and faculty holds for princely court.[139] "Court medicine" risks reifying the court and reducing it to a locus of patronage and high culture. The court was also a household (as in "la maison médicale du roi") with all the medical production, consumption, and communication that entailed.[140] Second, it was a unit of community healthcare. While a personal or first physician looked after sovereign and family, a court physician could be contracted to keep *everyone* at court healthy. His duty to treat "the humble as well as the great," their wives, children, and servants, echoed that of the town physician to treat rich and poor alike.[141] This community was informed, demanding, and contentious. It kept physicians like Mayerne very busy at their casebooks. Third, like a city, the court was a communications hub, such that historians have compared networked court physicians to networked town physicians.[142] Fourth, even taking care of the sovereign was not "private" but public practice, not because the king had two bodies, but because his corporeal body was a matter of dynastic and public concern, as was that of the queen or indeed the Pope, whose week-to-week or even day-to-day health could be followed in clinical detail in diplomatic dispatches and in news services like the *Avvisi di Roma*.[143] And, finally, the court was a center of territorial administration. Of course, this meant bureaucracy, surveillance, and (attempted) control, such as that of the *premier médecin du roi* over mineral waters, drugs, and the medical trades throughout the realm.[144] But especially in states smaller than France, it also meant the opposite: *consultation* by town councils, judges, bailiffs, and other local agencies needing to decide situations of uncertainty, disagreement, possible danger or injustice. This involved court physicians in the same sorts of cases, queries, and proceedings in which town physicians were involved —and thus the same practices of evaluating evidence, informed judgment, documenting, and translating.

In all these ways, civic medicine describes much more than what happened in the *civitas*. Concepts of civic medicine, public practice, and medical polity may be useful in the way medical marketplace has been for the past 30 years. They draw our attention instead to the collective and communal in past and present. And they signal the relation to knowledge and technique more than "welfare" has done and avoid the sectoring effect of histories of public health, charity, and poor relief. No doubt they have their own limitations to be explored.

3 **Civic Sci Rev?** Physicians comprised a large proportion of the membership of learned and scientific societies and generally of European communities of natural and "useful" knowledge. So much is well known, though little researched, and has even led historians to see doctors as the "cutting edge" of the Scientific Revolution, or at least its non-mathematical side.[145] Less remembered is that many of these physician-naturalists were civic doctors, in all of the ways explored here. Agricola in Chemnitz, Conrad Gesner in Zurich, Ulisse Aldrovandi in Bologna, the Bauhins of Basel, Nicolaes Tulp, immortalized by Rembrandt as

anatomist but also a magistrate of Amsterdam: these are only the big names, and the list could go on and on. Indeed, one such list was published regularly in its own time. It was the roster of contributors of *observationes* to the Leopoldina's *Miscellanea curiosa*: almost everyone appears as Archiater or Physicus or Poliater.[146] We have mathematical, Baconian, religious, political, artisanal, gentlemanly, legal, technological, state-building, imperial, humanist, courtly, commercial, and indeed medical narratives of early modern science. Any such account featuring physicians may turn out to be more civic than commercial in its shaping and driving forces, as much about polity as—via pharmacy, botany, and trade—about the market, which, moreover, was itself coming to be regulated for the good of the polity, above all by physicians.[147] And vice versa: any civic narrative of early modern science ought to feature physicians. There is a classic one, Eugenio Garin's *Science and Civic Life in Renaissance Italy*. It is almost forgotten in our preoccupation with court and market, patronage and shopping, as important as these were.[148] Garin grounds science in the ideal and attempted reality of the just and healthy *polis* and moves on to … Leonardo and Galileo, the latter now better known as heretic, courtier, engineer, and very serious joker than as civic natural philosopher.[149] Garin skips past medicine—as does the whole literature on civic humanism—and those key players in the story, the civic doctors.

4   **History of what?** If doctors were more than doctors and there was no such thing yet as modern science, then what are we writing the history of? This chapter is an attempt to address that question, and I hope to have shown it is worth asking. If the office of physician was—their communities made clear—an indispensable and public one and physicians' activity so varied, then historians are seeing only pieces of a larger puzzle by writing history of "medicine," or of "health," or the medical market, or medical learning, or of the sciences and disciplines in which physicians often led, from anatomy to chemistry to botany; or by writing histories of societies as though their university-educated knowers of the natural world hardly existed. Yet how can we define our object of study? One answer has been power. Research on practice, however, shows "power" to be far less apt than once assumed, even in the several knowledge-entangled forms explored in stimulating ways by Foucault and others since the 1960s. A more recent answer has been simply "knowledge." Its advantage turns out also to be its disadvantage: expansiveness. The challenge is how to think about this, if not in spaces and places or in categories like medicine or government or the household or the sciences and practical arts.[150] For knowing seems to happen athwart as much as within them, as the doctor's perspective so well shows. Moreover, knowing was rarely far from doing and the values associated with it. This was often a matter of making things. For physicians, it was a matter of working to sustain people and—in the

public dimension explored here—the polity. This required neither reform, nor altruism, but simply what it meant to be a polity with a *poliater*, a political community with its physician and all that this entailed.[151] How about history of that? This would be to build on urban histories of medicine and health pioneered in the 1980s and early 1990s but not to continue them into ever more detailed studies of urban medical systems.[152] Conclusions 5 to 9, below, suggest some directions.

5 **From bureaucracy to community.** Histories of science, technology, medicine, and more recently "expertise" in early modern polities have looked generally for the state, or princely court: as patron of science, user of expertise, and matrix for both.[153] What gets overlooked is governance where it mostly happened in social life: locally, case-by-case. For physicians in local governance, office meant serving people more than ruling them. And this meant two-way action and negotiation, unlike Foucault's unilateral "pastoral technology" of power/knowledge.[154] In values and practices, medical office meant community—with conflict, disagreement, and uncertainty to resolve—more than bureaucracy, certainly until the nineteenth century and in many places probably to the present.[155] And in knowledge, it meant knowing in cases more than knowing territory and population.[156] Cases were what—and how—physicians (and jurists) knew best. This is not only a descriptive difference but a difference in applicable history and theory. Applying Weber misleads. Foucault, with no eye for interaction and its effects, is not directly relevant and Habermas is only partly. Medical office was and was not Weberian bureaucratic. On the one hand, as early as 1500, candidates applied and competed according to generally known criteria, and holders swore impartiality. On the other hand, they were part-time, amateur administrators who also had a paying clientele. Moreover, physicians' activity such as documenting or certifying formed a continuum from office to unofficial public life, or civil society in Anglo-American parlance. This was, in turn, not Habermasian (universal, bourgeois, liberal, consumer-based), but (a) both translocal in its empirical rationality and relentlessly local in its purpose and problems; (b) more communal (with contention) than liberal in both its raison d'être and its mode of raisonnement in identifying and solving problems; and (c) extending far beyond bourgeois and aristocratic civility to encompass all citizens and inhabitants, including the sick poor who were examined by the town physician yet who themselves often initiated such examinations, actively shaped results, and negotiated for municipal care.[157] The problem is that study of interaction is, well, divided. Study of scholarly and scientific communication seldom concerns political sustainability and development.[158] And, vice versa, study of political community and communication usually conceives people as authorities and citizens or subjects, or as members of social strata, the

estates (*états*, *Stände*), or corporative groups, not as "knowers" making observations and exercising reasoned if also interested judgment. Putting the two stories together could therefore yield something other than a social history *of* knowledge: a knowledge history of polity, and perhaps also—to borrow from mainly environmental and economic parlance—of political sustainability.

6   **Kinds of public and practices that cut across them.** Public office, political community (mixing civil society and official functions), wider reading and writing publics, both vernacular and learned: these four kinds of *res publica* in which physicians acted in leading ways, possibly more consistently across all four than any other group in their societies, can be characterized as differently as they are in the politico-historical theories of Weber (office, bureaucracy), Aristotle (*polis*, political community), Habermas (public sphere), and Malinowski, Mauss, or Merton (gift exchange in the republic of letters, communalism of knowledge in scientific communities).[159] These are bigger differences than those usually identified in the now standard argument that there have been many publics rather than a single Habermasian public sphere.[160] They are differences of universality and locality, of kinds of rationality, of constructions of individual behavior and shared interest or commonality, of scope of action and duty, of openness and exclusivity, and historically were defined partly against each other. The surprising thing we can learn by looking at physicians, however, is that even these four different kinds of public life were nonetheless related through a set of interactive cross-cutting empirical rational practices whose genealogies, workings, and effects deserve to be explored.

7   **From differentiation to commonality.** Differentiation is likely to remain fundamental to describing modern societies, whether by occupation, functional system and "code" (rules specific to emerging systems like politics, religion, sport, economy, or science), division of labor, or otherwise. Differentiation is also likely to remain fundamental to describing modern knowledge, whether by lay/technical divide (and bridging thereof), disciplines and interdisciplinarity, specialization, sheer complexity, or at the meta level demarcating science from politics, what counts as science from non-science.[161] Yet despite modernity by differentiation, in physicians we see a single modernizing figure grow in functions. Empirical rational practice therefore grew as well.[162] It cut across most or all of these differentiations. The historical problem becomes not so much to show differentiation, or transition from one kind of differentiation to another,[163] or differentiation-based change like medicalization, but rather to identify cross-cutting empirical rational practices and describe their expansion and development. This can be done over a *longue durée* and across more domains than usually studied in any single field of history, including areas traditionally regarded as (and claiming to be) separate because they are learned,

scientific, technical, or specialized. These once invited investigation "in context." They are now often seen and studied as "expertise." Yet they may yield instead to the kind of analysis suggested here by studying physicians. They are not the timeless universals of structural anthropology to which Braudel was responding in 1958. Nor are they *mentalités* or intellectual traditions, such as Aristotelianism or the persistent idea of a crusade, which, in his view, were as exemplary of *longue durée* historical reality as were geography and economy. Instead, they comprised ends and means of knowing and doing.

8   **Ways of knowing, ways of living together.** It is easy enough to see early modern Europe, local and global, as a knowledge or information society.[164] It is rather harder to know what this means. This is difficult because expanding research has depended on keeping "knowledge" loosely defined and inclusive. It is difficult because, as Robert Darnton has written, "every age was an age of information, each in its own way, and ... communication systems have always shaped events."[165] And, finally, it is difficult because research is divided.[166] Most information history focuses on news, print, correspondence, and other media of communication.[167] Other histories explore the paper "little tools of knowledge" at work in "academic and bureaucratic" practices.[168] Scholarship has flourished on each of these—separately.[169] We now have histories of creating and managing scholarly information in books, notebooks, and libraries, which mainly bracket the knowledge question. And we have histories of states or other large administrative institutions (the church, religious orders, the East India companies) creating and managing information. Largely untold is the history of the enormous amount of information, information use, and knowing practice generated by the ways and problems of living together in communities, which, for all its conflicts and injustices, has never ceased. Yet to what extent were there separate scholarly and administrative written practices? Political, commercial, and other sorts? Shared ones? More fundamentally: are genres, media, paper technology, practices of writing and reading, of oral and written communication, of information and "data" ultimate units of inquiry for historical narrative, explanation, and meaning, or just preliminary ones? The latter seems more plausible. The gain from looking at physicians, especially civic doctors, is that they straddled all spheres of information (news, state, scholarly, local communal, domestic, juridical) and that they fulfilled communally defined purposes and obligations other than pursuit of knowledge or power. It seems unlikely that a knowledge/polity nexus will be found in shared genres like the protocol, or kinds of writing like *historia*, or in practices like visitation or filing or listing. More promising is crosscutting activity at a higher level—like evaluating evidence, testing, documenting, reasoning to judgment, translating (including translocation that transforms the locations and what is moved), and doubtless

others, from accounting to classifying to predicting. These were more complex. They were therefore more not less elemental of both knowledge and polity. This is because they included (and were *about*) public values and problems, standards and obligations, horizons of expectation and the unexpected, the not yet known. These kinds of activity did not belong specifically to "medicine" or "society" or "politics" or law or government or humanist scholarship or the liberal arts or the disciplines or the household or natural history or practical arts. Yet they were not, therefore, mere all-purpose communication and information practices. They would hardly exist without values and imperatives associated with justice and the common good. Finally, they were not bound to states or centers of calculation or even the library: individuals and groups across society engaged in them. Unlike early modern state surveys, which tended to "run aground" when it came to data-processing and use,[170] they "worked": integral to the day-to-day functioning and year-to-year sustainability of polities.

9 **Futures.** Exactly here, however, the tendency of historians and social scientists to look for order, legitimation, control, and consensus, or their disruption through conflict, disobedience, resistance, and revolution, falls short of the descriptive task. Documenting, evaluating, translating—none of these was novel, but all were newly and indeed explosively growing activities. All depended on principles and practices of collectivity in time as well as space or, as Gesner wrote to fellow physician-naturalist Leonhart Fuchs, each putting "in common his own observations" toward knowledge in a century to come.[171] And so, most interestingly, they belonged to what contemporaries sensed or pursued as the unfolding future of their societies. To characterize this collective anticipation and pursuit will require concepts more communal than those of state-building or economic development and more explicitly about knowing. This future unfolded through towns and cities slowly creating health and welfare systems around observing, evaluating, documenting, and translating led by learned physicians, overseeing yet also working far more together with barber-surgeons, midwives, and apothecaries—themselves often under oath and contract of civic duty—than usually assumed. This future unfolded through doctors' documenting and evaluating local resources and the "possibilities of the land"; through societies and schemes for improvement in which doctors usually predominated; through "good police," in its less petty and more practical and environmental regulations, as a means of maximizing "the creative energies and potential of a stable and harmonious society"; through physicians acting for "the preservation of the integrity of the civic polity" (*civitatis*)—as F. J. Baier put it, in publishing a collection of 30 medico-juridical cases—by developing empirical rational method around public situations of uncertainty or disagreement.[172] It is a combination of conservative and progressive worth contemplating.

The Long and Early Modern?

Aspects of the foregoing are usually associated with modernity—medical and wider—since the Enlightenment and the rise of the modern state and civil society. Yet looking through earlier doctors at the activities that intersected in their lives shows how far back patterns reach that defy these categories—and how far forward. This is despite the periodizations of medicine, science, politics, and the public, which typically posit transformation in the decades around 1800.

Professionalization, state-building, social disciplining, medicalization, biopolitics, disease becoming a political problem, scientization of medicine and of society, structural transformation of the public sphere and its implications for natural knowledge and expertise: these historical narratives of transformation, pivoting around 1800, are all either explicitly medical or involve health. Medicine may span more of them than does any other field of activity.[173] My purpose here is not to join the valid criticism that has already been made of these narratives. Such criticism has left an outline of sweeping change surprisingly intact. What we once thought was unilateral medicalization from above was in fact a two-way creation, driven equally from below, of a world of health overseen by academic physicians. What was once teleologically told as professionalization in fact involved a shift in kind (around 1800) from medieval corporative system to modern system of professions.[174] What all these share is that they construe polity as the national or territorial-administrative state, or simply take this as the unit of analysis. Looking instead at urban plural Europe in the *longue durée* permits a simple historiographical observation. A nation-state like France or a territorial state like Baden was not medically modern until 1850 or later; a city-state like Zurich was medically modern from 1550; a port like Rotterdam, from the 1640s; some Mediterranean cities, from as early as the 1300s.[175] Though lacking the civic medical offices and institutions of old plural Europe, early modern France looks considerably closer to it when described as cities rather than state and territory.[176] And perhaps the relative lack in early modern England of a real world of civic doctors and public medical systems helped make it unusually generative of projects and movements to reform natural knowledge and polity, usually with some form of public medicine at or near the center.[177] Tellingly, one such scheme that reached the Hartlib Circle was written by one of the few doctors to hold the post of town physician in early modern England. Historians have called these schemes and movements utopian; they might just as well be called European. If the "full health care program of enlightened absolutism was too radical for the French Revolution" and never got beyond debate in the Constituent Assembly, if it found expression in England mainly in seventeenth-century radical politics, that politics, minus both the radicalism and the absolutism, was everyday, often contractual community and governance in the rest of Europe.[178] The point here is not

merely to change scenes or push back the timeline (and it has been persua-
sively pushed back to the thirteenth century for precocious Florence and
for Aragon).[179] The point is that there is therefore another history than
those of these *-izations* to tell—namely, of what physicians did in and for
more or less medically modern polities over the past 500 years and of how
they knew what to do in public life and developed these capacities, notably
in the form of empirical rational activity like documenting, describing,
evaluating evidence, explaining, and translational knowing.

The long and early modernity manifested in the office and figure of the
civic physician ran from the Middle Ages to the twentieth century.
Seventeenth-century codifications of his functions, built on fifteenth-century
ones, were still being reprinted as their basis in the nineteenth century.[180]
We know the duties and the very names of the town physicians of, say, Bern
from 1266 to the twentieth century, some serving for a year or two, others
for as many as 60.[181] Though we may think rock (and what weathers it) is
the bedrock of *longue durée* history, the geography of civic medicine was
more stable than that of the land, which changed substantially, as we now
know from environmental histories. Far from spearheading a biopolitical
revolution after 1800, doctors in public office continued to carry out a set of
duties that had been growing for centuries on foundations that were essen-
tially those of medieval and indeed Aristotelian as well as Christian good
governance. Even the country furthest from having official town doctors,
England, now came to have them, with its massive new system of over 800
Medical Officers of Health, each a licensed physician overseeing a town or
parish. They were not paid to treat patients, but neither were continental
town and district physicians by this time.[182] Viewed against the background
sketched here, that "English revolution in social medicine" falls into place as
the late version of a centuries-long European evolution of knowledgeable
governance.[183] In this area, the English were late, perhaps for the same
reasons they were early in state-building and parliamentary government on
a supra-urban scale.

As polities grew in complexity, the few lines of a fifteenth-century contract
or oath specifying town physician duties swelled to the 1,216 pages of
a handbook like *The District Physician* around 1900, whose title nonetheless
underlined the persistence of one-man multifunctionality amid state sprawl
and differentiated bureaucratic government.[184] Primary care no longer
belonged officially to these functions, but de facto it often did, especially in
smaller towns where the medical officer might be virtually the only doctor or
the one attending physician in the local hospital. Far from stagnation, all this
meant continuing to develop the evidence base of medicine by building its
case literature as well as developing public health and epidemiology, medical
geography and demography, occupational health and legal medicine, not to
mention natural history and pharmacy. Moreover, modern medical officer
and civic doctor biographies take us immediately into leadership in education, local and national government, scientific academies, urban reform, and

"citizenship and the survival of civilization," all bound up with experimental, clinical, social, and mathematical inquiry. This multifaceted figure retained many facets and acquired new ones.[185] (The story is not all rosy, as one of the main new ones was eugenic.) In ways that suggest thinking far more *longue durée* about related groups such as jurists or even engineers, whom we usually think of as rising in modern times through professionalization,[186] the physicians do not "rise" in the nineteenth and twentieth centuries. Their golden age *as physicians* in public and scientific life was in the prior three centuries[187]—from the pioneering bedside observer, early quantifier of plague, and cultural chronicler Felix Platter as *Archiater*—chief physician—of Basel to Rembrandt's anatomizing Dr. Tulp as *Regent* of a global city (both authors of important collections of medical and natural-historical *observationes*), to hundreds or indeed thousands of forgotten town and district physicians and numerous doctor-mayors and physician-leaders of organized science. And as local as those activities and publics were, they were bridged by news, government messaging, and physicians' participation in both, their academic peregrinations, and their correspondence and publishing.[188] Nor does the western medico-political-epistemic complex emerge with cameralism, enlightened absolutism, and medical police in the late eighteenth century or with early industrializing states in the nineteenth century; it had been growing in local communities and sovereign cities—and their rapid learned and vernacular communications—for centuries. And, finally, even curative medicine in much of Europe had been as much a matter of knowledgeable citizens as of knowledgeable consumers centuries before the rise of the "political problem" of disease and the answer of national health and welfare from "Bismarck to Beveridge."[189] And since the civic doctors at the center of all this were also leading figures in the ongoing empirical renewal of medical and natural knowledge, it seems likely that this renewal formed one history with the polity.

In short: What we call public or national or even global health today *is* early modern medicine—not the market of which the physician had a slice, but the polity whose *Archiater* he could be.

Notes

1 On the variety of Agricola's activities, see the 53 papers in Friedrich Naumann (ed.), *Georgius Agricola, 500 Jahre* (Basel, 1994).
2 See Pomata, "A Sense of Place," Chapter 8 of this volume.
3 See Frank Trentmann (ed.), *Paradoxes of Civil Society: New Perspectives on Modern German and British History*, revised 2nd edn (New York, 2003); Lynn K. Nyhart and Thomas H. Broman (eds), *Science and Civil Society*, volume 17 of *Osiris* (Chicago, 2002).
4 Hence the title of this essay; for contrast, see Christopher Crenner, *Private Practice: In the Early Twentieth-Century Medical Office of Dr. Richard Cabot* (Baltimore, 2005).
5 On early modern making and knowing generally: Pamela H. Smith, Amy R. W. Meyers, and Harold J. Cook (eds), *Ways of Making and Knowing: The*

Material Culture of Empirical Knowledge (Ann Arbor, 2014); Pamela Long, *Artisan/Practitioners and the Rise of the New Sciences, 1400–1600* (Corvallis, 2011); and literature going back to Boris Hessen, Robert Merton, and Edgar Zilsel; John V. Pickstone, "Working Knowledges before and after circa 1800: Practices and Disciplines in the History of Science, Technology and Medicine," *Isis*, 98 (2007): 489–515. Commerce: Staffan Müller-Wille, *Botanik und weltweiter Handel: Zur Begründung eines natürlichen Systems der Pflanzen durch Carl von Linné (1707–78)* (Berlin, 1999); Pamela H. Smith and Paula Findlen (eds), *Merchants and Marvels: Commerce, Science and Arts in Early Modern Europe* (New York and London, 2002); Harold J. Cook, *Matters of Exchange: Commerce, Medicine, and Science in the Dutch Golden Age* (New Haven/London, 2007); Dániel Margócsy, *Commercial Visions: Science, Trade, and Visual Culture in the Dutch Golden Age* (Chicago, 2014). Historicizing economy and natural knowledge: Margaret Schabas and Neil De Marchi (eds), *Oeconomies in the Age of Newton* (Durham, NC, 2003). States: Charles Coulston Gillispie, *Science and Polity in France at the End of the Old Regime* (Princeton, 1980); Eric Brian, *La mesure de l'état: administrateurs et géomètres au XVIIIe siècle* (Paris, 1994); Peter Collin and Thomas Horstmann (eds), *Das Wissen des Staates: Geschichte, Theorie, Praxis*, Schriften zur Rechtspolitologie (Baden-Baden, 2004); Eric H. Ash (ed.), *Expertise: Practical Knowledge and the Early Modern State*, volume 25 of *Osiris* (Chicago, 2010); Ursula Klein, *Humboldts Preußen: Wissenschaft und Technik im Aufbruch* (Darmstadt, 2015). Colonial and trading empires: Londa Schiebinger, *Plants and Empire: Colonial Bioprospecting in the Atlantic World* (Cambridge, MA, 2004); Londa Schiebinger and Claudia Swan (eds), *Colonial Botany: Science, Commerce, and Politics in the Early Modern World* (Philadelphia, 2005); Miles Ogborn, *Indian Ink: Script and Print in the Making of the English East India Company* (Chicago, 2007); Arndt Brendecke, *Imperium und Empirie: Funktionen des Wissens in der spanischen Kolonialherrschaft* (Cologne, 2009); Pratik Chakrabarti, *Materials and Medicine: Trade, Conquest and Therapeutics in the Eighteenth Century* (Manchester, 2010); Daniela Bleichmar, *Visible Empire: Botanical Expeditions and Visual Culture in the Hispanic Enlightenment* (Chicago, 2012).

6   Related but different research possibilities include studying role direction of multifunctional physicians: Bruce T. Moran, "Prince-Practitioning and the Direction of Medical Roles at the German Court: Maurice of Hesse-Kassel and his Physicians," in Vivian Nutton (ed.), *Medicine at the Courts of Europe, 1500–1837*, The Wellcome Institute Series in the History of Medicine (London and New York, 1990): 95–116; or studying a physician's "multifaceted" activity "as a whole": Chiara Crisciani, "Histories, Stories, Exempla, and Anecdotes: Michele Savonarola from Latin to Vernacular," in Gianna Pomata and Nancy G. Siraisi (eds), *Historia: Empiricism and Erudition in Early Modern Europe* (Cambridge, MA, 2005): 297–324, p. 301.

7   Physicians were key communicators *about* making, as in the opening example of Agricola on mining, and some became active as makers, notably of drugs or, more unusually, anatomical specimens; see recently Margócsy, *Commercial Visions*.

8   See notes 15, 27–28 below.

9   Niklas Luhmann, *The Differentiation of Society*, trans. Stephen Holmes and Charles Larmore (New York, 1982); Thomas F. Gieryn, "Boundary-Work and the Demarcation of Science from Non-Science: Strains and Interest in Professional Ideologies of Scientists," *American Sociological Review*, 48 (1983): 781–95. For an introduction by a contributor to history of differentiation in

the natural sciences, see Rudolf Stichweh, "The History and Systematics of Functional Differentiation in Sociology," in Mathias Albert, Barry Buzan, Michael Zürn (eds), *Bringing Sociology to International Relations: World Politics as Differentiation Theory* (Cambridge, 2013): 50–70. For application in early modern historiography: Matthias Pohlig, "Drawing Boundaries between Politics and Religion: Early Modern Politics Revisited," in Willibald Steinmetz, Ingrid Gilcher-Holtey and Heinz-Gerhard Haupt (eds), *Writing Political History Today* (Frankfurt and New York, 2013): 155–73 and work summarized there.

10 See notes 30–32 below; Toby Gelfand, "The History of Medical Profession," in W. F. Bynum and Roy Porter (eds), *Companion Encyclopedia of the History of Medicine*, 2 vols. (London, 1994), ch. 47; Thomas Broman, "Rethinking Professionalization: Theory, Practice, and Professional Ideology in Eighteenth-Century German Medicine," *Journal of Modern History*, 67 (1995): 835–72; Robert A. Nye, "The Evolution of the Concept of Medicalization in the Late Twentieth Century," *Journal of the History of the Behavioral Sciences*, 39 (2003): 115–29.

11 Fernand Braudel, "Histoire et sciences sociales: La longue durée," *Annales: Histoire, Sciences Sociales*, 13 (1958): 725–53.

12 For the newest of these three (or four) models, see the graduate research program "Expertenkulturen des 12. bis 18. Jahrhunderts": www.uni-goettingen.de/de/100282.html; Hedwig Röckelein and Udo Friedrich (eds), *Experten der Vormoderne zwischen Wissen und Erfahrung*, special issue of *Das Mittelalter*, 17/2 (Berlin, 2012); Björn Reich, Frank Rexroth, and Matthias Roick (eds), *Wissen, massgeschneidert: Experten und Expertenkulturen im Europa der Vormoderne*, Historische Zeitschrift Beiheft, n.s., 57 (Munich, 2012).

13 Ole Peter Grell and Andrew Cunningham, "The Reformation and Changes in Welfare Provision in Early Modern Northern Europe," in Grell and Cunningham (eds), *Health Care and Poor Relief in Protestant Europe, 1500–1700* (London and New York, 1997): 1–41, p. 1; see Ole Peter Grell, Andrew Cunningham, and Jon Arrizabalaga (eds), *Health Care and Poor Relief in Counter-Reformation Europe* (London and New York, 1999).

14 Davis proposed an alternative model, of urban crisis and coalition, featuring "vocational experience" in business and law; "Poor Relief, Humanism, and Heresy," in Natalie Zemon Davis, *Society and Culture in Early Modern France* (Stanford, 1975): 17–64, pp. 59–61; classic statements of the opposing positions: Jerrold E. Seigel, "'Civic Humanism' or Ciceronian Rhetoric? The Culture of Petrarch and Bruni," *Past and Present*, 34 (1966): 3–48; Hans Baron, "Leonardo Bruni: 'Professional Rhetorician' or 'Civic Humanist'?" *Past and Present*, 36 (1967): 21–37; see James Hankins (ed.), *Renaissance Civic Humanism: Reappraisals and Reflections* (Cambridge, 2000).

15 In addition to examples cited throughout this essay around the physician as figure of intersection, a related node of intersection to be explored is the apothecary and his shop: on Venice in this regard, see Filippo de Vivo, "Pharmacies as Centres of Communication in Early Modern Venice," *Renaissance Studies*, 21 (2007): 505–21; Valentina Pugliano, "Specimen Lists: Artisanal Writing or Natural Historical Paperwork?" *Isis*, 103 (2012): 716–26.

16 Building on extensive research on women as medical practitioners, pioneered by Monica Green and others since the 1980s, recent expansions of history of medical knowing beyond physicians include: Katharine Park, *Secrets of Women: Gender, Generation, and the Origins of Human Dissection* (New York, 2006); Alisha Rankin, *Panaceia's Daughters: Noblewomen as Healers in Early Modern*

Germany (Chicago, 2013); bringing domestic medicine into the history of knowing: Elaine Leong, "Making Medicines in the Early Modern Household," *Bulletin of the History of Medicine*, 82 (2008): 145–68.

17 Hence Laurence Brockliss and Colin Jones, *The Medical World of Early Modern France* (Oxford, 1997) is part synthesis (quotation from p. 14 n.), part encyclopedia, as are Mary Lindemann, *Medicine and Society in Early Modern Europe*, New Approaches to European History, 16 (Cambridge, 1999); Mary Lindemann, *Health and Healing in Eighteenth-Century Germany* (Baltimore, 1996); Andrew Wear, *Knowledge and Practice in English Medicine, 1550–1680* (Cambridge, 2000); pluralism as organizing concept: David Gentilcore, *Healers and Healing in Early Modern Italy* (Manchester, 1998); market as organizing concept: Mark S. R. Jenner and Patrick Wallis eds, *Medicine and the Market in England and Its Colonies*, c. 1450 – c. 1850 (Basingstoke and New York, 2007). Synthetic on learned medicine and literate surgery: Nancy G. Siraisi, *Medieval and Early Renaissance Medicine: An Introduction to Knowledge and Practice* (Chicago, 1990); Michael R. McVaugh and Nancy G. Siraisi (eds), *Renaissance Medical Learning: Evolution of a Tradition*, volume 6 of *Osiris* (Philadelphia, 1991); Ian MacLean, *Logic, Signs, and Nature in the Renaissance: The Case of Learned Medicine*, Ideas in Context, 62 (Cambridge, 2002); for the end of the period: Thomas H. Broman, *The Transformation of German Academic Medicine, 1750–1820* (Cambridge, 1996).

18 Lindemann, *Medicine and Society*, ch. 7; Sharon T. Strocchia (ed.), *Women and Healthcare in Early Modern Europe*, special issue of *Renaissance Studies* 28 (2014); Leigh Whaley, *Women and the Practice of Medical Care in Early Modern Europe, 1400–1800* (Basingstoke and New York, 2011).

19 Spain's medical history appears to exemplify a third model between the plural and monarchical with protracted struggle and negotiation between an ambitiously centralizing crown and pre-existing municipal and corporative medical organization: Michele L. Clouse, *Medicine, Government and Public Health in Philip II's Spain: Shared Interests, Competing Authorities* (Farnham, 2011), especially the introduction and ch. 1; medieval Aragon exhibits aspects of the early modern story outlined here: see Michael McVaugh, *Medicine before the Plague: Practitioners and Their Patients in the Crown of Aragon, 1285–1345* (Cambridge, 1993), ch. 7.

20 See notes 58–63 below.

21 Margaret Pelling, *Medical Conflicts in Early Modern London: Patronage, Physicians, and Irregular Practitioners, 1550–1640*, with Frances White (Oxford, 2003), p. 16, 20; Harold J. Cook, *The Decline of the Old Medical Regime in Stuart London* (Ithaca, 1986); Christopher Lawrence, "Incommunicable Knowledge: Science, Technology and the Clinical Art in Britain 1850–1914," *Journal of Contemporary History*, 20 (1985): 503–20; but see Harold J. Cook, "Policing the Health of London: The College of Physicians and the Early Stuart Monarchy," *Social History of Medicine*, 2 (1989): 1–33. Contrasting with London, early modern English towns present a more civic medical world, though with few learned physicians: Margaret Pelling, *The Common Lot: Sickness, Medical Occupations, and the Urban Poor in Early Modern England: Essays* (London, 1998).

22 Andrew W. Russell (ed.) *The Town and State Physician in Europe from the Middle Ages to the Enlightenment*, Wolfenbütteler Forschungen, 17 (Wolfenbüttel, 1981); brief survey: Brockliss and Jones, *Medical World*, 11–14; best overview for eighteenth-century Germany: Lindemann, *Health and Healing*, ch. 2 "The Physici"; toward the present volume: Ruth Schilling, Sabine

Schlegelmilch, and Susan Splinter, "Stadtarzt oder Arzt in der Stadt? Drei Ärzte der Frühen Neuzeit und ihr Verständnis des städtischen Amtes," *Medizinhistorisches Journal*, 46 (2011): 99–133.

23 Only a handful of early modern English towns are known to have employed physicians on an ad hoc or retainer basis for treating the poor; see Margaret Pelling, "Healing the Sick Poor: Social Policy and Disability in Norwich, 1550–1640," *Medical History*, 29 (1985): 115–37, pp. 122–24; David Harley, "Pious Physic for the Poor: The Lost Durham County Medical Scheme of 1655," *Medical History*, 37 (1993): 148–66, pp. 148–50. In times of plague in the eighteenth century, some French cities contracted with doctors but, when danger had passed, were denied central funding to continue these positions; Brockliss and Jones, *Medical World*, pp. 746–47; for practitioners on retainer by medieval French towns, see Danielle Jacquart, *Le milieu médical en France du XIIe au XVe siècle* (Geneva, 1981), "Le service des villes," pp. 131–40, 285–86.

24 See, however, Werner Paravicini and Jörg Wettlaufer (eds), *Der Hof und die Stadt: Konfrontation, Koexistenz und Integration in Spätmittelalter und Früher Neuzeit*, Residenzenforschung, 20 (Ostfildern, 2006); Caspar Hirschi, "Höflinge der Bürgerschaft—Bürger des Hofes: Zur Beziehung von Humanismus und städtischer Gesellschaft," in Gernot Michael Müller (ed.), *Humanismus und Renaissance in Augsburg: Kulturgeschichte einer Stadt zwischen Spätmittelalter und Dreissigjährigem Krieg* (Berlin, 2010): 31–60.

25 Physicians at court or in royal or ducal service appearing in this chapter are: Agricola, Baldini, Handsch, Mayerne, Erndtel; see generally Nutton, *Medicine at the Courts of Europe*.

26 Heinrich Deichert, *Geschichte des Medizinalwesens im Gebiet des ehemaligen Königreichs Hannover: Ein Beitrag zur vaterländischen Kulturgeschichte* (Hannover and Leipzig, 1908), p. 8; on the multifunctionality of court physicians: Vivian Nutton, "Introduction," in Nutton, *Medicine at the Courts of Europe*: 1–14, p. 4 and 11; Moran, "Prince-Practitioning"; Crisciani, "Histories, Stories, Exempla"; Hugh Trevor-Roper, *Europe's Physician: The Various Life of Sir Theodore de Mayerne, 1573–1655* (New Haven, 2006).

27 Exemplary of elaborate, evolving, *longue durée* "municipal midwifery systems" are those of the south German cities: Merry Wiesner, "The Midwives of South Germany and the Public/Private Dichotomy," in Hilary Marland (ed.), *The Art of Midwifery: Early Modern Midwives in Europe*, Wellcome Series in the History of Medicine (London, 1993): 77–94, quotation from p. 80; Sibylla Flügge, *Hebammen und heilkundige Frauen: Recht und Rechtswirklichkeit im 15. und 16. Jahrhundert* (Frankfurt, 1998).

28 Among the few works to examine public reporting functions of all four groups is Esther Fischer-Homberger, *Medizin vor Gericht: Gerichtsmedizin von der Renaissance bis zur Aufklärung* (Bern, 1983), esp. pp. 31–52 on barber-surgeons, pp. 53–68 on midwives; for public functions of surgeons in France, see Christelle Rabier, "Surgery, Professional Conflicts and Legal Powers in Paris and London Courtrooms, 1760–1790," in Christelle Rabier (ed.), *Fields of Expertise: A Comparative History of Expert Procedures in Paris and London, 1600 to Present* (Newcastle-upon-Tyne, 2007): 85–114, pp. 91–92 for extension of Paris system throughout the realm; for earlier Iberian midwife testimony: Debra Blumenthal, "Domestic Medicine: Slaves, Servants and Female Medical Expertise in Late Medieval Valencia," *Renaissance Studies*, 28 (2014): 515–32.

29 Katharine Park, *Doctors and Medicine in Early Renaissance Florence* (Princeton, 1985), pp. 13, 16–17; McVaugh, *Medicine before the Plague*, esp. ch. 7; Brockliss and Jones, *Medical World*, esp. chs. 3 and 8, pp. 8–9, 818–26; and in England their troubles: Cook, *Decline*; Pelling, *Medical Conflicts*.

30 Quoting Brockliss and Jones, *Medical World*, p. 9. Classic: George Rosen, *From Medical Police to Social Medicine: Essays on the History of Health Care* (New York, 1974), which was a key starting point for this phase of Michel Foucault's work; see generally for the earlier period: Carlo M. Cipolla, *Public Health and the Medical Profession in the Renaissance* (Cambridge, 1976); David Gentilcore, "All That Pertains to Medicine: Protomedici and Protomedicati in Early Modern Italy," *Medical History*, 38 (1994): 121–42; Clouse, *Medicine, Government and Public Health in Philip II's Spain*; for the later period: Ute Frevert, *Krankheit als politisches Problem 1770–1880: Soziale Unterschichten in Preußen zwischen medizinischer Polizei und staatlicher Sozialversicherung*, Kritische Studien zur Geschichtswissenschaft, 62 (Göttingen, 1984); Bettina Wahrig and Werner Sohn (eds), *Zwischen Aufklärung, Policey und Verwaltung: Zur Genese des Medizinalwesens 1750–1850*, Wolfenbütteler Forschungen, 102 (Wiesbaden, 2003).

31 Classic point of reference in English for medicalization is *Journal of Contemporary History*, 20/4 (1985), special issue: "Medicine, History and Society," esp. Claudia Huerkamp, "The History of Smallpox Vaccination in Germany: A First Step in the Medicalization of the General Public," 617–35; Ute Frevert, "Professional Medicine and the Working Classes in Imperial Germany," 637–58; see texts from 1974–1978 in Michel Foucault, *Power: Essential Works of Foucault, 1954–1984*, Volume 3 (ed.) James D. Faubion, 3 vols. (London, 2015); Colin Jones and Roy Porter (eds), *Reassessing Foucault: Power, Medicine and the Body* (London and New York, 1994); recently Claudia Stein, "The Birth of Biopower in Eighteenth-Century Germany," *Medical History*, 55 (2011): 331–37 and references there; the most in-depth, archive-based study remains Francisca Loetz, *Vom Kranken zum Patienten: "Medikalisierung" und medizinische Vergesellschaftung am Beispiel Badens, 1750–1850* (Stuttgart, 1993), which also reviews the historiography in which "medicalization" intersects with "social disciplining," historian Gerhard Oestreich's concept that shaped a generation of historical research; see Stefan Breuer, "Sozialdisziplinierung: Probleme und Problemverlagerungen eines Konzepts bei Max Weber, Gerhard Oestreich und Michel Foucault," in Christoph Sachße and Florian Tennstedt (eds), *Soziale Sicherheit und soziale Disziplinierung: Beiträge zu einer historischen Theorie der Sozialpolitik* (Frankfurt am Main, 1986): 45–69. Also relevant here is the large literature on early modern criminality and sexuality, which includes work on constructing deviance as disease.

32 Cautionary tale: Mary Nagle Wessling, "Official Medicine and Customary Medicine in Early Modern Württemberg: The Career of Christoph Friedrich Pichler," *Medizin, Gesellschaft und Geschichte*, 9 (1990): 21–44; Loetz, *"Medikalisierung" und medizinische Vergesellschaftung*, esp. pp. 85–87, 144–69; similarly critical of older "police state" and "rationalization" histories: Lindemann, *Health and Healing*, esp. pp. 72–73, 138–42; Brockliss and Jones, *Medical World*, p. 32. Fresh challenges to medicalization narratives include Blumenthal, "Domestic Medicine," and recent extensions of the concept include "medicalization of domestic life": Sandra Cavallo and Tessa Storey, *Healthy Living in Late Renaissance Italy* (Oxford, 2013), p. 272 and see their discussion on p. 11.

33 Classic in English: Marc Raeff, "The Well-Ordered Police State and the Development of Modernity in Seventeenth- and Eighteenth-Century Europe: An Attempt at a Comparative Approach," *American Historical Review*, 80 (1975): 1221–43; widely cited, arguing from examples beginning in the eighteenth century: James C. Scott, *Seeing Like a State: How Certain Schemes to Improve the Human Condition Have Failed* (New Haven, 1998); critical reassessment: Andre Wakefield, *The Disordered Police State: German Cameralism as Science and Practice* (Chicago, 2009); on punishment: Michel Foucault, *Discipline and Punish: The Birth of the Prison* (New York, 1977), Part 1; Richard J. Evans, *Rituals of Retribution: Capital Punishment in Germany, 1600–1987* (Oxford, 1996), chs. 1–2.

34 This large complex of literatures can be approached in English through André Holenstein, Wims Blokmans, Jon Mathieu (eds), *Empowering Interactions: Political Culture and the Emergence of the State in Europe, 1300–1900* (Farnham, 2009); Rudolf Schlögl (ed.), *Urban Elections and Decision-Making in Early Modern Europe, 1500–1800* (Newcastle-upon-Tyne, 2009); Peter Blickle (ed.), *Resistance, Representation and Community* (Oxford, 1997), which is the relevant volume of "The Origins of the Modern State in Europe, 13th to 18th Centuries," a seven-volume series edited by Wim Blockmans and Jean-Philippe Genet (Oxford University Press, 1995–2000); Jason P. Coy, Benjamin Marschke, David W. Sabean (eds), *The Holy Roman Empire, Reconsidered* (New York, 2010); John Brewer and Eckhart Hellmuth (eds), *Rethinking Leviathan: The Eighteenth-Century State in Britain and Germany* (Oxford UP 1999). Several of the key lines of research have been developed mainly in German historiography: (1) since the mid-1980s, an urban history of "republicanism" in ideal and practice, led especially by Heinz Schilling, in Continental European cities and towns, and a rural as well as urban history of "communalism" led esp. by Peter Blickle, both contrasting with old histories of "absolutist" princely political order "from above": overview: Wolfgang Mager, "Genossenschaft, Republikanismus und konsensgestütztes Ratsregiment" in Luise Schorn-Schütte (ed.), *Aspekte der politischen Kommunikation im Europa des 16. und 17. Jahrhunderts*, Historische Zeitschrift Beihefte, n.s., 39 (Munich, 2004): 13–122; classic essays: Helmut G. Koenigsberger (ed.), *Republiken und Republikanismus im Europa der Frühen Neuzeit* (Munich, 1988); (2) since the mid-1990s, a new history of "police" (*Policey, police,* later *Polizei*) and of juridical processes in practice rather than only in theory and statute, led especially from the Max Planck Institut für europäische Rechtsgeschichte and the Arbeitskreis Policey/ Polizei im vormodernen Europa (www.univie.ac.at/policey-ak/), which has produced many monographs and collective volumes: see Michael Stolleis (ed.), *Policey im Europa der frühen Neuzeit* (Frankfurt am Main, 1996); André Holenstein et al. (eds), *Policey in lokalen Räumen: Ordnungskräfte und Sicherheitspersonal in Gemeinden und Territorien vom Spätmittelalter bis zum frühen 19. Jahrhundert* (Frankfurt am Main, 2002); Peter Blickle, Peter Kissling and Heinrich Richard Schmidt (eds), *Gute Policey als Politik im 16. Jahrhundert: die Entstehung des öffentlichen Raumes in Oberdeutschland* (Frankfurt am Main, 2003); and see Paolo Napoli, *Naissance de la police moderne: Pouvoir, normes, société* (Paris, 2003); (3) since around 2000, two schools of research on political communication *besides* news and print (which have been the main focus of history of communication): one at Münster led by Barbara Stollberg-Rilinger focusing on ceremony and symbolic communication and one at Constance led by Rudolf Schlögl focusing on oral and handwritten communication in urban politics: see Barbara Stollberg-Rilinger (ed.), *Vormoderne*

politische Verfahren (Berlin, 2001); Rudolf Schlögl (ed.), *Interaktion und Herrschaft: die Politik der frühneuzeitlichen Stadt* (Constance, 2004); combining oral and handwritten with print communication: Filippo de Vivo, *Information and Communication in Venice: Rethinking Early Modern Politics* (Oxford, 2007). Also relevant is the critical historiography dismantling "absolutism," which is now discussed mainly as a "myth" or, contradicting the concept in a more empirically productive way, a permanent debate, even for France: Fanny Cosandey and Robert Descimon, *L'absolutisme en France: histoire et historiographie* (Paris, 2002).

35 Brockliss and Jones, *Medical World*, p. 25: "the Europe of Enlightened Despotism"; Christopher Hamlin, "Forensic Cultures in Historical Perspective: Technologies of Witness, Testimony, Judgment (and Justice?)," *Studies in History and Philosophy of Biological and Biomedical Sciences*, 44 (2013): 4–15, p. 9: "the inquisitorial systems of jurisprudence of continental states (authoritarian, reactionary states)"; Pelling, *Medical Conflicts*, p. 21: "absolutism may be intrinsic to any system of medical police."

36 Michaela Hohkamp, *Herrschaft in der Herrschaft: Die vorderösterreichische Obervogtei Triberg von 1737 bis 1780* (Göttingen, 1998); Lars Behrisch, *Städtische Obrigkeit und soziale Kontrolle: Görlitz 1450–1600* (Epfendorf, 2005); and see notes 38 and 55 below.

37 On political ideals and values: Blickle, Kissling, and Schmidt, *Gute Policey als Politik*, Part 3, citing secondary literature since the early twentieth century; in the 1970s in English, Raeff, "Well-Ordered Police State," which assumed that practice followed principle; also in the 1970s, Foucault's clearest positioning, Michel Foucault, "'*Omnes et Singulatim*': Toward a Critique of Political Reason," in Foucault, *Power: Essential Works*, vol. 3; more recently Herfried Münkler and Harald Bluhm (eds), *Gemeinwohl und Gemeinsinn: historische Semantiken politischer Leitbegriffe* (Berlin, 2001); Thomas Simon, "*Gute Policey*": *Ordnungsleitbilder und Zielvorstellungen politischen Handelns in der Frühen Neuzeit* (Frankfurt am Main, 2004); Wakefield, *Disorderly Police State*, showing practice contradicted principle, but focused on state finance rather than local governance and "good police" of morals, health, environment, food supply, safety, education, agricultural and craft production, and community finance, on which the most in-depth case study is André Holenstein, "*Gute Policey*" *und lokale Gesellschaft im Staat des Ancien Régime: Das Fallbeispiel der Markgrafschaft Baden(-Durlach)*, 2 vols. (Tübingen, 2003); all of which shares vocabulary with, but contrasts with, "reason of state": see Peter Burke, "Tacitism, Scepticism, and Reason of State" in J. H. Burns (ed.), *The Cambridge History of Political Thought 1450–1700* (Cambridge, 1991): 479–98; Maurizio Viroli, *From Politics to Reason of State: The Acquisition and Transformation of the Language of Politics, 1250–1600* (Cambridge, 1992), esp. ch. 2; Horst Dreitzel, "Reason of State and the Crisis of Political Aristotelianism: An Essay on the Development of 17th-Century Political Philosophy," *History of European Ideas*, 28 (2002): 163–87.

38 Patrick Boucheron and Nicolas Offenstadt (eds), *L'espace public au Moyen âge: débats autour de Jürgen Habermas* (Paris, 2011) including bibliography of work since the 1970s on medieval *Öffentlichkeit*; Martin Kintzinger and Bernd Scheidmüller (eds), *Politische Öffentlichkeit im Spätmittelalter* (Ostfildern, 2011); James Van Horn Melton (ed.), *Cultures of Communication from Reformation to Enlightenment: Constructing Publics in the Early Modern German Lands* (Aldershot, 2002); de Vivo, *Information and Communication*

in Venice; Peter Lake and Steve Pincus (eds), *The Politics of the Public Sphere in Early Modern England* (Manchester, 2008); Bronwen Wilson and Paul Yachnin (eds), *Making Publics in Early Modern Europe* (Routledge, 2010); Gerd Schwerhoff (ed.), *Stadt und Öffentlichkeit in der frühen Neuzeit* (Cologne, 2011).

39 James A. Secord, "Knowledge in Transit," *Isis*, 95 (2004): 654–72; Cook, *Matters of Exchange*; Pamela H. Smith, "Science on the Move: Recent Trends in the History of Early Modern Science," *Renaissance Quarterly*, 62 (2009): 345–75; Anthony Grafton, *Worlds Made by Words: Scholarship and Community in the Modern West* (Cambridge, MA, 2009); Kaspar von Greyerz, Silvia Flubacher, and Philipp Senn (eds), *Wissenschaftsgeschichte und Geschichte des Wissens im Dialog—Connecting Science and Knowledge* (Göttingen, 2013); Elizabeth Yale, *Sociable Knowledge: Natural History and the Nation in Early Modern Britain* (Philadelphia, 2016).

40 Mary Fissell and Roger Cooter, "Exploring Natural Knowledge: Science and the Popular," in Roy Porter (ed.), *The Cambridge History of Science, Volume 4: Eighteenth-Century Science* (Cambridge, 2003): 129–58; Katherine Park and Lorraine Daston (eds), *The Cambridge History of Science, Volume 3: Early Modern Science* (Cambridge, 2006), chs. 7–9: Londa Schiebinger, "Women of Natural Knowledge," 192–205; William Eamon, "Markets, Piazzas, and Villages," 206–23; Alix Cooper, "Homes and Households," 224–37.

41 See Schlögl, *Interaktion und Herrschaft*; de Vivo, *Information and Communication in Venice*; Alexander Schlaak, "Overloaded Interactions: Effects of the Growing Use of Writing in German Imperial Cities, 1500–1800," in Coy, Marschke, and Sabean, *Holy Roman Empire*: 35–48; all of this work contrasts with media and communication histories focused on print: see Brendan Dooley and Sabrina A. Baron (eds), *The Politics of Information in Early Modern Europe* (London and New York, 2001); James Van Horn Melton, *The Rise of the Public in Enlightenment Europe* (Cambridge, 2001); and see note 97 below.

42 Chiara Crisciani, "Ethique des consilia et de la consultation: à propos de la cohesion morale de la profession médicale (XIIIe-XIVe siècles)," *Médiévales*, 46 (2004): 23–44, p. 25, though emphasizing "la figure du médecin de cour" as "la manifestation la plus éclatante de cet assemblage de compétences variées."

43 See John Harley Warner and Frank G. Huisman (eds), *Locating Medical History: The Stories and Their Meanings* (Baltimore, 2004), esp. Roger Cooter, "Framing the End of the Social History of Medicine," 309–37.

44 Jacob Soll, "Healing the Body Politic: French Royal Doctors, History and the Birth of a Nation, 1560–1634," *Renaissance Quarterly*, 55 (2002): 1259–86; Silvia De Renzi, "Medical Competence, Anatomy and the Polity in Seventeenth-Century Rome," *Renaissance Studies*, 21 (2007): 551–67, esp. pp. 558–61.

45 Sheila Jasanoff, *States of Knowledge: The Co-Production of Science and Social Order* (London, 2004); Steven Shapin and Simon Schaffer, *Leviathan and the Air-Pump: Hobbes, Boyle, and the Experimental Life* (Princeton, 1985); Vera Keller, *Knowledge and the Public Interest, 1575–1725* (Cambridge, 2015).

46 As it is here: Stolberg, "The Many Uses of Writing," Chapter 2 of this volume. The only recent overview of premodern physicians is written mainly from this perspective: Roger K. French, *Medicine before Science: The Rational and Learned Doctor from the Middle Ages to the Enlightenment* (Cambridge, 2003).

47   On scholars' behavior in domestic life: Gadi Algazi, "Scholars in Households: Refiguring the Learned Habitus, 1480–1550," *Science in Context*, 16 (2003): 9–42; in academic life: William Clark, *Academic Charisma and the Origins of the Research University* (Chicago, 2006); Marian Füssel, *Gelehrtenkultur als symbolische Praxis: Rang, Ritual und Konflikt an der Universität der frühen Neuzeit* (Darmstadt, 2006); Richard Kirwan, *Scholarly Self-Fashioning and Community in the Early Modern University* (Ashgate, 2013); Marian Füssel, "'On the Means of Becoming Famous in the Learned World': Practices of Scholarly Status Constitution and the Emergence of Moral Economy of Knowledge in the 18th Century," in André Holenstein et al. (eds), *Scholars in Action: The Practice of Knowledge and the Figure of the Savant in the 18th Century*, 2 vols. (Leiden, 2013), vol. 1: 123–43.

48   Sixteenth-century example: Stolberg, "The Many Uses of Writing," Chapter 2 of this volume; eighteenth-century example: Lisa Wynne Smith, "Secrets of Place: The Medical Casebooks of Vivant-Augustin Ganiare," in Elaine Leong and Alisha Rankin (eds), *Secrets and Knowledge in Medicine and Science, 1500–1800* (Farnham, 2011): 213–31.

49   Johann Jacob Baier, *Introductio in medicinam forensem et responsa eiusdem argumenti; tam ordinis sui nomine quam propria autoritate data in publicum proponuntur a Ferd. Iac. Baiero, filio* (Frankfurt, 1748), pp. 36–195: 30 cases with responsa, 1705–1735; on the Baiers and the Leopoldina: Marion Mücke and Thomas Schnalke, *Briefnetz Leopoldina: Die Korrespondenz der Deutschen Akademie der Naturforscher um 1750* (Berlin, 2009), pp. 609–10 and passim.

50   Jack Goody, *The Domestication of the Savage Mind* (Cambridge, 1977); Jack Goody, *The Logic of Writing and the Organization of Society* (Cambridge, 1986).

51   Limited to scholars acting among themselves, despite the promising title: Holenstein et al., *Scholars in Action*; but see Christian Jacob (ed.), *Lieux de savoir*, 2 vols. (Paris, 2007–2011).

52   Stolberg, "The Many Uses of Writing," Chapter 2 of this volume; Michael Stolberg, "Learning from the Common Folks: Academic Physicians and Medical Lay Culture in the Sixteenth Century," *Social History of Medicine*, 27 (2014): 649–67; see note 97 below.

53   Or Jews, including female medical practitioners: Joseph Shatzmiller, *Jews, Medicine, and Medieval Society* (Berkeley, 1994), pp. 112–18.

54   My discussion here builds on Schlegelmilch, "Promoting a Good Physician," Chapter 3 of this volume; see generally Michael Stolleis, "Grundzüge der Beamtenethik, 1550–1650," in Roman Schnur (ed.), *Die Rolle der Juristen bei der Entstehung des modernen Staates* (Berlin, 1986): 273–302; Bernhard Siegert and Joseph Vogl (eds), *Europa: Kultur der Sekretäre* (Zurich, 2003).

55   Peter Blickle (ed.), *Gemeinde und Staat im Alten Europa*, Historische Zeitschrift Beiheft, n.s., 25 (Munich, 1998); David Zaret, *Origins of Democratic Culture: Printing, Petitions, and the Public Sphere in Early Modern England* (Princeton, 2000); Friso Ross and Achim Landwehr (eds), *Denunziation und Justiz: Historische Dimensionen eines sozialen Phänomens* (Tübingen, 2000); Lex Heerma van Voss (ed.), *Petitions in Social History*, International Review of Social History Supplement, 9 (Amsterdam, 2001); Michaela Hohkamp and Claudia Ulbrich (eds), *Der Staatsbürger als Spitzel: Denunziation während des 18. und 19. Jahrhunderts aus europäischer Perspektive* (Leipzig, 2001); Cecilia Nubola and Andreas Würgler (eds), *Suppliche e gravamina: politica, amministrazione, giustizia in Europa (secoli XIV–XVIII)* (Bologna, 2002).

56   See Dross, "De Officiis," Chapter 4 of this volume.

57 Peter Blickle and André Holenstein (eds), *Der Fluch und der Eid: Die meta-physische Begründung gesellschaftlichen Zusammenlebens und politischer Ordnung in der ständischen Gesellschaft* (Berlin, 1993); Paolo Prodi (ed.), *Glaube und Eid: Treueformeln, Glaubensbekenntnisse und Sozialdisziplinier-ung zwischen Mittelalter und Neuzeit* (Munich, 1993).

58 Pomata, "A Sense of Place," Chapter 8 of this volume; Pugliano, "Account-ability, Autobiography, and Belonging," Chapter 7 of this volume; Vivian Nutton, "Continuity or Rediscovery? The City Physician in Classical Antiquity and Mediaeval Italy," in Russell, *Town and State Physician*: 9–46, pp. 31–33; Richard Palmer, "Physicians and the State in Post-Mediaeval Italy," in ibid.: 47–62.

59 Palmer, "Post-Mediaeval Italy," p. 56; information is mostly in older over-views and local studies; for Germany: Alfons Fischer, *Geschichte des deutschen Gesundheitswesens*, 2 vols. (Berlin, 1933); extensive bibliographies in Manfred Stürzbecher, "The Physici in German-Speaking Countries from the Middle Ages to the Enlightenment," in Russell, *Town and State Physician*: 123–30; Huldrych Koelbing, "The Town and State Physicians in Switzerland from the 16th to 18th Centuries" in ibid.: 141–55; for Dutch town phys-icians, see the example of Pieter van Foreest: H. L. Houtzager (ed.), *Pieter van Foreest: Een Hollands medicus in de zestiende eew* (Amsterdam, 1989); Henriette A. Bosman-Jegelrsma (ed.), *Petrus Forestus Medicus* (Amsterdam, 1996).

60 Gentilcore, "All That Pertains to Medicine"; Clouse, *Medicine, Government*; Di Giammatteo and Mendelsohn, "Reporting for Action," Chapter 5 of this volume.

61 Palmer, "Post-Mediaeval Italy," p. 59; Cipolla, *Public Health*. None of this is meant to idealize office, which could be a means of personal gain, profes-sional status, and dominance over competing practitioner groups; see Gentil-core, "All That Pertains to Medicine"; Brockliss and Jones, *Medical World*, ch. 10.

62 Lindemann, *Health and Healing*, ch. 2; Fischer, *Geschichte des deutschen Gesundheitswesens*, vol. 1: 329–31; vol. 2: 55–57; and detailed in the many regional studies listed in Stürzbecher, "Physici."

63 Fischer, *Geschichte des deutschen Gesundheitswesens*, vol. 2, pp. 37–38, 113–20, 143; Stürzbecher, "Physici," pp. 126–27; see Alix Cooper, *Inventing the Indigenous: Local Knowledge and Natural History in Early Modern Europe* (Cambridge, 2007), pp. 180–82.

64 This point can be viewed as an important result of the research for this volume: for the examples given here, see Chapter 5 for Tadino, Chapter 7 for Bianchi, Chapter 8 for Ferdinando, Chapter 9 for Erndtel, Chapter 11 for Nuremberg collegium.

65 For Ruysch and Tulp: Cook, *Matters of Exchange*, ch. 4; Margócsy, *Commer-cial Visions*; Sebastian A. C. Dudok van Heel (ed.), *Nicolaes Tulp: The Life and Work of an Amsterdam Physician and Magistrate in the 17th Century* (Amsterdam, 1998); for Magirus and similar examples: Schilling, Schlegel-milch, and Splinter, "Stadtarzt"; for Aldrovandi: Paula Findlen, *Possessing Nature: Museums, Collecting, and Scientific Culture in Early Modern Italy* (Berkeley, 1996), ch. 6 and passim; for Gesner as public instructor-examiner: Gustav Adolf Wehrli, *Die Krankenanstalten und die öffentlich angestellten Ärzte und Wundärzte im alten Zürich* (Zurich, 1934), pp. 39–40 (of mid-wives), 43–44 (natural philosophy and other subjects); and for context and textbook of midwifery in Zurich: Hildegard Elisabeth Keller and Hubert Steinke, "Jakob Ruf's *Trostbüchlein* and *De conceptu* (Zurich 1554):

A Textbook for Midwives and Physicians," in Emidio Campi et al. (eds), *Scholarly Knowledge: Textbooks in Early Modern Europe* (Geneva, 2008): 307–32; for Stadtärzte as instructors in Schleusingen: Carl Gottlob Dietmann, *Kurzgefasste Kirchen- und Schulgeschichte der gefürsteten Graffschaft Henneberg, Kurfürstlich-Sächsischen Antheils* (Gotha, 1781), p. 152; for Leopoldina rosters, see note 146 below.

66 Vernacular publishing by physicians: see the following section. Case study of news networks and disease: Christine Werkstetter, "Die Pest in der Stadt des Reichstags: Die Regensburger 'Contagion' von 1713/14 in kommunikationsgeschichtlicher Perspektive," in Johannes Burkhardt and Christine Werkstetter (eds), *Kommunikation und Medien in der Frühen Neuzeit*, Historische Zeitschrift Beihefte, n.s., 41 (Munich, 2005): 267–92. Physicians and learned published news: Kinzelbach and Ruisinger, "Trading Information," Chapter 11 of this volume; see generally Sven Dupré and Sachiko Kusukawa (eds), *The Circulation of News and Knowledge in Intersecting Networks*, volume 18 of *History of Universities* (New York, 2008). Learned medical correspondence and medical republic of letters: Hubert Steinke and Martin Stuber (eds), *Medical Correspondence in Early Modern Europe*, special issue of *Gesnerus*, 61/3–4 (2004); Ian MacLean, "The Medical Republic of Letters before the Thirty Years War," *Intellectual History Review*, 18 (2008): 15–30; Nancy G. Siraisi, *Communities of Learned Experience: Epistolary Medicine in the Renaissance* (Baltimore, 2013); Mücke and Schnalke, *Briefnetz Leopoldina*.

67 Among them physicians, such as Symphorien Champier in Lyon: see Davis, "Poor Relief, Humanism, and Heresy," pp. 28–31, 55, 61–62; on historiography since Davis and the question of the relative importance of civic, Christian humanist, Reformation, and Catholic impulses, see Ole Peter Grell, "The Protestant Imperative of Christian Care and Neighbourly Love," in Grell and Cunningham, *Health Care and Poor Relief in Protestant Europe*: 42–63.

68 An opposite story, of community resistance, can be found in eighteenth-century territorial states seeking to impose official medicine by centrally appointed medical officers: Wessling, "Official Medicine and Customary Medicine."

69 Wehrli, *Krankenanstalten*, p. 32, 76–78.

70 Valentin Lötscher (ed.), *Felix Platter: Tagebuch (Lebensbeschreibung) 1536–1567* (Basel and Stuttgart, 1976), appendix.

71 Candice Delisle, "Accessing Nature, Circulating Knowledge: Conrad Gessner's Correspondence Networks and his Medical and Naturalist Practices," *History of Universities*, 18 (2008): 35–58, pp. 35–36.

72 Wessling, "Official Medicine and Customary Medicine."

73 Ole Peter Grell, "Conflicting Duties: Plague and the Obligations of Early Modern Physicians towards Patients and Commonwealth in England and the Netherlands," in Andrew Wear et al. (eds), *Doctors and Ethics: The Earlier Historical Setting of Professional Ethics* (Amsterdam, 1993): 131–52.

74 Robert Black, "Humanism," in Christopher Allmand (ed.), *The New Cambridge Medieval History VII, c. 1415 – c. 1500* (Cambridge, 1998): 243–77, esp. pp. 274–77; Hankins, *Renaissance Civic Humanism*; Hirschi, "Höflinge der Bürgerschaft—Bürger des Hofes."

75 See generally Helmut Zedelmaier, *Bibliotheca Universalis und Bibliotheca Selecta: Das Problem der Ordnung des gelehrten Wissens in der Frühen Neuzeit*, Beihefte zum Archiv für Kulturgeschichte, 33 (Cologne, Weimar, Vienna, 1992); Peter Becker and William Clark (eds), *Little Tools of Knowledge: Historical Essays on Academic and Bureaucratic Practices* (Ann Arbor, 2001); special issue on "Early Modern Information Overload," *Journal of the*

History of Ideas 64/1 (2003); Elisabeth Décultot, *Lire, copier, écrire: les bib-liothèques manuscrites et leurs usages au XVIIIe siècle* (Paris, 2003); Arndt Brendecke, Markus Friedrich, and Susanne Friedrich (eds), *Information in der Frühen Neuzeit: Status, Bestände, Strategien*, Pluralisierung & Autorität, 16 (Berlin, 2008); Delphine Gardey, *Ecrire, calculer, classer: comment une révo-lution de papier à transformé les sociétés contemporaines (1800–1940)* (Paris, 2008); Ben Kafka, "Paperwork: The State of the Discipline," *Book History*, 12 (2009): 340–53; Ann Blair, *Too Much to Know: Managing Scholarly Information before the Modern Age* (New Haven, 2010); Ann Blair and Rich-ard Yeo (eds), *Note-Taking in Early Modern Europe*, special issue of *Intellec-tual History Review*, 20/3 (2010); Volker Hess and J. Andrew Mendelsohn, "Paper Technology und Wissensgeschichte," *NTM: Zeitschrift für Geschichte der Wissenschaften, Technik und Medizin* 21 (2013): 1–10; Lisa Gitelman, *Paper Knowledge: Toward a Media History of Documents* (Durham, NC, 2014).

76 Deaths and injuries: recent overviews include Katherine D. Watson, *Forensic Medicine in Western Society* (New York, 2011), chs. 2–3; Silvia De Renzi, "Medical Expertise, Bodies, and Law in Early Modern Courts," *Isis*, 98 (2007): 315–22. Danger to others: Guenter B. Risse, *Mending Bodies, Saving Souls: A History of Hospitals* (New York, 1999), ch. 4 and references there to literature on leprosy inspection. Evaluating for charitable care: Claudia Stein, *Negotiating the French Pox in Early Modern Germany* (Aldershot, 2009), ch. 3; Mitchell L. Hammond, "Medical Examination and Poor Relief in Early Modern Germany," *Social History of Medicine*, 23 (2010): 1–16. Impotence: Pierre Darmon, *Trial by Impotence: Virility and Marriage in Pre-Revolutionary France* (London, 1985); Edward Behrend-Martinez, *Unfit for Marriage: Impotent Spouses on Trial in the Basque Region of Spain, 1650–1750* (Reno, 2007); Joseph Bajada, *Sexual Impotence: The Contribu-tion of Paolo Zacchia (1584–1659)* (Rome, 1988). Evaluating naturalia, mate-ria medica, environments: see notes 77, 87–88 below.

77 But see now Alexa Geisthövel and Volker Hess (eds), *Medizinisches Gutach-ten: Geschichte einer neuzeitlichen Praxis* (Berlin, 2017).

78 For recent nuanced formulation of the problem of definition and origins, see Joël Chandelier and Marilyn Nicoud, "Entre droit et médecine: les origines de la médecine légale en Italie (XIIIe–XIVe siècles)," in Joël Chandelier and Aur-élien Robert (eds), *Les frontières des savoirs en Italie à l'époque des premières universités (XIIIe–XVe siècles)* (Rome, 2015): 233–93. On Zacchia: Silvia De Renzi, "Witnesses of the Body: Medico-Legal Cases in Seventeenth-Century Rome," *Studies in the History and Philosophy of Science*, 33 (2002): 219–42; Jacalyn Duffin, "Questioning Medicine in Seventeenth-Century Rome: The Consultations of Paolo Zacchia," *Canadian Bulletin of Medical History*, 28 (2011): 149–70. Noting the wide range of issues beyond deaths and injuries: Catherine Crawford, "Medicine and the Law," in Bynum and Porter, *Com-panion Encyclopedia*, vol. 2: 1619–40, p. 1624; De Renzi, "Witnesses of the Body," p. 226; Hamlin, "Forensic Cultures," p. 7; Duffin, "Questioning Medicine."

79 Matthew Ramsey, "Traditional Medicine and Medical Enlightenment: The Regulation of Secret Remedies in the Ancien Regime," in Jean-Pierre Goubert (ed.), *La médicalisation de la société française, 1770–1830*, special issue of *Historical Reflections/Réflexions historiques*, 9/1–2 (1982): 215–32, p. 225, 230–31; Caroline Hannaway, *Medicine, Public Welfare and the State in Eighteenth-Century France: The Société royale de médecine of Paris, 1776–1793* (Ph.D. Diss., Johns Hopkins University, 1974); see generally

Andreas-Holger Maehle, *Drugs on Trial: Experimental Pharmacology and Therapeutic Innovation in the Eighteenth Century*, Clio Medica, 53 (Amsterdam, 1999); and recently: Saskia Klerk, *Galen Reconsidered: Studying Drug Properties and the Foundations of Medicine in the Dutch Republic, ca. 1550–1700* (Utrecht, 2015).

80 Classically in leprosy inspection and in impotence trial; see note 76 above.

81 See many examples in Fischer-Homberger, *Medizin vor Gericht.*

82 Geisthövel and Hess, *Medizinisches Gutachten*; see Jole Agrimi and Chiara Crisciani, *Les "consilia" médicaux*, Typologie des sources du moyen age occidental, 69 (Turnhout, 1994).

83 On the rise of written medical certification from as early as the thirteenth century: Shatzmiller, *Jews, Medicine*, pp. 3–5, on wide variety of reasons for certificates; Andreas Meyer, "Lepra und Lepragutachten aus dem Lucca des 13. Jahrhundert," in Andreas Meyer and Jürgen Schulz-Grobert (eds), *Gesund und krank im Mittelalter*, Marburger Beiträge zur Kulturgeschichte der Medizin (Leipzig, 2007): 145–210; literature on leprosy certificates goes back to a series of articles by Karl Sudhoff beginning with "Lepraschaubriefe aus dem 15. Jahrhundert," *Archiv für Geschichte der Medizin*, 4–5 (1910): 370–78; example in English in Risse, *Mending Bodies*, ch. 4; early oral medical testimony: Allessandro Simili, "The Beginnings of Forensic Medicine in Bologna" and Peter Volk and Hans Jürgen Warlo, "The Role of Medical Experts in Court Proceedings in the Medieval Town," in Heinrich Karplus (ed.), *International Symposium on Society, Medicine and Law* (Amsterdam, 1973): 91–100, 101–16; Joseph Shatzmiller, *Médecine et justice en Provence médiévale: documents de Manosque, 1262–1348* (Aix-en-Provence, 1989); oral and written: Wendy J. Turner and Sara Butler (eds), *Medicine and the Law in the Middle Ages* (Leiden, 2014).

84 Kinzelbach, "Negotiating on Paper," Chapter 6 of this volume.

85 Di Giammatteo and Mendelsohn, "Reporting for Action," Chapter 5 of this volume.

86 Political prudence in relation to medicine and law: Burke, "Tacitism," p. 482; Pomata, "Sharing Cases," pp. 231–32; medico-political counsel to rulers: Soll, "Healing the Body Politic"; De Renzi, "Medical Competence," pp. 559–61.

87 For an example of evaluation by the Roman College of Physicians, the *protomedico*, other Roman physicans, and apothecaries in a protracted case of merchant dispute over a shipment of medicinal wood: Nancy G. Siraisi, *History, Medicine, and the Traditions of Renaissance Learning* (Ann Arbor, 2007), pp. 173–74.

88 On mineral spring analysis, see most recently Alix Cooper, "Die Begutachtung der Natur: Frühmodernes medizinisches Berichten am Beispiel von 'Judicia' über Mineralwässer in Friedrich Hoffmanns *Medicina consultatoria*," in Geisthövel and Hess, *Medizinisches Gutachten*: 145–65; mineral spring analysis for government as early as the fourteenth century: Park, *Doctors and Medicine*, p. 97; relation to development of natural knowledge: Katharine Park, "Natural Particulars: Medical Epistemology, Practice, and the Literature of Healing Springs," in Anthony Grafton and Nancy Siraisi (ed.), *Natural Particulars: Nature and the Disciplines in Renaissance Europe* (Cambridge, MA, 1999): 347–67, emphasizing aristocratic patronage, though noting role of municipalities, pp. 349–50. Evaluating potability of Tiber river: Nancy G. Siraisi, "Historiae, Natural History, Roman Antiquity, and Some Roman Physicians," in Pomata and Siraisi, *Historia*: 325–54. Privileges of inspecting waters were important enough to be fought over, as for example in France

between medical faculties and royal physicians and, during its relatively brief existence, the Société royale de médecine: Hannaway, *Medicine, Public Health and the State*; Pascale Cosma-Muller, "Entre science et commerce: les eaux minérales en France à la fin de l'Ancien Régime," in Goubert, *La médicalisation*: 249–62; Brockliss and Jones, *Medical World*, pp. 769–79. Evaluating airs came later in the period: Simon Schaffer, "Measuring Virtue: Eudiometry, Enlightenment and Pneumatic Medicine," in Andrew Cunningham and Roger French (eds), *The Medical Enlightenment of the Eighteenth Century* (Cambridge, 1990): 281–318.

89 See notes 30, 33–34, 37 above.
90 Cooper, *Inventing the Indigenous*, pp. 91, 101.
91 Findlen, *Possessing Nature*, ch. 6, esp. pp. 261–72.
92 Pomata, "Sharing Cases," pp. 226–30, emphasizing the practitioner profile of town and court physicians and being on the periphery of university medicine; see Brian K. Nance, *Turquet de Mayerne as Baroque Physician: The Art of Medical Portraiture*, Clio Medica, 65 (Amsterdam and New York, 2001), ch. 2; Michael Stolberg, "Formen und Funktionen medizinischer Fallberichte in der Frühen Neuzeit (1500–1800)," in Johannes Süßmann, Susanne Scholz, and Gisela Engel (eds), *Fallstudien: Theorie—Geschichte—Methode*, Frankfurter Kulturwissenschaftliche Beiträge (Berlin, 2007): 81–95.
93 Simona Cerutti and Gianna Pomata (eds), *Fatti: storie dell'evidenza empirica*, special issue of *Quaderni storici*, 108/3 (2001); Gianna Pomata, "Praxis Historialis: The Uses of *Historia* in Early Modern Medicine," in Pomata and Siraisi, *Historia*: 105–46; Katharine Park, "Observation in the Margins, 500–1500" and Gianna Pomata, "Observation Rising: Birth of an Epistemic Genre, 1500–1650," in Lorraine Daston and Elizabeth Lunbeck (eds), *Histories of Scientific Observation* (Chicago, 2011): 15–44, 45–80.
94 Schilling, "Physical City," Chapter 9 of this volume.
95 Pomata and Siraisi, *Historia*; Michael Niehaus and Hans-Walter Schmidt-Hannisa (eds), *Das Protokoll: Kulturelle Funktionen einer Textsorte* (Frankfurt am Main, 2005); Blair and Yeo, *Note-Taking*; James Delbourgo and Staffan Müller-Wille, "Listmania: Introduction," *Isis*, 103 (2012): 710–15.
96 On the reductive power of cataloguing and lists in long-term historical transformations of knowledge of nature: Cooper, *Inventing the Indigenous*, pp. 72–80, 171–72; on specific long-term knowledge effects of indexing, commonplacing, administrative recordkeeping, and paper organization of work in institutions: Volker Hess and J. Andrew Mendelsohn, "Case and Series: Medical Knowledge and Paper Technology, 1600–1900," *History of Science*, 48 (2010): 287–314; effects of commonplacing on early modern medical knowledge: Michael Stolberg, "Medizinische Loci Communes: Formen und Funktionen einer ärztlichen Aufzeichnungspraxis im 16. und 17. Jahrhundert," *NTM: Zeitschrift für Geschichte der Wissenschaften, Technik und Medizin*, 21 (2013): 37–60.
97 Miles Ogborn, "Talking Plants: Botany and Speech in Eighteenth-Century Jamaica," *History of Science*, 51 (2013): 1–32; Cooper, *Inventing the Indigenous*, esp. ch. 5; Martha Baldwin, "Expanding the Therapeutic Canon: Learned Medicine Listens to Folk Medicine," in Van Horn Melton, *Cultures of Communication*: 239–56; Wear, *Knowledge and Practice*, ch. 2, esp. pp. 56–67; Elaine Leong and Alisha Rankin, "Introduction: Secrets and Knowledge," in Leong and Rankin, *Secrets and Knowledge*: 1–20.
98 Case study of mobility and correspondence: Delisle, "Accessing Nature"; more generally on travel and correspondence in making "matters of fact":

David S. Lux and Harold J. Cook. "Closed Circles or Open Networks?: Communicating at a Distance during the Scientific Revolution," *History of Science*, 36 (1998): 179–211.

99   Stolberg, "Learning from the Common Folks."

100 Natalie Zemon Davis, "Printing and the People" and "Proverbial Wisdom and Popular Errors," in her *Society and Culture in Early Modern France* (Stanford, 1975): 189–226 and 227–67, esp. p. 224.

101 Schilling, "Physical City," Chapter 9 of this volume.

102 On medicine's second-hand empiricism, see J. Andrew Mendelsohn, "Empiricism in the Library: Medicine's Case Histories," in Lorraine Daston (ed.), *Science in the Archives: Pasts, Presents, Futures* (Chicago, 2017): 85–109.

103 Surveying this variety: Siraisi, *History, Medicine*.

104 Siraisi, *History, Medicine*, pp. 95, 184–87; Siraisi, "*Historiae*, Natural History."

105 Smith, "Secrets of Place," pp. 214–15.

106 Cavallo and Storey, *Healthy Living*, p. 79.

107 Mirko D. Grmek, "Géographie médicale et histoire des civilisations," *Annales: Économies, Sociétés, Civilisations*, 18 (1963): 1071–97, pp. 1075–78; Jan Brügelmann, "Observations on the Process of Medicalisation in Germany, 1770–1830, Based on Medical Topographies," in Goubert, *La médicalisation*: 131–49; Conevery Bolton Valencius, "Histories of Medical Geography," in Nicolaas A. Rupke (ed.), *Medical Geography in Historical Perspective*, Medical History Supplement, 20 (London, 2000): 3–28, p. 12.

108 See Gianna Pomata, "The Recipe and the Case: Epistemic Genres and the Dynamics of Cognitive Practices," in von Greyerz, Flubacher and Senn, *Wissenschaftsgeschichte*: 131–54; on commentary as well as case, Gianna Pomata, "The Medical Case Narrative: Distant Reading of an Epistemic Genre," *Literature and Medicine*, 32 (2014): 1–23 and references there; on textbooks: Campi et al., *Scholarly Knowledge*.

109 Dross, "De Officiis," Chapter 4 of this volume.

110 Shatzmiller, *Jews, Medicine*, pp. 124–31, on Provence; Marius J. van Lieburg, "Die medizinische Versorgung einer Stadtbevölkerung im 17. Jahrhundert: Die Quellen- und Forschungssituation für Rotterdam," in Wolfgang Eckart and Johanna Geyer-Kordesch (eds), *Heilberufe und Kranke im 17. und 18. Jahrhundert: Die Quellen- und Forschungssituation: Ein Arbeitsgespräch*, Münstersche Beiträge zur Geschichte und Theorie der Medizin, 18 (Tecklenburg, 1982): 29–48, pp. 35–36; Gianna Pomata, *Contracting a Cure: Patients, Healers, and the Law in Early Modern Bologna* (Baltimore, 1998); Constitutio Criminalis Carolina, Art. 134; thinking broadly about physicians, responsibility, and error, see Mariacarla Gadebusch Bondio (ed.), *Medical Ethics: Premodern Negotiations between Medicine and Philosophy* (Stuttgart, 2014); Mariacarla Gadebusch Bondio and Agostino Paravicini Bagliani (eds), *Errors and Mistakes: A Cultural History of Fallibility* (Florence, 2012).

111 Nance, *Turquet de Mayerne*, p. 53, 65, and ch. 2 generally.

112 Pugliano, "Accountability, Autobiography, and Belonging," Chapter 7 of this volume.

113 For accounting in medical practice records, see Volker Hess and Sabine Schlegelmilch, "Cornucopia Officinae Medicae: Medical Practice Records and Their Origin," in Martin Dinges et al. (eds), *Medical Practice, 1600–1900: Physicians and Their Patients*, Clio Medica, 96 (Leiden, 2016): 11–38, p. 23, 26, 29–30. Though historians have long used hospital financial records as sources, historical study of accounting and medicine is a new field: see Enrico Bracci, Laura Maran, and Emidia Vagnoni, "Saint Anna's Hospital in Ferrara, Italy: Accounting and Organizational Change during the Devolution,"

Accounting History, 15 (2010): 463–504; Andy Holden, Warwick Funnell, and David Oldroyd, "Accounting and the Moral Economy of Illness in Victorian England: The Newcastle Infirmary," *Accounting, Auditing & Accountability Journal*, 22 (2009): 525–52.

114 See the classic study by Michael T. Clanchy, *From Memory to Written Record: England, 1066–1307* (Cambridge, 1979); on "writing and responsibility," see Goody, *Logic of Writing*, pp. 124–26.

115 Brockliss and Jones, *Medical World*, esp. ch. 3 and ch. 8, acknowledging both sides but emphasizing the former; monopoly and hierarchy in alliance with the state, pp. 8–9; "neo-corporatist," p. 826; reviewing literature on other places, pp. 11–14; for England: Cook, *Decline*; Cook, "Policing"; Pelling, *Medical Conflicts*; in Germany, medical collegia arose in closer relation to government: Fischer, *Geschichte des deutschen Gesundheitswesens*, vol. 1: pp. 171–72, 183–87, 328–31; vol. 2: pp. 63–70; Broman, *Transformation*.

116 Pelling, *Medical Conflicts*, pp. 26–33, quotation on p. 30 from the College Annals of 1599; see Margaret Pelling, "Public and Private Dilemmas: The College of Physicians in Early Modern London," in Steve Sturdy (ed.), *Medicine, Health, and the Public Sphere in Britain, 1600–2000* (London, 2002): 27–42.

117 Park, *Doctors and Medicine*, ch. 1 and ch. 3, esp. pp. 87–99.

118 For striking examples of this richness of medical translation, see Luke Demaitre, "Medical Writing in Transition: Between Ars and Vulgus" in William Cosgrove (ed.), *The Vernacularization of Science, Medicine, and Technology in Late Medieval Europe*, special issue of *Early Science and Medicine*, 3/2 (1998): 88–102; Crisciani, "Histories, Stories, Exempla"; Mechthild Habermann, *Deutsche Fachtexte der frühen Neuzeit: Naturkundlich-medizinische Wissensvermittlung im Spannungsfeld von Latein und Volkssprache* (Berlin, 2001).

119 For a similar suggestion, see Keller and Steinke, "Jakob Ruf's *Trostbüchlein*," pp. 318–19; on the problem, see Luke Demaitre, "Theory and Practice in Medical Education at the University of Montpellier in the Thirteenth and Fourteenth Centuries," *Journal of the History of Medicine and Allied Sciences*, 30 (1975): 103–23; Danielle Jacquart, "Theory, Everyday Practice, and Three Fifteenth-Century Physicians," *Osiris*, 6 (1990): 140–60; Siraisi, *Medieval and Early Renaissance Medicine*; Broman, *Transformation*.

120 Ash, *Power and Knowledge*; Simon Schaffer et al. (eds), *The Brokered World: Go-Betweens and Global Intelligence, 1770–1820* (Sagamore Beach, MA, 2009); see also note 39 above.

121 Andreas Deutsch, "Klagspiegel und Laienspiegel—Sebastian Brants Beitrag zum Ruhm zweier Rechtsbücher," in Klaus Bergdolt et al. (eds), *Sebastian Brant und die Kommunikationskultur um 1500* (Wiesbaden, 2010): 75–98.

122 Karen Meier Reeds, "Renaissance Humanism and Botany," *Annals of Science*, 33 (1976): 519–42; Anthony Grafton, *New Worlds, Ancient Texts: The Power of Tradition and the Shock of Discovery*, with April Shelford and Nancy G. Siraisi (Cambridge, MA, 1992), ch. 4; Findlen, *Possessing Nature*, esp. pp. 163–70, 179–84; Brian W. Ogilvie, *The Science of Describing: Natural History in Renaissance Europe* (Chicago, 2006); Cooper, *Inventing the Indigenous*, ch. 1.

123 Georg Agricola, *Georgii Agricolae Medici Bermannvs sive De Re Metallica* (Basel, 1530).

124 Most recently: Margócsy, *Commercial Visions*, ch. 1.

125 Joachim Telle, "Wissenschaft und Öffentlichkeit im Spiegel der deutschen Arzneibuchliteratur: Zum deutsch-lateinischen Sprachenstreit in der Medizin des

16. und 17. Jahrhunderts," *Medizinhistorisches Journal*, 14 (1979): 32–52, pp. 34–35 and bibliography, for Uffenbach and earlier Stadtarzt Adam Lonicer.

126 Mary Fissell, "The Disappearance of the Patient's Narrative and the Invention of Hospital Medicine," in Roger French and Andrew Wear (eds), *British Medicine in an Age of Reform* (New York, 1991): 92–109, p. 103.

127 Quoted in Telle, "Wissenschaft und Öffentlichkeit," p. 34, from a 1603 preface by Uffenbach.

128 Institut für Stadtgeschichte, Frankfurt am Main, Städtisches Archiv, Criminalia 853, fol. 6.

129 Peter Stallybrass, "'Little Jobs': Broadsides and the Printing Revolution," in Sabrina Alcorn Baron, Eric N. Lindquist, and Eleanor Shevlin (eds), *Agent of Change: Print Culture Studies after Elizabeth L. Eisenstein* (Amherst, 2007): 315–41; Lauren Kassell, "Almanacs and Prognostications," in Joad Raymond (ed.), *The Oxford History of Popular Print Culture, Volume One: Cheap Print in Britain and Ireland to 1660* (Oxford, 2011): 431–42; overview of sources and literature on writing in almanacs: Harald Tersch, *Schreibkalender und Schreibkultur: Zur Rezeptionsgeschichte eines frühen Massenmediums* (Graz, 2008).

130 Sabine Schlegelmilch, "Vom Nutzen des Nebensächlichen: Paratexte in den Kalendern des Johannes Magirus," in Klaus-Dieter Herbst (ed.), *Astronomie— Literatur—Volksaufklärung: Der Schreibkalender der Frühen Neuzeit mit seinen Text- und Bildbeigaben* (Bremen, 2012): 393–411, p. 404 for his use of *observationes*.

131 See Tersch, *Schreibkalender*, pp. 9–11, 91–92, and references there.

132 As was the case in Zurich from the sixteenth to the eighteenth century and included almanac production by leading physician-naturalists; Wehrli, *Krankenanstalten*, pp. 43–44.

133 Kinzelbach and Ruisinger, "Trading Information," Chapter 11 of this volume; physician-entrepreneurs in anatomical publishing: Margócsy, *Commercial Visions*.

134 Leong, "Transformative Itineraries and Communities of Knowledge in Early Modern Europe," Chapter 10 of this volume; see Mary Fissell, "Popular Medical Writing," in Raymond, *Oxford History of Popular Print Culture*: 417–30; Paul Slack, "Mirrors of Health and Treasures of Poor Men: The Uses of the Vernacular Medical Literature of Tudor England," in Charles Webster (ed.), *Health, Medicine and Mortality in the Sixteenth Century* (Cambridge, 1979): 237–73; see note 118 above.

135 Cited in Peter Burke, "Cultures of Translation in Early Modern Europe," in Peter Burke and R. Po-chia Hsia (eds), *Cultural Translation in Early Modern Europe* (Cambridge, 2007): 7–38, p. 8.

136 Quoted in Leong, "Transformative Itineraries and Communities of Knowledge in Early Modern Europe," Chapter 10 of this volume; such a medical commonwealth already existed to some extent in provincial urban England: Pelling, *Common Lot*.

137 See the four-volume series *Cultural Exchange in Early Modern Europe* (Cambridge, 2006–07).

138 For the model of "state as client": Park, *Doctors and Medicine*, pp. 87–99; Pelling, "Healing the Sick Poor," pp. 121–26 (ad hoc and retainer contracts in which "the city exercised consumer choice," p. 122); for practices of community within competition: James E. Shaw and Evelyn S. Welch, *Making and Marketing Medicine in Renaissance Florence*, Clio Medica, 89 (Amsterdam,

2011), p. 23; for other problems with "the medical marketplace model": Wear, *Knowledge and Practice*, pp. 28–29.

139 See note 26 above.

140 Alexandre Lunel, *La maison médicale du roi, XVIe-XVIIIe siècles: Le pouvoir royal et les professions de santé (médecins, chirurgiens, apothicaires)* (Seyssel, 2008); Gabriele Wacker, *Arznei und Confect: Medikale Kultur am Wolfenbütteler Hof im 16. und 18. Jahrhundert*, Wolfenbütteler Forschungen, 134 (Wiesbaden, 2013).

141 See, for example, Peter Bahl, *Der Hof des Grossen Kurfürsten: Studien zur höheren Amtsträgerschaft Brandenburg-Preussens* (Cologne, 2001), pp. 76–77, quotation on p. 77 from a 1654 certificate of appointment; my thanks to Marion Mücke and Molly Taylor-Polesky for introducing me to the intricacies of medicine at the Brandenburg court.

142 Nutton, "Introduction," p. 11.

143 Richard Palmer, "Medicine at the Papal Court in the Sixteenth Century," in Nutton, *Medicine at the Courts of Europe*: 49–78, pp. 60–61; popular *Affiches* circulating news on the health of the French royal family: Brockliss and Jones, *Medical World*, p. 649.

144 Focusing on this is Lunel, *La maison médicale du roi*.

145 Harold J. Cook, "The Cutting Edge of a Revolution? Medicine and Natural History near the Shores of the North Sea," in J.V. Feld and Frank A.J.L. James (eds), *Renaissance and Revolution: Humanists, Scholars, Craftsmen and Natural Philosophers in Early Modern Europe* (Cambridge, 1993): 45–61; along with Cook's many pathbreaking papers on the subject, major studies emphasizing the shaping of early modern scientific culture by medicine and physicians include Findlen, *Possessing Nature*, esp. ch. 6; Cooper, *Inventing the Indigenous*; see also Park, "Observation in the Margins" and Pomata, "Observation Rising," in which medicine is central.

146 In addition to the lists of *observationes* contributors published in each volume of the *Miscellanea*, see membership rosters such as "Catalogus S.R.I. Academiae Naturae Curiosorum Collegarum omnium" in *Miscellanea Curiosa sive Ephemeridum Medico-Physicarum Germanicarum Academiae Naturae Curiosorum, Decuriae II, Annus Primus, Anni MDCLXXXII* (1683); contributors and members listed as professors were often also official town physicians as were those with court appointments.

147 Though they fit neatly into the history of commerce and naturalia, physician-entrepreneurs may be unusual rather than typical; see most recently Margócsy, *Commercial Visions*.

148 Eugenio Garin, *Science and Civic Life in the Italian Renaissance*, trans. Peter Munz (Garden City, NY, 1969 [orig. 1965]), with title word "civile" appropriately given as "civic" rather than "civil." In contrast, historiography of early modern science has focused on the driving and shaping force of *civility* as part of courtly and patrician culture: see Findlen, *Possessing Nature*, pp. 15–16, ch. 3, passim; Mario Biagioli, *Galileo, Courtier: The Practice of Science in the Culture of Absolutism* (Chicago, 1993), ch. 2, pp. 154–56. Recently on Renaissance consumption and medical market: Evelyn S. Welch, *Shopping in the Renaissance: Consumer Cultures in Italy 1400–1600* (New Haven, 2005); Shaw and Welch, *Making and Marketing Medicine*, cautioning that the early modern "medical marketplace" was neither impersonal nor free (pp. 22–23); see Cavallo and Storey, *Healthy Living*.

149 Pietro Redondi, *Galileo, Heretic*, trans. Raymond Rosenthal (Princeton, 1987); Biagioli, *Galileo, Courtier*; Matteo Valleriani, *Galileo, Engineer* (Dordrecht,

2010); Paula Findlen, "Jokes of Nature and Jokes of Knowledge: The Playfulness of Scientific Discourse in Early Modern Europe," *Renaissance Quarterly*, 43 (1990): 292–331.

150 On places and spaces, recent overviews include Jacob, *Lieux de savoir*; Sabrina Brevaglieri and Antonella Romano (eds), *Produzione di saperi, costruzione di spazi* (Bologna, 2013).

151 Recently on reform: Keller, *Knowledge and the Public Interest*; Margaret Pelling and Scott Mandelbrote (eds), *The Practice of Reform in Health, Medicine, and Science, 1500–2000: Essays for Charles Webster* (Aldershot, 2005).

152 See note 175 below.

153 Overview in Bruce T. Moran, "Courts and Academies," in Park and Daston, *Cambridge History of Science*, ch. 11; Ash, *Expertise*; recent: Klein, *Humboldts Preußen*.

154 Foucault, "'*Omnes et Singulatim*'."

155 See for example the essays in Sturdy, *Medicine, Health, and the Public Sphere*.

156 Jacques Revel, "Knowledge of the Territory," *Science in Context*, 4 (1991): 133–62; Brian, *La mesure de l'état*; Andrea A. Rusnock, *Vital Accounts: Quantifying Health and Population in Eighteenth-Century England and France* (Cambridge, 2002); Susanne Friedrich, "'Zu Nothdürfftiger Information': Herrschaftlich veranlasste Landeserfassungen des 16. und 17. Jahrhunderts im Alten Reich," in Brendecke, Friedrich, and Friedrich, *Information in der Frühen Neuzeit*: 301–34; Justus Nipperdey, *Die Erfindung der Bevölkerungspolitik: Staat, politische Theorie und Population in der Frühen Neuzeit* (Göttingen, 2012).

157 On negotiating: Kinzelbach, "Negotiating on Paper," Chapter 6 of this volume; Stein, *Negotiating the French Pox*; Hammond, "Medical Examination." Habermas: see note 38 above; understandably Habermas applies better to published science and academic medicine in the Enlightenment: Broman, *Transformation*; Thomas Broman, "The Habermasian Public Sphere and 'Science in the Enlightenment'," *History of Science*, 36 (1998): 123–49. For the turn away from Weberian histories of the early modern state: Holenstein, Blokmans, and Mathieu, *Empowering Interactions*; Brewer and Hellmuth, *Rethinking Leviathan*.

158 See note 39 above; but see now Keller, *Knowledge and the Public Interest*, on political aims and ideals in and around early modern natural knowledge; and Yale, *Sociable Knowledge*, showing how a human and natural "Britannia" was constructed by naturalists and antiquaries communicating and collaborating by correspondence.

159 On applying Marcel Mauss and Robert Merton, see most recently Margócsy, *Commercial Visions*, pp. 6–8, and references there; on coexistence of gift and commodity exchange in knowledge circulation, see Smith and Findlen, *Merchants and Marvels*.

160 See note 38 above; Johannes Arndt and Esther-Beate Körber (eds), *Das Mediensystem im Alten Reich der Frühen Neuzeit (1600–1750)* (Göttingen, 2010); Werner Faulstich, *Geschichte der Medien*, 5 vols. (Göttingen, 1996–2004) is organised around the concept of "Teilöffentlichkeiten," systems of them at any given time, and changes in their dominance.

161 See note 9 above; Gieryn, "Boundary-Work"; Shapin and Schaffer, *Leviathan*, p. 342: "The language that transports politics outside of science is precisely what we need to understand and explain"; Martin Mulsow and Frank Rexroth (eds), *Was als wissenschaftlich gelten darf: Praktiken der Grenzziehung in Gelehrtenmilieus der Vormoderne* (Frankfurt and New York, 2014);

but see Bruno Latour, *We Have Never Been Modern*, trans. Catherine Porter (Cambridge, MA, 1993).

162 This is analogous to the persistent multifunctionality of the town council, which poses a problem for the argument that functional differentiation of government was crucial for political legitimation and stabilization, which can be answered by noticing older yet still-growing politically stabilizing social practices, such as those of mercy and leniency: Franz-Josef Arlinghaus, "Gnade und Verfahren: Kommunikationsmodi in spätmittelalterlichen Stadt-gerichten," in Schlögl (ed.), *Interaktion und Herrschaft*: 137–62.

163 Most importantly from "stratifying to functional"; see Pohlig, "Drawing Boundaries," p. 167, quoting Rudolf Schlögl and with reference to Luhmann.

164 Burke, *Social History of Knowledge*; Richard van Dülmen and Sina Rauschen-bach (eds), *Macht des Wissens: Die Entstehung der modernen Wissensge-sellschaft* (Cologne, 2004).

165 Robert Darnton, "An Early Information Society: News and the Media in Eighteenth-Century Paris," *American Historical Review*, 105 (2000): 1–35, p. 1.

166 Burke, *Social History of Knowledge*, covers many of them but in separate chapters.

167 Exemplary: Darnton, "An Early Information Society"; see Dooley and Baron, *Politics of Information*; Dupré and Kusukawa, *Circulation of News and Knowledge*.

168 Becker and Clark, *Little Tools*; see note 75 above.

169 An exception is Jacob Soll, *The Information Master: Jean-Baptiste Colbert's Secret State Intelligence System* (Ann Arbor, 2009), which is about both.

170 Brendecke, *Imperium und Empirie*, pp. 22–23; Marie-Nöelle Bourguet, *Déchiffrer la France: La statistique départementale à l'époque napoléoni-enne* (Paris, 1989); for an example in which large amounts of gathered data were processed and used, see J. Andrew Mendelsohn, "The World on a Page: Making a General Observation in the Eighteenth Century" in Daston and Lunbeck, *Histories of Scientific Observation*: 396–420; on traces and modes of use: Friedrich, "Herrschaftlich veranlasste Landeserfas-sungen," pp. 323–26.

171 Gesner to Fuchs, 1556, quoted in Delisle, "Accessing nature," p. 36.

172 Examples of physicians as improvers of urban polities: Findlen, *Possessing Nature*, esp. chs. 3 and 6 on Aldrovandi; Cook, *Matters of Exchange*, ch. 4 on Tulp; physicians on local natural resources: Cooper, *Inventing the Indigenous*, chs. 3–4; quotation from Raeff, "Well-Ordered Police State," p. 1227; opposing view: Lindemann, *Health and Healing*, ch. 2, p. 139, 142; balanced review: Holenstein, *"Gute Policey" und lokale Gesellschaft*, pp. 25–32, 832–36; Baier, *Introductio in medicinam forensem*, p. 2; on desiderata: Keller, *Knowledge and the Public Interest*; on reform, see note 151 above and note 177 below.

173 All discussed above except "scientization," as in medicine becoming scientific through the "birth of the clinic" around 1800: see for example Brockliss and Jones, *Medical World*, Conclusion, pp. 826–34; Werner Sohn, "Von der Policey zur Verwaltung: Transformationen des Wissens und Veränderungen der Bevölkerungspolitik um 1800," in Wahrig and Sohn, *Zwischen Aufklär-ung, Policey und Verwaltung*: 71–89, p. 86: "Verstaatlichung und Verwis-senschaftlichung der Medizin."

174 For medicalization critiqued and rewritten, Loetz, *"Medikalisierung" und medizinische Vergesellschaftung*; for professionalization critiqued and rewrit-ten, Brockliss and Jones, *Medical World*; Broman, *Transformation*.

175 By modern here, I mean simply having many of the features discussed in this chapter and the literature cited, such as an elaborate and enduring

public–private system of healthcare and allocation to it; notarial or juridical or corporative mechanisms—or all three—for agreeing and monitoring care and resolving disagreements or investigating "error"; medical office and "police," in both its narrower (professional) and wider (environmental) regulatory functions; expert medical counsel in government. Rotterdam: van Lieburg, "Die medizinische Versorgung einer Stadtbevölkerung"; Zurich: Wehrli, *Krankenanstalten*. Old plural Europe's medical systems have been detailed in local histories over the past century which await re-reading and synthesis; see bibliographies in Russell, *Town and State Physician*. For Italian cities: Cipolla, *Public Health*; Park, *Doctors and Medicine*; Pomata, *Contracting a Cure*; Elisa Andretta, *Roma medica: anatomie d'un système médical au XVIe siècle* (Rome, 2011); Marilyn Nicoud, "Formes et enjeux d'une médicalisation médiévale: réflexion sur les cités italiennes (XIIIe-XVe siècles)," *Genèse*, 82 (2011): 7–30; west German cities: Robert Jütte, "Die medizinische Versorgung einer Stadtbevölkerung im 16. und 17. Jahrhundert am Beispiel der Reichsstadt Köln," *Medizinhistorisches Journal*, 22 (1987): 173–84; south German cities: Annemarie Kinzelbach, *Gesundbleiben, Krankwerden, Armsein in der frühneuzeitlichen Gesellschaft: Gesunde und Kranke in den Reichsstädten Überlingen und Ulm, 1500–1700* (Stuttgart, 1995); Stein, *Negotiating the French Pox*; Low Countries: Frank G. Huisman, *Stadsbelang en standsbesef: gezondheiszorg en medisch beroep in Groningen, 1500–1730* (Rotterdam, 1992); and see generally Grell and Cunningham, *Health Care and Poor Relief in Protestant Europe*; Grell, Cunningham, and Arrizabalaga, *Health Care and Poor Relief in Counter-Reformation Europe*.

176 Urban corporative medical organization in France regulated healthcare to an extent, included some municipal pharmacopoeia from as early as in plural Europe and much earlier than in France as a whole, and is hard to distinguish on the local level from the "regulated, neo-corporatist" model that emerged after 1800; Brockliss and Jones, *Medical World*, ch. 3, p. 197 (pharmacopoeia), pp. 818–26, quotation p. 826.

177 Harley, "Pious Physic for the Poor," pp. 149–50; see Pelling, "Healing the Sick Poor," pp. 116–17; Charles Webster, *The Great Instauration: Science, Medicine and Reform, 1626–1660* (London, 1975); Paul Slack, *From Reformation to Improvement: Public Welfare in Early Modern England* (Oxford, 1999).

178 Quotation from George D. Sussman, "Enlightened Health Reform, Professional Medicine and Traditional Society: The Cantonal Physicians of the Bas-Rhin, 1810–1870," *Bulletin of the History of Medicine*, 51 (1977): 565–84; Dora B. Weiner, *The Citizen-Patient in Revolutionary and Imperial Paris* (Baltimore, 1993); Brockliss and Jones, *Medical World*, pp. 802–19.

179 Park, *Doctors and Medicine*; for Aragon, see McVaugh, *Medicine before the Plague*, ch. 7, and recently Blumenthal, "Domestic Medicine."

180 For the Prussian example of this continuity, see Physicus instructions and related official texts reprinted in Ludwig von Rönne and Heinrich Simon, *Das Medicinal-Wesen des preußischen Staates*, 2 vols. (Breslau, 1844–46), vol. 1, pp. 118–261; for a well-documented example of evolving written specification of town physician duties from the fifteenth century, see Yvonne Thurnheer, *Die Stadtärzte und ihr Amt im alten Bern* (Bern, 1944), pp. 6–8, 15–16, passim; generally Fischer, *Geschichte des deutschen Gesundheitswesens*, vol. 1, pp. 75–92; vol. 2, pp. 55–57, 374–76.

181 Thurnheer, *Stadtärzte*, passim.

182 Fundamental on the MOH system is still Dorothy E. Watkins, *The English Revolution in Social Medicine, 1889–1911* (Ph.D. Diss. University of London, 1984); Anne Hardy "Public Health and the Expert: The London Medical Officers of Health, 1856–1900," in Roy M. MacLeod (ed.), *Government and Expertise: Specialists, Administrators, and Professionals, 1860–1919* (Cambridge, 1988): 128–42. Inspection and disease notification, standard in many European towns and cities from the sixteenth century, developed in England in the second half of the nineteenth: Graham Mooney, "Public Health versus Private Practice: The Contested Development of Compulsory Infectious Disease Notification in Late-Nineteenth Century Britain," *Bulletin of the History of Medicine*, 73 (1999): 238–67; Christopher Hamlin, "Nuisances and Community in Mid-Victorian England: The Attractions of Inspection," *Social History*, 38 (2013): 346–79.

183 At a time when England looked to German models for health, welfare, national public science, and technical education; Watkins, *English Revolution*; E.P. Hennock, *British Social Reform and German Precedents: The Case of Social Insurance, 1880–1914* (Oxford, 1987); E.P. Hennock, "Technological Education in England, 1850–1926: The Uses of a German Model," *History of Education*, 19 (1990): 299–331.

184 Isak Schlockow, Arthur Leppmann, and Emanuel Roth, *Der Kreisarzt: (Neue Folge von: Der preußische Physikus) Anleitung zur Kreisarztprüfung, zur Geschäftsführung der Medizinalbeamten und zur Sachverständigen-Thätigkeit der Aerzte*, 6th edn, 2 vols. (Berlin, 1906). George Rosen missed this range and growth of functions in his classic statement on the reduction of medical police to controlling communicable disease: Rosen, "The Fate of the Concept of Medical Police, 1780–1890" (1957), reprinted in *Centaurus*, 50 (2008): 46–62, with illuminating commentary by Christopher Hamlin, pp. 63–69.

185 This list is compiled from the following examples. Multifaceted figures we usually think of on a national or international stage worked from a civic base: Max von Pettenkofer, *The Value of Health to a City: Two Lectures Delivered in 1873*, trans. Henry Sigerist (Baltimore, 1941). Exemplary of the significance and scope of the scientific and political activity of modern German district physicians and civic doctors are figures such as Robert Koch, Adolf Gottstein, and Alfred Grotjahn: see Paul Weindling, *Health, Race and German Politics between National Unification and Nazism, 1870–1945* (Cambridge, 1989); Paul Weindling, "Medical Practice in Imperial Berlin: The Casebook of Alfred Grotjahn," *Bulletin of the History of Medicine*, 61 (1987): 391–410. English medical officers of health with biographies rich in contribution to knowledge and polity: Terrie M. Romano, *Making Medicine Scientific: John Burdon Sanderson and the Culture of Victorian Science* (Baltimore, 2002); John M. Eyler, *Sir Arthur Newsholme and State Medicine, 1885–1935* (Cambridge, 1997); Steve Sturdy, "Hippocrates and State Medicine: George Newman Outlines the Founding Policy of the Ministry of Health," in Christopher Lawrence and George Weisz (eds), *Greater than the Parts: Holism in Biomedicine, 1920–1950* (New York, 1998): 112–34; quotation from George Newman, *Citizenship and the Survival of Civilization* (New Haven, 1928).

186 Hélène Vérin, *La gloire des ingénieurs: l'intelligence technique du XVIe au XVIIIe siècle* (Paris, 1993); Antoine Picon, "Engineers and Engineering History: Problems and Perspectives," *History and Technology*, 20 (2004): 421–36, p. 426. Jurists in late medieval and early modern public life: Rainer Christoph Schwinges (ed.), *Gelehrte im Reich: Zur Sozial- und Wirkungsgeschichte akademischer Eliten des 14. bis 16. Jahrhunderts*, Zeitschrift für

historische Forschung Beiheft 18 (Berlin, 1996); Schnur, *Rolle der Juristen*; David A. Bell, *Lawyers and Citizens: The Making of a Political Elite in Old Regime France* (New York, 1994).

187 Influential accounts of rise in the nineteenth century are Claudia Huerkamp, "The Making of the Modern Medical Profession, 1800–1914: Prussian Doctors in the Nineteenth Century," in Geoffrey Cocks and Konrad H. Jarausch (eds), *German Professions, 1800–1950* (New York, 1990): 66–84, summarizing her work in German; Paul Starr, *The Social Transformation of American Medicine* (New York, 1982).

188 See Ole Peter Grell, Andrew Cunningham, and Jon Arrizabalaga (eds), *Centres of Medical Excellence? Medical Travel and Education in Europe, 1500–1789* (Farnham, 2010); Dupré and Kusukawa, *Circulation of News and Knowledge*; on relations between news, knowledge-making, medical peregrination, and medical correspondence: Delisle, "Accessing Nature."

189 The phrases are from Henry E. Sigerist, "From Bismarck to Beveridge: Developments and Trends in Social Security Legislation," *Bulletin of the History of Medicine*, 13 (1943): 365–88; and Frevert, *Krankheit als politisches Problem*; see Weiner, *Citizen-Patient*.

Part I
Scholar in Town, Scholar in Office

2 The Many Uses of Writing

A Humanist Physician in Sixteenth-Century Prague

Michael Stolberg

In one of the notebooks of the Bohemian physician Georg Handsch (1529–1578?), a strange list of terms catches the reader's eye: "poeta," "orator," "arithmeticus," "musicus," "grammaticus," "[lector?] de variis rebus," "medicus," "organista," "nigromanticus."[1] Later, Handsch added further terms, with a different quill and in a different ink, such as "dialecticus" and "praestigiator." Other somewhat more detailed entries on the following pages shed light on the meaning of this list. His *magister*, we read, intended to recommend him for work as an *arithmeticus* in the metal works of a certain Herr Gendorf. He wished the Lord would help him become a *lector* at Prague University. "Stadtschreiber werden," "become a town scribe" he noted in German. There can be little doubt that Handsch, at that time a young man of about 20 years,[2] was pondering the options for his professional future. Medicine was only one of them and by no means on top of the list. In hindsight, it was, by all appearances, thanks to a stroke of good fortune that he eventually became a physician. He had made friends with Julius Gallus, the son of one of the personal physicians to the Archduke Ferdinand, Andreas Gallus. It seems that the latter wanted Handsch to accompany Julius to study medicine in Padua and was prepared to pay for it.[3]

The range of professional options on Handsch's list reminds us of a simple but often neglected fact: some physicians' sons may be an exception, but most future physicians were not destined since childhood for a medical career. Quite to the contrary, they frequently decided to study medicine only at the end of a liberal arts course, and some future physicians even spent years in other fields before they turned to medicine. Nevertheless, historians have tended to study early modern physicians primarily as members of the medical profession, as medical practitioners, medical authors, or professors.[4] In doing so, they have implicitly drawn on a modern understanding of what it means to "be" a physician. By all appearances, most early modern physicians eventually made their living almost exclusively by treating patients.[5] We risk arriving at an overly narrow, one-sided picture, however, if we study the lives and works of early modern physicians based on modern notions of professional identity

DOI: 10.4324/9781315554693-4

and treat their other, non-medical scholarly interests and activities as pre-liminary or accessory. For, as I will argue in this chapter for the sixteenth century—the long-term changes remain to be studied in more detail—phys-icians were perceived and perceived themselves as medical men much less exclusively than today. Their self-fashioning, their social standing and even their careers as medical practitioners, were based on, and reflected to a considerable degree, their mastery of a wide range of scholarly skills.

The range of careers young Handsch envisaged is revealing in this respect. It may seem broad at first glance. Yet, with the possible exception of the "magician" ("praestigiator"),[6] they all had one thing in common: they called for skills and knowledge associated with the liberal arts, that is with grammar, rhetoric and dialectics plus the *quadrivium* of natural phil-osophy (including natural magic), arithmetic, geometry and music theory. By their early twenties, most future physicians were well versed in these areas. They had at least a decade of training in the liberal arts and the *studia humanitatis* behind them. They had learned Latin and possibly some Greek as well. Moreover, they were familiar with the cultural heritage of ancient Greece and Rome, with the works of the major classical authors and with the whole range of classical genres from poetry and letter writing to historical narratives and fables. In addition, they mastered important practical skills. They knew how to speak and write with style, how to extract useful quotes and knowledge from a rapidly growing number of books,[7] and how to hold their own in learned debates about all sorts of issues. This was the crucial embodied cultural capital, to use Pierre Bour-dieu's well-known term, with which they embarked on their careers.[8]

Many of these skills were also useful for the medical practitioner. Sabine Schlegelmilch argues in her contribution to this volume that this mastery of basic learned skills was even an important reason why town authorities in the sixteenth century came to prefer academically trained physicians to barber-surgeons when they appointed town physicians. As Handsch's list nicely illustrates, however, medicine was only one out of a range of differ-ent professions to which a liberal arts education equipped young men at the time. Even if they eventually turned to medicine, their fundamental *habitus* was that of the learned scholar.[9] They continued to interact, in their respective towns, with other scholars, with and without medical train-ing. There were physicians who devoted themselves extensively and with considerable success to non-medical scholarly interests, to numismatics, for example, to history, to genealogy, to archaeology,[10] and some, like Nico-laus Copernicus, Johannes Posthius and Petrus Lotichius, are known today primarily as astronomers or poets. By all appearances, many physicians also had the necessary time. The few surviving diaries and casebooks of sixteenth- and early seventeenth-century physicians suggest that they usu-ally only saw a few patients a day.[11]

A scholarly *habitus* also allowed them to distance themselves from the many non-academic healers with whom they competed in the highly contested early modern medical marketplace. They were "doctors," a term which, in the end, became synonymous with the university-trained physician. Visual evidence underscores this scholarly self-presentation. Early modern genre painting almost inevitably showed the physician as a medical practitioner, usually examining a patient's urine or feeling the pulse at the sickbed. In striking contrast to this iconographic tradition, I do not know of a single personal portrait of an individual, named, early modern learned physician that shows him as a medical practitioner. When physicians had control over the way they were represented, as in author's portraits, they preferred to be shown in their study, surrounded by books and other symbols of learned, scholarly activity.[12]

If we take this humanist habitus and scholarly self-fashioning seriously, the figure of the sixteenth-century physician appears in a distinctly different light. Medicine was far less a "profession" in the modern sense. It was, in many ways, one of several means by which a young man with a solid training in the liberal arts could find his place in society and make a living, and medical practice frequently combined with other activities that underlined his learned status and helped promote his social standing. If we approach the lives and careers of sixteenth-century physicians from this perspective, we need to examine not only their strictly medical works, however, which many physicians never published in the first place, but everything they wrote and did in order to assert their scholarly status and to establish themselves as members of the cultural elite. In particular, we have to broaden the focus from the medical republic of letters, which was only one of several stages on which physicians moved, and the medical marketplace, in which they competed, to embrace the local context: the city or town to which many physicians moved as strangers with little else to rely on but their scholarly training.

It is from this perspective that I want to study, in this chapter, the different ways in which one specific young scholar who eventually became a physician—the above-mentioned Georg Handsch—used his learning and more specifically a range of humanist writing and note-taking skills to make his way in one of the major cities of his time. My analysis will draw on Handsch's voluminous manuscript *Nachlass* in the Österreichische Nationalbibliothek in Vienna. A rare finding for this period, it also comprises writings from Handsch's early adulthood, before he studied medicine. This makes it possible to also examine to which degree and in what way his writing and note-taking changed once he turned to medicine and sought to make a living as a medical practitioner.

Georg Handsch

Georg Handsch came from a fairly affluent, but provincial, background.[13] He grew up and received his first schooling in Leipa, a small town some 60 miles north of Prague. His father then sent him to Valentin

Trotzendorf's *schola* in the Silesian town of Goldberg, one of the most renowned famous Latin schools of the time.

When he left the school and moved to Prague in 1545/46, his future was wide open.[14] Prague must have been an exciting place for an ambitious young man from the Bohemian provinces. It was the capital of the kingdom, residence of the Imperial *Statthalter* Archduke Ferdinand II and one of the principal economic and cultural centers of Europe. The powers of the civic authorities had recently been crushed by the Catholic Habsburg rulers, but the flourishing economy continued to attract merchants from all over Europe and many of the richest and most powerful families of Bohemia had their palaces in the city's boroughs.[15]

Handsch may have begun to study the liberal arts at Charles University, which Matthaeus Collinus and his circle had recently turned into a stronghold of humanism,[16] but his name does not appear in the register of those who received a bachelor's degree, so it may be that he had private instruction instead.[17] His father, who had remarried after the early death of Handsch's mother, seems to have no longer given him sufficient financial support. In this situation, his excellent education in Goldberg may have proved crucial for his economic survival and his future career. Probably thanks to the support of his teacher, Johannes Schentygar,[18] Collinus gave him work as a teaching assistant in his private school for boys from high-ranking families in the Angel's Garden, in Prague's New Town.[19] Handsch's involvement with the school and the Prague humanists opened other doors, in turn, and paved the way to his gradual social and professional ascent. In particular, Collinus introduced him to the rich *mecenas* of the Prague humanists, the former vice-judge of Bohemia, Johannes Hoddeovinus, who had large estates in the countryside and a stately palace in the Malá Strana, in Prague.[20]

Handsch lived, worked and studied for four or five years in Prague before he went to Padua. With time, he developed a growing interest in medicine. He began to see patients with a local physician, Ulrich Lehner, and called himself an "iatrophilos," a "lover of medicine," in his notebooks. As one of his poems shows, he had come to the conclusion that medicine ultimately was more lucrative.[21] After his return from Italy, he acted as a kind of *famulus* or apprentice physician to Andreas Gallus. He lived in his house and accompanied him and other physicians, including the famous botanist and court physician Pierandrea Mattioli, on their visits. Occasionally, he treated patients of his own, but was apparently unable to establish a successful practice, and Gallus' death deprived him of his most important mentor. Over the following years, he strengthened his ties with Mattioli and obtained his permission to translate his highly successful commentaries on Dioscorides into German.[22] It was only in the 1560s, however, more than a decade after he had received his doctorate, that he could secure some modest financial security. Probably thanks to a recommendation from Mattioli, Handsch was appointed personal physician to Archduke Ferdinand. He moved with Ferdinand from Prague to Innsbruck where the Archduke took his residence in the nearby castle of Ambras. Handsch died in his hometown Leipa on February 25, 1578. The last entries in his surviving manuscripts date from 1576 or 1577.

Poetry

By far the most important kind of writing by which Handsch initially sought to establish himself had little to do with medicine, but it was at the very heart of the humanist enterprise: poetry.[23] He had already acquired the necessary skills as a student in Goldberg where reading and reciting classical poetry and composing poems was part of the curriculum.[24] Dozens of Handsch's poems have survived in a manuscript collection he compiled in 1559.[25] Later, in the early 1560s, some of these poems appeared in print, in the *Farragines poematum*, a four-volume edition of poems dedicated to Johannes Hoddeovinus.[26]

Handsch exercized his skills in a large variety of poetic genres, from elegies and *idyllia* to *hodeoporica* (commemorating journeys) and *epithalamia* (celebrating weddings). He wrote little *distycha*, epitaphs and playful poems such as chronograms (in which the capitalized Ms, Ds, Cs, Ls, Xs, Vs and Is gave the year of an important event described in the poem) and *acrostycha* (in which the first letters of each line, read downward, revealed a word or name).[27] He was particularly productive and, to some degree, successful in this field and the little recent historical work on Handsch has largely focused on his poetry.[28] He was not all that exceptional, however. Many scholars wrote poems at the time—including physicians. In medical treatises and printed dissertations we frequently find poetic eulogies, which the author's friends wrote for him, and even physicians' entries in the popular *Alba amicorum* reveal poetic aspirations.[29]

Today, we tend to associate poetry with a superior artistic sensitivity, with a particular gift to express emotions, moods, and experiences in a condensed form. This view does not do justice to the essence of humanist poetry. Poetry was, above all, a skill. The poet had to master elegant Latin and the complex rules of Latin poetic metrology and he needed to be familiar with the classical heritage in order to spice his poems with allusions to Greek and Roman mythology and literature. Even more importantly in our context, poetry was to a considerable extent a means of communication and public self-fashioning. It was a tool by which humanists could acquire social capital[30] and raise their status among the educated circles of their respective town.

In Handsch's case, this instrumental role of poetry is obvious. His poems allowed him to demonstrate his poetic skills and to prove that he was a worthy member of the circle of Prague humanists and deserved his place among the city's cultural elite. His personal notes reveal a spirit of competition and emulation, in fact, in matters of poetry. They underline that poems were not just a literary genre, but also played an important part in convivial gatherings, as an entertainment at dinner tables, and as an opportunity for improvised exhibitions of poetic skills. In his notes, Handsch repeatedly even mentions little poetic contests, in which the host or someone else invited the guests to improvise *ex tempore* poems on a set topic, such as "Natura nihil facit frustra."[31]

What is more, most of Handsch's poems served a very specific communicative purpose. For good reasons, Handsch, at one point, referred to "epistolas meas poeticas": he addressed many of his poems to a specific person. Like letters, some carried the date and place of writing, others offered very concrete and personal news, or addressed the relationship between Handsch and the man to whom he was writing.[32]

Among the recipients of these "epistolary poems" we find mostly members of the circle of humanists in Prague with whom Handsch also interacted personally: Matthaeus Collinus, Martin Hanno, Johannes Schentygar, Thomas Mitis[33] and, most important of all, Johann Hoddeovinus, the *mecenas* of the Prague humanists. Handsch introduced himself to Hoddeovinus with a poem. He used poems to apologize or to express his gratitude to him or, writing on a range of topics, simply to please Hoddeovinus or upon his request. His efforts quite literally paid off, as Hoddeovinus rewarded the poets of his circle financially for their poems.[34] In 1556, he even procured a title of nobility for Handsch and his friend Thomas Mitis. Handsch could now proudly call himself "Georgius Handschius a Limuso."[35]

In a few of his poems, Handsch also put the city of Prague itself into the limelight, underlining his place in and allegiance to the city in this manner.[36] He wrote a poem on the big church bell donated by Ferdinand I.[37] When Ferdinand I crushed the uprising of the Bohemian estates and the burghers of Prague, in 1547, Handsch responded with a poem on the impact of the war and on the downfall of the "republic"—the burghers of Prague had lost many of their former prerogatives[38]—in which the first lines all started with a "P" for "pax" (peace).[39] In another poem on the great fire in the castle of Prague, Handsch emulated J. Orpheus' poem on the same topic, 'De conflagratione inclytae arcis Pragensis.'[40] Most remarkably, finally, in an epistolary poem addressed to his friend Thomas Caesar, he resorted to some of the typical elements of the humanist *laus urbis*, the praise of the city,[41] which tended to refer to the walls of the city (a symbol of its political independence and power), its site on the banks of one or several rivers, its buildings and its outstanding political and economic importance.[42]

The place of poetry in Handsch's career and writings changed very markedly in the course of his life, in line with its varying importance as a means of securing status and support. The manuscript collection of his poems compiled in 1559 contains only five that he wrote as a medical student in Italy,[43] including one addressing Musa Brasavola in Ferrara, one of the foremost medical humanists of the time, on the occasion of his doctoral exam.[44] In one of his notebooks, he also mentioned his earlier plan to write a poem in praise of Brasavola, whose favor and trust he needed in order to be admitted to the doctoral exam in Ferrara. For, as he revealed in his notebook, he had to pretend (among other things by obtaining letters which addressed him as "magister") that he possessed the necessary master's degree from Prague, which he had never obtained.[45]

Back in Prague when he began to work as a physician, Handsch continued to write poems, above all for Hoddeovinus. Around 1560, he spent nine months in Hoddeovinus's castle in Rzepice devoting himself entirely to the preparation of the above-mentioned four-volume *Farrago*, a collection of poems written by himself, Collinus, Schentygar, Mitis, Hanno, and other Prague humanists and dedicated to Hoddeovinus.[46] From then on, his poetic activities seem to have declined rapidly. He never stopped altogether, as the manuscript collection of his own poems, which he started in 1559, concludes with a poem written in August 1576, on the occasion of the death of the captain of the Archducal castle in Ambras and with an epitaph for himself. However, only about 30 pages, at the very end of the 650-page manuscript, offer poems written after 1560. Tellingly, they reflect a marked reorientation away from the educated elites of Prague toward his new employer, the Habsburg Court. The poems no longer addressed Hoddeovinus and the members of the circle of Prague humanists. They dealt with the Emperors Ferdinand and Rudolf, celebrated the marriage of Duke August of Saxonia's court musician, commented on a portrait of the Archduke's principal administrator Count Franz von Thurn, or offered epitaphs for ladies of the court and their families, such as Virginia Loxan, the daughter of the Archduke's aunt Katharina.[47]

Letters

In addition to his "poetic epistles," Handsch, like most scholars and physicians of his time, also wrote ordinary letters. Letters were an important means of self-fashioning and networking, at the time, and physicians played a major role in early modern epistolary networks.[48] Letters were not only a major medium of communication in the early modern *res publica litteraria*, in which books, theories and new findings were discussed, in which scholars informed each other about events in their personal and professional lives and about political and religious conflicts, and through which they sought to live up to the humanist ideal of *amicitas*. Similar to poems, letters also allowed writers to demonstrate their elegant style and their knowledge of the cultural heritage of ancient Greece and Rome.[49] Those to whom famous scholars addressed their letters began to keep them or indeed collect them and some of these letters—including those of some of the most famous physicians[50]—began to appear in print.

Only a small selection of Handsch's letters have come down to us.[51] Handsch copied them into a little manuscript volume,[52] and corrections in the text suggest that he hoped to publish them (though he never did). By that time, in the early 1560s, he had been a physician for almost a decade. Yet the letters he selected point again to his self-fashioning as a humanist scholar rather than a medical man. There is a letter from his time as a pupil in Goldberg. A number of letters were addressed to relatives and acquaintances in Leipa, and others to fellow students and scholars of the circle around Hoddeovinus and Collinus. Only a minority of the letters dealt primarily with medical issues and even here we sometimes find typical humanist elements. In a letter to the podagric Collinus, for example, Handsch gave the dietetic advice suitable for a famous scholar—to avoid working at bad hours (presumably at night) because it affected his "nerves"—and added the adage of an unknown *avicennista* that the name of Minerva, the patron goddess of the arts, was derived from the Latin *minuo*: "Minerva quia minuit nervos."[53]

Only in some of the later letters, can we identify new, medical ways of writing, especially in the typical epistolary genre of the practicing physician, the *consilium*.[54] A letter to Viderinus offered detailed instructions on the treatment of his chronic disease. In view of the current constellation of the moon, the planets and Sirius, the patient was to take his medicines on Saturday only.[55] In a letter to a certain Sebastian Wingler, Handsch expressed his opinion on a patient, probably Ulrich von Eyczing, and regretted that he could not pronounce his judgment on the color of the patient's urine because the glass (which presumably had been sent to him) had been damaged.[56] Handsch also included three of his letters to the well-known Saxonian physician, Johann Neefe, concerning the sick Frau von Wartenberg, discussing among other things the use of hellebore dilutions and pointing out a prescription for *succus helleborinus* in the *Thesaurus Evonymi Philiatri* attributed to Conrad Gessner.[57] It was hardly coincidental that he selected these letters. They showed him as a physician in whom some of the highest-ranking families of the kingdom put their trust—and as someone who communicated on an eye-to-eye level with some of the most famous physicians of the time.

Writing for the Printing Press

As we have seen, Handsch did not write his poems for a general reading public. Those that were eventually published appeared only at a later date. Nonetheless, like other scholars and physicians of his time, Handsch also conceived works for the printing press. Most of them never made it into print. It was not easy, especially for a young man with few credentials, to find a publisher. The surviving texts offer an idea of the ways, however, in which Handsch hoped to address his readership.

Books were an important means to gain reputation in the *res publica litteraria*. A successful medical writer was also more likely to become known to and consulted by affluent patients and their ordinary physicians elsewhere and to be preferred to others when a town or court physician was to be appointed. Especially in the case of medical works, printed publications also promised a positive impact on the author's standing in his own city or town, in the place where he practiced or sought to establish himself. Certain kinds of medical writing, such as health advice on how to escape the plague or other epidemics, might even be penned for the specific situation and the health concerns in a specific city or town. Likewise, astrological calendars, one of the most successful products of the early modern printing press, which often focused on health issues and were frequently written by physicians, had to be based on astronomical calculations made for the respective geographical longitude and latitude of their town.[58] In addition, books also promised more immediate, financial rewards. It was common practice that physicians dedicated their work either to princes or to their respective town authorities and received some money, in return, as a sign of recognition.[59]

From the time before he went to Padua to study medicine, only one major work that Handsch clearly prepared for publication has survived. It belonged to a genre better known as a typical paper technology of the humanist scholar, but which sometimes also appeared in print.[60] On more than 1,100 pages, Handsch's *Promptuarium sive loci communes latinitatis* offered a huge compilation of definitions and commonplaces or *loci communes* taken from the works of the major writers of antiquity.[61] Grouped under different headings, they covered the whole range of the knowable, from God, the sky, the earth and the times to regions, towns and places to the anatomy and the diseases of the human bodies to agricultural tools. Handsch advertised the work as a useful repository for whoever wrote in Latin, including schoolboys.[62] He may well have thought of the boys he was teaching at the time, in Collinus's private school in Prague. Certainly, the very first text written by Handsch to make it into print had such a didactic impetus. It was a so-called *cisioianus*, a mnemonic calendar, that appeared in 1550 in a Latin and Czech grammar book Matthaeus Collinus issued for use in his private school.[63]

Around 1560, Handsch still prepared the above-mentioned collections of his letters and poems for publication and curated the four-volume poetic *Farragines*. In the following years, however, we can identify a shift of focus in the kind of works he conceived, away from the circle of humanists in Prague to the medical republic of letters and the court. In 1563, his German translation of Mattioli's herbal appeared in Prague, with a short preface by Handsch and some additions of his own to the body of the text. The last work that Handsch carefully prepared for publication was a five-volume *Historia animalium*.[64] Just as Mattioli was doing with botany, writers like Conrad Gessner and Ulisse Aldrovandi were complementing the writings of ancient authors like Aristotle and Pliny with more recent empirical findings.[65] Handsch's work, by contrast, was largely a scholarly compilation from the works of others. His only major original contribution was an account of fish and fishing in the river Elbe.[66] Rather than joining the ranks of contemporary naturalists, Handsch seems to have sought to impress Archduke Ferdinand, who probably commissioned the work to underline his own status as a benefactor of the arts and the sciences.[67] It was never published.

Personal Notes

The bulk of Handsch's extant writing was not addressed to others but is found in his personal notebooks. As a student and as a young physician, Handsch was an extremely prolific note-taker. From the late 1550s, his zeal waned considerably, but his notebooks extend to the very last years of his life.

His two earliest surviving notebooks were devoted entirely to humanist aspirations. They were similar in character to the *Promptuarium* with its countless commonplaces taken from classical authors, but they clearly served as personal working tools. The first one, to which Handsch himself gave the Greek title *Rhapsodia*, seems to have been assembled at a somewhat later stage from smaller fascicles or indeed loose sheets of paper.[68] After a few dozen pages with miscellaneous notes on all kinds of topics, from *coelum* and *eclipsis* to *lachrimae* and *timor*, the note-taking method changes to a fairly widespread subtype of commonplacing[69] based on alphabetical order: Handsch assigned the pages in advance to the different letters of the alphabet. He then made his entries on individual topics on the page reserved for topics with the corresponding initial letter.[70] The remaining pages of the notebook are filled with a detailed index to Ovid's fables, a collection of synonyms and some notes on letter writing and the art of poetry.

Begun in 1547, Handsch's *Adversaria sacra et profana ex varia lectione collecta* offers a similar *cornucopia* of entries, though natural-philosophical topics take a more prominent place. Notes on major works such as Pico della Mirandola's famous critique of divinatory astrology and examples for the importance of the number "3" stand next to more practical advice, for example on how to use one's fingers to calculate the time just from the sun's position in the sky.[71]

At first glance, the title of another of Handsch's manuscripts, *Proverbia, dicteria ad politicum usum congesta*, suggests a further collection of humanist *loci communes* and some of the pages are in fact pre-assigned to entries on certain "topics" such as *charitas* or *humanus*.[72] It starts with numerous Latin proverbs, moralist adages and aphorisms, such as "Honores mutant mores, sed raro in meliores" ("Honors change the habits, but rarely to the better").[73] Some entries reflect humanist traditions of misogyny and reservations against the hazards of married life (though, at the time, marriage became increasingly common among humanist scholars): "Mulier quantum formosa, tantum venenosa" ("The more beautiful a woman, the more poisonous"), he noted, and quoted an Italian saying "Uxorem duxi, libertatem vendidi" ("I took a wife, I sold my freedom").[74]

There is a crucial difference, however, between this manuscript and the collections of commonplaces presented above. Handsch did not just compile passages from the works of the ancient poets and historians. He was mostly writing about his own world, his own society. An alternative, German title written on the first page of the manuscript— possibly by Handsch himself—comes much closer to the character of this compilation: *Weltbüchle*, that is, "little book of the world." While Handsch usually took his notes in Latin, large parts of the manuscript are devoted to German proverbs and idiomatic expressions, and numerous changes in ink and quill suggest that he collected them over a long period of time or, in fact, throughout his life. Under the heading "cor" ("heart") we find, for example, the German term *Herczeleid* ("heart ache") and expressions such as "das Hercz ym Leibe weinet mir" ("the heart is shedding tears inside me"), "ich hab nicht eyn steynern Hercz" ("I do not have a heart of stone") or "das Hercze lacht ym ym Leib" ("the heart is laughing inside him").[75] In the second part of the manuscript he also recorded little "popular stories" or *historiae vulgares*.

Handsch's interest in German proverbs, vernacular ways of saying and "popular stories" probably must be seen, among others, in the light of another major aspect of the humanist endeavor. Taking the poets and writers of ancient Rome as their model, leading humanists, sometimes with markedly patriotic undertones, called for a sustained interest in the language and customs of the ordinary people and in the influence of location and climate on their "character."[76] The famous humanist poet Konrad Celtis in particular, author of a description of Nuremberg and of a poem that compared Prague with ancient Rome, contrasted the endeavors of other scholars who boasted of their travels to distant countries with his own. He, the German scholar, was familiar instead with "the limits and terms of his native language, and of the various rites, laws, languages, religions, habitus and affections of the people, and the lineaments and the figures of their bodies [...]."[77]

Handsch's Prague was a city in which two "national" cultures coexisted side by side and were not always in harmony, to say the least. Many merchants and artisans were Czech, and members of noble families tended to be bilingual, at least. Parts of the population and, in particular, the Habsburg Court, on the other hand, privileged German.[78] Handsch's allegiance was clear. He spoke Czech and even taught it to others, but in his manuscripts he consistently referred to himself as a *Germano-Bohemus*,[79] fashioning himself as a representative of the Germanic culture to which his *Weltbüchle* was almost exclusively devoted.

Resembling Handsch's use of poems in this respect, proverbs and adages as well as little stories and anecdotes were also of considerable interest for a very different reason for someone like Handsch. They were entertaining. He could use them in conversations, at the dinner table, and in other kinds of social gatherings, to improve his social graces, to make himself a welcome guest and to secure his standing as a learned and resourceful participant in urban sociability.[80] Handsch's notes on the stories or remarkable ways of saying that he heard, in turn, from others, underline the value that educated people attributed to this kind of entertainment. Sometimes Handsch even mentioned the occasion, for example a dinner conversation, or the person who told him.[81] From this perspective, his *Weltbüchle*—and the same goes to some degree for his collections of commonplaces—was a convenient mnemonic tool for oral communication. In fact, some entries are so short and incomprehensible that they could only serve to help him remember the rest. One entry, for example, reads "De incantatione. De balneatore Lippense, qui pro digito accepit totum corpus" ("On incantation. The barber-surgeon in Leipa who accepted a whole body for a finger"), and another "De annulo diaboli pro zelotypo" ("On a devil's ring for a man suffering from zelotypia [morbid jealousy]").[82]

Handsch's remaining notebooks, by contrast, reflect his growing interest in medicine. His years as a medical student in Padua, unsurprisingly, resulted in several volumes with lecture notes and excerpts from his medical readings.[83] In addition, he filled a whole series of notebooks, with altogether about 4,000 pages, with notes on medical practice. Some go back to the late 1540s, when he started seeing patients with Ulrich Lehner in Prague.[84] The large majority reflect his experiences with different patients, diseases and medicines as a medical student in Padua and as a fledgling physician in Prague, in the years up to about 1560.[85] In other words, he wrote them before he curated the *Farragines*, at a time, when he was also still trying to put his poetic skills to use.

As in his other notebooks, Handsch organized most of his medical notes by means of commonplacing, the quintessential note-taking technique of the humanist scholar, but in this case he privileged a different approach to commonplacing.[86] He did not assign individual pages to pre-established headings, as in a textbook, based on a systematic structure, or to different letters of the alphabet for topics starting with the same initial. He simply filled his medical notebooks from the first page to the last.[87] He did maintain the crucial characteristic of commonplacing, however: to every single entry he made he added a prominent "heading" in the margin. In most cases, this heading referred to the disease or drug to which the entry was devoted and/or the name of the patient. Thanks to these headings in the margins he could later quickly retrieve entries on a specific topic (or patient), all the more easily if he compiled an index from them, as he usually did.

This sequential—rather than systematic/structured or alphabetical—approach to commonplacing was particularly suitable for note-taking in medicine and natural philosophy. From the late fifteenth century, these fields underwent a marked shift, from universals to particulars and from theory to empirical observation. The focus of Handsch's notes is almost entirely on the personal observations that he and his colleagues made on individual patients and/or on the effects of various drugs he witnessed or that others communicated to him. Occasionally only, we find a series of entries, as in a diary, on one particular patient whom Handsch saw over days or weeks, sometimes with the corresponding dates.[88] In one of his medical notebooks, he also wrote a fairly extensive account of a devastating outbreak of the plague in Prague in 1562/63.[89] Handsch recorded the cases of individual plague victims, examined how they might have been infected and carefully noted the prophylactic and therapeutic effects of different drugs and quintessences. Most entries are very short, however, often comprising no more than three or four lines. Many of them highlight only a single, particularly noteworthy aspect of the case in question or the effect of a medicine in a certain disease. Instead of compiling quotes and other noteworthy passages on all kinds of issues from the writings of major classical authors, Handsch assembled little snippets of information and empirical observations. He collected quotes from the "book of Nature" so to speak.

The little stories and anecdotes found in Handsch's *Weltbüchle*, in turn, offered an equivalent of the medical case histories of varying length that he recorded in his medical notebooks, among numerous other notes on all kinds of topics and findings. Already as a medical student in Padua, he recorded *observationes*—the histories of individual patients he saw with his professors, in the patients' homes or in the local Ospedale di San Francesco.[90] In the second half of the sixteenth century, such medical *observationes* on individual patients rapidly gained importance as a new and highly popular genre of medical writing.[91] Several series of case histories in Handsch's notebooks are, at present, the earliest known instance of such *observations*, which are explicitly recorded as such under titles like *Tercia observatio de hydrope ex retentis menstruis*, about a dropsical woman from the countryside, though it is unlikely that young Handsch actually coined that usage of the term.[92]

Other entries are reminiscent, in turn, of the vernacular expressions he noted in his *Weltbüchle*. Handsch frequently recorded—in German and sometimes verbatim—what he heard from patients, relatives or acquaintances about popular medical beliefs and practices. When ordinary people wanted to know, Handsch noted, for example, whether an infant or child suffered from worms, they poured some brandy on the belly button and if bubbles formed this was thought to indicate the presence of worms.[93]

By all appearances, the principal purpose of these notes on ordinary people's medical beliefs and practices was quite different from his notes on popular stories and expressions. They followed the same rationale that informed Handsch's notes on medical practice in general: he collected all kinds of information and experiences that might help him become a more successful practitioner. Just as he frequently recorded the validity of certain diagnostic signs and the effects of certain remedies that other learned physicians had observed, he was prepared to take the observations, experiences and practices of ordinary people seriously as a source of useful knowledge, including that of "old women," "Jews" and "empirici." He repeatedly even used expressions like "didici" in this context, which he had "learned" from ordinary folks.[94]

There was also another reason for taking note of "popular" medical beliefs and expressions: the desire or indeed need to use the appropriate language when dealing with patients and their relatives. This is underlined by the fact that he sometimes also noted Czech equivalents of certain medical terms—not everyone in sixteenth-century Prague understood German. Watching the physicians around him and from his own experience, Handsch seems to have come to the realization that a physician, in the highly competitive medical market of a city like Prague, could not afford to hide behind his learned Latin terminology. In order to win the trust of patients and families in his expertise and in the validity of his prescriptions, he had to provide the patients and their families with a plausible explanation of the causes of the disease and the rationale of his treatment. His words had to make sense to them. Hence it was indispensable that he acquainted himself with their ideas, with their medical language, with their preferred diagnostic and therapeutic practices.

It was clearly for this reason that Handsch also recorded numerous vernacular German expressions, in turn, which he and other physicians could profitably use or actually had used at the sickbed. Occasionally, he even added a "placuit" ("it pleased") or "non displicuit" ("it did not displease"), presumably with the idea of using a similar expression also on other patients.[95]

Conclusion

As I hope to have shown in this chapter, Handsch's writings were pervasively shaped by a scholarly, humanist habitus. From his early twenties, medicine acquired an increasingly important place in his life and in his writings, but it did not simply replace his previous learned, humanist interests and activities. They coexisted and his note-taking and writing practices in these various fields had much in common. Commonplacing remained his principal paper tool—but the sequential, chronological approach to commonplacing largely superseded the alphabetical and the systematic approach (with empty pages pre-assigned to certain letters or topics) he had initially used. In certain respects, notes on empirical observations, quotations from the book of Nature, only took the place of quotations and commonplaces from classical texts.[96] His interest in popular proverbs and expressions was paralleled by his interest in the medical beliefs and practices of ordinary people. The entertaining stories and anecdotes he collected had their equivalent in the brief medical case histories or *observationes* he gathered from his own experience and from other physicians. What ultimately links all his writings is that they served concrete, practical purposes. They were, each in their own way, useful tools by which Handsch sought to secure a place in the city in which he spent most of his adult life, to acquire social status, reputation and—even if he was not particularly successful in this respect—a lucrative medical practice.

With all his efforts, one may wonder, in hindsight, why Handsch ultimately was not particularly successful as a physician and might well have ended in poverty if he had not eventually obtained a modest position as a personal physician to the Archduke. Most patients he mentioned as having been treated by him alone, were either members of his family or they belonged to Collinus's school in the Angel's Garden. Was medicine not the right choice, after all, for a man who confessed, in his personal notebooks, that he could not watch a blood-letting?[97] Did he taint his reputation by making the two fundamental mistakes of which he repeatedly accused himself in his notes, namely treating incurable patients and being too audacious in his prognostic judgments? Did his affiliation with the Catholic physicians of the Habsburg Court keep local patients away? Were there rumors that Handsch, who never married, had sexual relations with other men, as his notebooks reveal?[98] We will probably never know.

To what degree was Handsch representative of the typical "ordinary" scholar-turned-physician of his time? The lack of similarly rich documentation for other early modern physicians makes it difficult to arrive at a clear answer. The sheer volume of Handsch's scholarly writing certainly does suggest a somewhat exceptional status. At a very early age he seems to have perceived scholarly work as a potential means to make a living and to pave the way to a career. The list of possible professional options that he drew up as a young man was complemented by a similar list of possible works which, in the end, he never seems to have written. They range from the plan to translate a history of Bohemia from Czech into German, to write "a comedy or some dialogue" and to edit Valentin Trozendorf's letters to the idea of writing a work on drunkenness, a "praise of the donkey" or a "praise of the rooster" (in Latin: "gallus") for Dr Gallus whose support eventually proved crucial for his medical career.[99]

We probably should not underestimate the time and effort, however, which many other ordinary physicians devoted to non-medical, scholarly interests. It is quite possible that their writings simply did not survive. After all, there is much evidence that almost every student in the sixteenth century took copious lecture notes—yet they have rarely come down to us. In the few cases, on the other hand, in which the papers of an early modern physician have been preserved at least to some extent, we are quite likely to find a fairly wide range of scholarly interests and quite different kinds of writings. The papers of Felix Platter, which include poems and the famous "description" of his life come to mind, or those of Johannes Magirus, physician in Berlin and Zerbst, who also took notes on English kings and Chinese letters.[100] Certainly the numerous sixteenth-century physicians whose letters are still extant amply attest to the pervasive impact of the scholarly, humanist *habitus* they had acquired from their early school years. The same goes for the publications of the minority of physicians who were successful enough to see their works printed, especially if we look at dedicatory letters and other paratexts. All this suggests that the figure of sixteenth-century physician cannot easily be equated with that of the physician in the twentieth and twenty-first centuries. His status and professional identity was defined much less by his being part of a collective professional body and much more by the standing he acquired, as an individual, in his respective urban context—as a medical practitioner and as a member of the educated urban elites with whom he shared a common educational background and who, ideally, would ensure his social and economic future in a city into which he had, like Handsch, typically moved as a stranger.

Notes

1 Österreichische Nationalbibliothek, Vienna (henceforth: ÖNB), Cod. 9666, fol. 1r.
2 The manuscript carries the date 23 September 1547, but Handsch probably wrote this list later, on the first pages that he had initially left free. He must have written the list, however, before he went to study medicine in Padua, in the autumn of 1550.
3 Handsch's few biographers have so far assumed that he had found a noble benefactor, but among the same notes on his professional future (ÖNB, Cod. 9666, fol. 1v) we also find: "Doctor Gallus vult me mittere in Italiam cum filio suis sumptibus" ("Doctor Gallus wants to send me to Italy with his son at his own expense").
4 See, however, Nancy G. Siraisi, "Oratory and Rhetoric in Renaissance Medicine," *Journal of the History of Ideas*, 65 (2004): 191–211; eadem, *History, Medicine and the Traditions of Renaissance Learning* (Ann Arbor, 2007).
5 This results from a biographical database of physicians from the German speaking lands, which we have established in Würzburg to supplement our research on early modern physicians' letters (see www.aerztebriefe.de). The database currently lists more than 4,000 physicians for the period from 1500 to 1700.
6 According to a later entry, he had learned some magicians' tricks with numbers and cards (ÖNB, Cod. 9666, foll. 134v–135r).
7 See Ann M. Blair, *Too Much to Know: Managing Scholarly Information Before the Modern Age* (New Haven and London, 2010).
8 Pierre Bourdieu, "The Forms of Capital," in John. G. Richardson (ed.), *Handbook of Theory and Research for the Sociology of Education* (New York, 1986): 241–60.
9 On the humanist *habitus* see Harald Müller, "'Specimen eruditionis': Zum Habitus der Renaissance-Humanisten und seiner sozialen Bedeutung," in Frank Rexroth (ed.), *Beiträge zur Kulturgeschichte der Gelehrten im späten Mittelalter* (Ostfildern, 2010): 117–51; Gadi Algazi, "Food for Thought:

Hieronymus Wolf Grapples with the Scholarly Habitus," in Dekker Rudolf (ed.), *Egodocuments and History: Autobiographical Writing in Its Social Context Since the Middle Ages* (Hilversum, 2002): 21–44; idem, "Eine gelernte Lebensweise: Figurationen des Gelehrtenlebens zwischen Mittelalter und Früher Neuzeit," *Berichte zur Wissenschaftsgeschichte*, 30 (2007): 107–18.

10 See Gianna Pomata and Nancy G. Siraisi (eds), *Historia: Empiricism and Erudition in Early Modern Europe* (Cambridge, MA, 2005).

11 See, for example, Biblioteca Vaticana, Rome Cpl. 1895–1; Stadtbibliothek Nürnberg, Ms. Cent. V. 10b; Germanisches Nationalmuseum Nürnberg 8° Hs 100.822, Nuremberg casebooks of Johann Magenbuch 1526–1528 and 1530–1534 and Georg Palma 1568–1570 and 1583–1591; Kungliga Biblioteket, Stockholm, Ms. X 101 *Medicinisches Receptur-Diarium* by Petrus Kirstenius, 1612–1616; Universitätsbibliothek Marburg, Ms. 96, *Diarium medicum* of Johannes Magirus; see Philipp Klaas, Hubert Steinke and Alois Unterkircher, "Daily Business: The Organization and Finances of Doctors' Practices," in Martin Dinges, Kay Peter Jankrift, Sabine Schlegelmilch and Michael Stolberg (eds), *Medical Practice, 1600–1900: Physicians and Their Patients* (Leiden, 2016).

12 Kitti Jurina, *Vom Quacksalber zum Doctor medicinae: Die Heilkunde in der deutschen Graphik des 16. Jahrhunderts* (Cologne, 1985); Susanne Fürst, *Das Arztporträt in der Frühen Neuzeit*. Unpublished medical dissertation (Regensburg, 2009).

13 For biographical information see Leopold Senfelder, "Georg Handsch von Limus: Lebensbild eines Arztes aus dem XVI. Jahrhundert," *Wiener klinische Rundschau* (1901): 495–99; 514–16; 533–35; Josef Smolka and Marta Vaculínová, "Renesanční lékař Georg Handsch (1529–1578)," *DVT – Dějiny věd a techniky*, 43 (2010): 1–26. The date of his death is given in a letter by the Mayor of Leipa to Archduke Ferdinand (Tiroler Landesarchiv Ferdinandea 164, 6 April, 1579).

14 On the Goldberg school see Gustav Bauch, *Valentin Trozendorf und die Goldberger Schule* (Berlin, 1921).

15 Jiří Pešek, "Prague between 1550 and 1650," in Eliška Fučíková et alii (eds), *Rudolf II and Prague: The Court and the City* (London, 1997), 252–86; Peter Demetz, *Prague in Black and Gold: Scenes from the Life of a European City* (New York, 1997), pp. 173–79.

16 For an overview of Bohemian humanism see Hans-Bernd Harder and Hans Rothe (eds), *Studien zum Humanismus in den böhmischen Ländern* (Vienna, Cologne, 1988); Lucie Storchová, *Bohemian School of Humanism and Its Editorial Practices (ca. 1550-1610)* (Turnhout, 2014); on Collinus and his Wittenberg connection see Josef Hejnic, "Filip Melanchton, Matouš Collinus a počátky měšťanského humanismu v Čechách," *Listy filologické*, 87 (1964): 361–79.

17 *Liber decanorum fac. phil. ab anno 1367, usque ad annum 1585. Pars secunda* (Prague, 1832).

18 See ÖNB, Cod. 9807, foll. 77v–78v (a poem by Handsch, asking Schentygar to support his wish to find employment as Collinus' *famulus*); on Schentygar see Josef Hejnic, *Dva humanisté v roce 1547 (Jan Šentygar a Bohuslav Hodějovský)* (Prague, 1957).

19 Martin Holý, "Soukromá škola Matouše Kollina z Chotěřiny v Praze a její šlechtičtí žáci," in Eva Semotanová (ed.), *Cestou dějin. K poctě prof. PhDr. Svatavy Rakové, CSc* (Prague, 2007): 159–84.

20 On Hoddeovinus and the circle of poets he supported, see Lucie Storchová, *Paupertate styloque connecti: Utváření humanistické učenecké komunity v českých zemích* (Prague, 2011), pp. 110–82.

21 Handsch, *Secunda farrago*, foll. 212r–v, "Grammaticus, rhetor, dialecticus, astrologusque, Aut nihil, aut precium vile laboris habent [...]. Arteficem medicina suum sustentat ubique" ("The grammarian, the orator, the dialectician and the astrologer receive nothing or a meagre pay for their work. [...] Medicine supports its practitioner everywhere").

22 Pietro Andrea Mattioli, *New Kreutterbuch mit den allerschönsten und artlichsten Figuren aller Gewechsz, dergleichen vormals in keiner Sprach nie an Tag kommen* (Venice, 1563).

23 On the performative aspects of humanist writing as a means of self-presentation and their importance among Bohemian humanists, in general, see Storchová, *Paupertate styloque connecti*, which also has a brief chapter on Handsch, in particular (ibid., pp. 97–100).

24 His earliest surviving poem dates from 1545 (ÖNB, Cod. 9821, fol. 1r–v).

25 ÖNB, Cod. 9821.

26 Georg Handsch (ed.), *Secunda farrago elegiarum et idylliorum ab aliquot studiosis poeticae bohemis scriptorum diversis temporibus ad nobilem et clarissimum virum D. Ioannem Seniorem Hoddeiovinum ab Hoddeiova* (Prague, 1561); the other three volumes appeared under very similar titles in 1561/62.

27 For example, ÖNB, Cod. 9821, 216v, on Emperor Charles.

28 Julie Nováková, "Rytmické kalendarium Jiřího Handsche," *Listy filologické*, 89 (1966): 315–20; Storchová, *Paupertate styloque connecti*.

29 See, for example, National Library of Medicine, Bethesda, Ms. E 77, *Album amicorum* of Conrad Gessner; Marienbibliothek, Halle, Ms. 92, *Album amicorum* of Joachim Oelhafen, with various entries by physicians.

30 Bourdieu, "Forms of Capital."

31 ÖNB Cod. 9821, fol. 254r: "Ex tempore apud coenam." Handsch came up with: "Omnia quae peperit rerum natura genitrix/Haec nec fine suo, nec ratione carent" ("Whatever Nature, the mother of things, has brought forth/ lacks neither reason nor end").

32 ÖNB, Cod. 9650, frontispiece.

33 ÖNB, Cod. 9807, fol. 63r.

34 Matthaeus Collinus et alii, *Quarta farrago poematum ab aliquot studiosis poeticae bohemis scriptorum* (Prague, 1562), foll. 617v–618v.

35 Staatsarchiv, Vienna, repertory on *Adelsakten*, refers to the nobility conferred, in Prague, to "Georg Hanczl," 4 May 1556 – undoubtedly a misspelling.

36 On the important role of "place" in early modern physicians' medical writings, see Pomata, "A Sense of Place," Chapter 8 of this volume.

37 ÖNB Cod. 9807, foll. 63v–64v.

38 Pešek, "Prague."

39 ÖNB Cod. 9807, foll. 113v–114v.

40 Modern edition in Hana Jechova-Voisine/Jacques Voisine (eds), *Poésie latine en Bohème – Renaissance et Manièrisme*, Paris 2002, 40–43 (Latin and French); my thanks to Ulrich Schlegelmilch, Würzburg, for pointing this out to me.

41 Nikolaus Thurn, "Deutsche neulateinische Städtelobgedichte: Ein Vergleich ausgewählter Beispiele des 16. Jahrhunderts," *Neulateinisches Jahrbuch*, 4 (2002): 253–69 (with extensive bibliography).

42 ÖNB, Cod. 9821, foll. 65r–66r.

43 ÖNB, Cod. 9821, foll. 243r–246r: "Quae in Italia scripsi Anno 1551 & 52. 53" ("What I wrote in Italy in the years 1551 & 52.53").

44 ÖNB, Cod. 9821, foll. 243r–v.

45 ÖNB, Cod. 11240, fol. 151r.

46 Handsch, *Secunda farrago*, foll. 192v–193r, "Cras sum discessurus ab arce/In qua novem menses fui" ("Tomorrow I will depart from the castle/in which I have spent nine months").

47 ÖNB, Cod. 9821, foll. 309v–321v.

48 Our Würzburg database of physicians' correspondences in the German-speaking territories in the sixteenth and seventeenth centuries (www.aerztebriefe.de) currently contains the records of about 40,000 letters; some 15,000 more have already been identified.

49 Giuseppe Olmi, "Molti amici in vari luoghi: Studio della natura e rapporti epistolari nel XVI secolo," *Nuncius*, 6 (1991): 3–31; Toon van Houdt et al. (eds), *Self-Presentation and Social Identification: The Rhetoric and Pragmatics of Letter Writing in Early Modern Times* (Leuven, 2002).

50 Nancy G. Siriasi, *Communities of Learned Experience: Epistolary Medicine in the Renaissance* (Baltimore, 2013).

51 Handsch repeatedly mentioned other letters, for example, ÖNB, Cod. 9650, fol. 24r, "Multas scripsi ad Doctorem Gallum nec non M. Ulricum [Lehnerum]" ("I have written many [letters] to Doctor Gallus and to M. Ulrich [Lehner]"); ibid., foll. 27v–28, on letters he sent to Tremenus in Poland; ibid., fol. 30v "Multas epistolas scripsi, quas huc referre neglexi, ad M. Schentigarum et M. Winkelmannum plures medicinales" ("I have written many letters to M. Schentygar and several medical ones to M. Winkelmann that I have left aside").

52 ÖNB, Cod. 9650; a few of these letters were published in Czech translation in Dana Martínková, *Poselství ducha. Latinská próza českých humanistů* (Prague, 1975); for detailed German summaries of all the letters in the manuscript see the database of early modern physicians' letters in Würzburg (www.aerztebriefe.de).

53 ÖNB, Cod. 9650, fol. 33v; the letter is not dated; Collinus died in 1556.

54 Jole Agrimi and Chiara Crisciani, *Consilia médicaux* (Turnhout, 1994).

55 ÖNB, Cod. 9650, foll. 31v–33r, 18 July 1556.

56 ÖNB, Cod, 9821, foll. 51r–52r, 12 April 1559.

57 Ibid., foll. 59v–60r, 24 October 1559.

58 See Brendan Dooley (ed.), *A Companion to Astrology in the Renaissance* (Leiden, 2014).

59 See Sabine Schlegelmilch, "Vom Nutzen des Nebensächlichen: Paratexte in den Kalendern des Arztes Johannes Magirus (1615–1697)," in Klaus-Dieter Herbst (ed.), *Astronomie, Literatur, Volksaufklärung: Der Schreibkalender der Frühen Neuzeit mit seinen Text- und Bildbeigaben* (Bremen, 2012): 393–411.

60 Wilhelm Schmidt-Biggemann, *Topica universalis: Eine Modellgeschichte humanistischer und barocker Wissenschaft* (Hamburg, 1983); Ann Moss, *Printed Commonplace-Books and the Structuring of Renaissance Thought* (Oxford, 1996); eadem, "Power and Persuasion: Commonplace Culture in Early Modern Europe," in David Cowling and Mette B. Bruun (eds), *Commonplace Culture in Western Europe in the Early Modern Period* (Leuven, Paris, Walpole, MA, 2011): 1–17.

61 ÖNB, Cod. 9550, foll. 2r–569v. The careful handwriting, headings in a different ink and, above all, Handsch's addressing the anticipated *lector* directly on the very first page, leave no doubt that this was not a personal notebook but a manuscript destined for publication.

62 The full title reads: *Promptuarium sive loci communes latinitatis ex eius selectissimis authoribus digesti ac adeo luculenter elaborati, ut etiam puero quacunoque de re latine scripturo vocabula et phrases in calamine exinde fluere possint.*

63 Nováková, "Rytmické kalendarium."

64   ÖNB, Cod. 11130, Cod. 11141, Cod. 11142, Cod 11143 and Cod. 11153.

65   On the background, see for example, William Eamon, *Science and the Secrets of Nature: Books of Secrets in Medieval and Early Modern Culture* (Princeton, 1994); Brian W. Ogilvie, *The Science of Describing: Natural History in Renaissance Europe* (Chicago, London, 2006).

66   Modern edition by Ottokar Schubert: Georg Handsch, *Die Elbefischerei in Böhmen und Meißen* (Prague, 1933).

67   See Madelon Simons, *"Een Theatrum van Representatie?" Aartshertog Ferdinand van Oostenrijk, stadhouder in Praag tussen 1547 en 1567.* PhD Diss. (Amsterdam, 2009), especially pp. 141–54.

68   ÖNB, Cod. 9607.

69   On different approaches to commonplacing, see Michael Stolberg, "Medizinische *Loci communes*: Formen und Funktionen einer ärztlichen Aufzeichnungspraxis im 16. und 17. Jahrhundert," *NTM – Zeitschrift für Geschichte der Wissenschaften, Technik und Medizin*, 21 (2013): 37–60; idem, "Medical Note-Taking in the Sixteenth and Seventeenth Centuries, in Alberto Cevolini (ed.). *Forgetting Machines: Knowledge Management Evolution in Early Modern Europe* (Leiden, Boston, 2016): 243–64.

70   ÖNB, Cod. 9607, foll. 48r–97v and foll. 107v–25v.

71   ÖNB, Cod. 9666; the title refers to the first part only, which is dated 23 September 1547; it is bound together with a short second manuscript, which is not in Handsch's handwriting and was owned by Christophorus Tauffkircher in 1554.

72   ÖNB, Cod. 9671.

73   Ibid., fol. 7v, fol. 8r and fol. 8v.

74   Ibid., fol. 12v.

75   Ibid., fol. 53v.

76   Erich Ludwig Schmidt, *Deutsche Volkskunde im Zeitalter des Humanismus und der Reformation* (Berlin, 1904) (= chapter 2, § 1 of his PhD dissertation, Berlin 1904).

77   Konrad Celtis, *Quattuor libri amorum secundum quattuor latera Germaniae. Germania generalis. Accedunt carmina aliorum ad libros amorum pertinentia.* Ed. by Felicitas Pindter (Leipzig, 1934), p. 7 (preface): "qui patriae suae linguae fines et terminos gentiumque in ea diversos ritus, leges, linguas, religiones, habitum denique et affectiones corporumque varia lineamenta et figura viderit et observavit"; see Hermann Wiegand, "Volkskunde und Ethnographie bei Konrad Celtis," in Franz Fuchs (ed.), *Konrad Celtis in Nürnberg (= Pirckheimer Jahrbuch für Renaissance- und Humanismusforschung, 9)* (Wiesbaden, 2004): 51–73.

78   Helmut Glück, *Deutsch als Fremdsprache in Europa vom Mittelalter bis zur Barockzeit* (Berlin, New York, 2002), pp. 345–50.

79   For example, ÖNB, Cod. 11006, frontispiece.

80   On urban sociability and the importance of oral communication in the emergence of an urban "public," see Susanne Rau and Gerd Schwerhoff (eds), *Zwischen Gotteshaus und Taverne: Öffentliche Räume in Spätmittelalter und Früher Neuzeit* (Cologne, 2004); Gerd Schwerhoff (ed.), *Stadt und Öffentlichkeit in der Frühen Neuzeit* (Cologne, Weimar, Vienna, 2011); Bronwen Wilson and Paul Yachnin (eds), *Making Publics in Early Modern Europe: People, Things, Forms of Knowledge* (New York, London, 2010).

81   ÖNB, Cod. 11006, fol. 121v.

82   ÖNB, Cod. 9671, fol. 124v.

83   See ÖNB, Cod. 11209, Cod. 11210, Cod. 11224, Cod. 11225, Cod. 11226, Cod. 11231.

84 They list, above all, patients from different ranks of society treated by Lehner; Handsch probably compiled them from Lehner's notes.
85 An exception is Handsch's diary of a journey he took with the Archduke and his wife to a spa (ÖNB, Cod. 11204).
86 See Stolberg, "Loci communes."
87 He did keep two separate notebooks, however, for medical recipes and "proven" *experimenta* (ÖNB, Cod. 11200 and ÖNB, Cod. 11251).
88 For example, ÖNB, Cod. 11183, fol. 174v, on the sick Daniel Buchhalter.
89 ÖNB, Cod. 11183, foll. 143r–46r.
90 Michael Stolberg, "Empiricism in Sixteenth-Century Medical Practice: The Notebooks of Georg Handsch," *Early Science and Medicine*, 16 (2013): 487–516.
91 Gianna Pomata, "*Praxis historialis*: The Uses of *Historia* in Early Modern Medicine," in Gianna Pomata and Nancy G. Siraisi (eds), *Historia: Empiricism and Erudition in Early Modern Europe* (Cambridge, MA, 2005): 105–46; Michael Stolberg, "Formen und Funktionen ärztlicher Fallbeobachtungen in der Frühen Neuzeit (1500–1800)," in Johannes Süßmann, Susanne Scholz and Gisela Engel (eds), *Fallstudien: Theorie – Geschichte – Methode* (Berlin, 2007): 81–95; Gianna Pomata, "Observation Rising: Birth of an Epistemic Genre, 1500–1600," in Lorraine Daston and Elizabeth Lunbeck (eds), *Histories of Scientific Observation* (Chicago, London, 2011): 45–80.
92 ÖNB, Cod. 11238, foll. 115r–118v; a further, shorter section of the same notebook is entitled "Ex praxi D. Comitis de Monte observata" (ibid., foll. 124v–25v).
93 ÖNB, Cod. 11183, fol. 206r; for a physician's notes on his exchanges with members of very different cultures, see Pugliano, "Accountability, Autobiography, and Belonging," Chapter 7 of this volume.
94 See Michael Stolberg, "Learning from the Common Folks: Academic Physicians and Medical Lay Culture in the Sixteenth Century," *Social History of Medicine*, 27 (2014): 649–67.
95 See Michael Stolberg, "'You Have No Good Blood in Your Body': Oral Communication in Sixteenth-Century Physicians' Medical Practice," *Medical History*, 59 (2015): 63–82.
96 See Stolberg, "Loci communes."
97 ÖNB, Cod. 11183, fol. 85r.
98 For example, ibid., fol. 59v, "Ter manuduxi cum Venceslao Sseliha" ("manuductio" was Handsch's standard term for masturbation).
99 ÖNB, Cod. 9666, foll. 1v–2v.
100 Felix Platter, *Tagebuch (Lebensbeschreibung) 1536–1567*, ed. Valentin Lötscher (Basel, 1976); Sabine Schlegelmilch, "Johannes Magirus: Stadtarzt in Zerbst (1651–1656)," *Mitteilungen des Vereins für Anhaltische Landeskunde*, 20 (2011): 9–30.

3 Promoting a Good Physician

Letters of Application to German Civic Authorities, 1500–1700

Sabine Schlegelmilch

Unlike in England and France, free towns and cities in the German-speaking world established the office of town physician (*Stadtarzt*) as an integral part of their autonomous health systems.[1] This civic medical office, or *Stadtphysikat*, with its often modest but regular salary and additional benefits, such as partial exemption from certain taxes and citizen duties, was seen as an attractive position by most physicians.[2] It offered the possibility to gain a foothold in an urban environment that could provide well-paying patients and benevolent patrons. To apply successfully for this office, candidates above all had to convince town authorities through a formal letter of application, a requirement even when they had already applied by word of mouth.[3] Among the records of German city archives, such letters of application often comprise a considerable share of all surviving documents regarding health. They are usually preserved in chronological order and classified as "concerning civic medical office" (*das Physikat betreffend*). Given their large number and wide dissemination, these letters invite us to draw on them not only as a source of biographical information. They also allow us to examine conventions in style and argumentation characterizing a specific genre of official writing. This is because the physicians who wrote them—usually in their own hand—did not compose them freely but made use of elements and patterns known from another type of document belonging to the sphere of communication between sovereign and subject: the supplication.[4]

In structure and style, physicians' applications for office can be classified as a variation of early modern supplications,[5] the most characteristic feature of which is to stress one's own (superficially) subservient attitude.[6] Supplicants were expected to speak a special "language of entreaty,"[7] and they did so by using longwinded and stereotypical salutatory addresses,[8] by intensifying their wishes with (often standardized) begging formulas in the *petitio* and *conclusio*,[9] and by amassing a wealth of words and images in the *subscriptio* to express their wishes of blessing and promises of loyalty. We find an example of this in Wolfgang Rinckler's verbal genuflection:

DOI: 10.4324/9781315554693-5

Hereby I commend the Noble, Honorable, Honest, Cautious and Wise [members of the city council] to the almighty sublime hand of God so that he may give blessed well-being and successful government, while [I also recommend] myself to the authorities' lasting deep favor and benevolence, subserviently and obediently as Your honorable, honest, cautious, subservient, obedient citizen Dr. Wolfgang Rincklerus.[10]

The physician repeatedly mentions and thereby emphasizes his subservience and obedience, but at the same time he assigns to himself some of the attributes he has ascribed to the members of the council: namely, being "honorable, honest, cautious." He thereby invoked a common set of values on which to base his argument while simultaneously submitting himself to the established hierarchy. Rinckler's letter thus shows a feature characteristic of the supplications in our sample: the contradiction between rhetorical form and communicative message.[11] The pleas, albeit suitably subservient in form and humble in tone, often call subtly on an *obligation* of political authorities to provide for deserving subjects—in this case, physicians—and thus to behave in accordance with Christian ethics. This allies such application letters with a specific kind of supplication, the supplication for mercy (*Gnadensupplikation*) which, in contrast to the supplication for justice (*Justizsupplikation*), puts forward a moral claim.[12] As to hierarchy, physicians and town authorities unanimously shared the understanding that anyone who submitted such a letter was to be seen as a supplicant. Johann Ulrich Oeler—to name just one—accordingly signed his letter as "most subservient supplicant" (*underthänigster supplicant*),[13] and when the members of the Collegium Medicum of Augsburg wrote to the city council concerning the case of the physician Johann Caspar Helbling, they called his application letter a supplication (*Supplikation umb eine Physikatsstell*).[14]

Yet the applications differ from supplications as usually understood by historians because the physicians were not only supplicants but had something to offer in return. Regarding this offer, town authorities expected competitors to state their cases convincingly and to explain why they should be preferred over others for appointment as town physician. What kinds of information did physicians consider important to include in these letters? What lines of argumentation did they follow to persuade authorities to see them as the best choice and to show common ground with authorities' expectations? As the following analysis of 140 letters of application to 11 cities and towns in the German-speaking world in the sixteenth and seventeenth centuries[15] will show, recurring patterns of argumentation can be found.[16] These not only illustrate how physicians saw and fashioned themselves as prospective town physicians, but also reveal the expectations on both sides—that of the physicians as well as that of the authorities.

Academic Training and Practical Knowledge

The position of town physician in Germany was usually filled by a university-trained academic.[17] Therefore applicants often referred to their formal academic qualifications, while offering to provide certification of their university degree. Johannes Husanus, who applied to become town physician in Altenburg, tried to forestall doubts about his qualification—which he was unable to prove by a doctoral diploma—by promising to hand in a testified *curriculum* of his academic career including the names of the universities he had visited.[18] It was not unusual for students to leave university without a doctorate. In such cases, they could obtain *testimonia* that were seen as proof of "diligence, academic socialization, virtuousness and ability for social integration, [...] abilities and qualities that were supposed to characterize a student quasi per definitionem," as Ulrich Rasche puts it.[19] Issued by the principal of the university or a faculty dean and officially sealed, these certificates not only confirmed their holders' learning, but also his *"vera religio* and good manners and, as a rule, ended with a recommendation to accept him with honors at his future place of work."[20] The fact that academic diplomas and testimonies contained strong moral connotations—a student in 1542 even labeled a doctoral degree not only a testimony *"de studiis,"* but also *"de moribus"*[21]—is seldom noticed by historians, as academic study is usually seen as preparation for the academic or scholarly aspects of doctors' lives. This view neglects the purposes of the many students who would turn their backs on the academic world after leaving the university as well as the purposes of universities themselves. The statutes of universities such as the Viadrina in Frankfurt on the Oder spelled out that only persons of integrity should be allowed to receive academic *testimonia*, "so that the authorities [*herrschaften*] may always know how each [applicant] can best be used with regard to his qualities by churches and schools as well as within administration and for other kinds of common benefit."[22] If we compare this claim of the university to produce useful academics for employment in municipal or state offices with the learned habitus that the same academics were eager to display in urban educated circles,[23] we discover the existence of at least two very different sets of expectations and values concerning university education and its utility in the polity—values that could be held by the same or different groups and actors.

In addition to listing their places of study—one applicant referred to Altdorf, Strasbourg, Jena, and Basel[24]—physicians often stressed that they had accomplished their studies with great care and thoroughness by providing the exact duration of their academic training (in this case, 11 years). Further studies at foreign universities were mentioned to enhance the applicant's reputation and show his cosmopolitanism. This is why a doctor named Petrus Scipio specified in his letter each stage of his academic career and proudly announced that he had studied without boasting: not only in Germany, at Strasbourg, at Wittenberg, and Basel; but also in foreign countries at great expense, efforts and labor: in Louvain in Brabant, in Douai in Artois, in Paris, in Orléans and finally in Padua and Bologna.[25]

It is questionable whether such an impressive enumeration was needed to meet the expectations of the council of a comparatively small town like Kitzingen. Authorities were more likely to suspect that an applicant with such broad academic connections would consider office in a small town as a temporary position and leave before long.

Although academic training was seen as a necessary requirement for office, it played a minor role among the arguments used in applications. Education alone was insufficient to convince city authorities of a physician's capability: theoretical knowledge had to be met by practical experience. This conforms to the requirements that many German universities defined very early on for gaining a diploma, as "most statutes lay down qualifications for practical experience before a license or a degree is to be granted."[26] However, "statutes tell us what ought to be done, not what is being done," as Vivian Nutton rightly points out.[27] No regular teaching structures for practical training were implemented in German universities until the eighteenth century. This may well be the reason why applicants took great pains to prove their individual experience, especially because physicians, unlike craft-trained barber-surgeons, were not usually taught practical skills at university at all. A university medical degree could shed favorable light on a candidate's social skills but did not tell the authorities whether its holder had ever seen a patient. This is why Wilhelm Günther Brügge, in his application, explicitly named two practitioners, Dr. Thielen in Wittenberg and Dr. Ortlob in Leipzig, as having given him "private information" (*privat information*) so that he now had the knowledge to practice himself.[28] Another physician, Eucharius Rößlin the Younger, wrote that his father had trained him as a physician from childhood on and, in addition, had paid for most of his studies. In his case, instruction by the father (himself a town physician, in Frankfurt on the Main) probably was a substantial argument for the city council when looking for a physician with practical experience.[29] Accordingly, Christopherus Romanus, in a letter following his application, was quick not only to promise to send the testimony of his studies for which the council members of Salzwedel had asked, but above all to assure that he would impress them by his daily practice.[30]

That there indeed existed clear expectations on the part of town authorities can be deduced from the fact that the description of one's practical knowledge (*experientia*) stands out as a major feature of applications in comparison to other features. Physicians never went into detail about what exactly they had done but usually claimed, in a more general way, to have served major or minor nobility,[31] or to have practiced (without having yet held civic medical office, but of course successfully) either in a foreign country or in another town or even in the same town.[32] Some offered written testimony of their practicing activity, similar to their academic certificates.[33] Archives in Rome still hold copies of such testimonies: for example, one from 1614 for a Swiss physician by the name of Rudolph Hager who evidently had traveled to Rome on his *peregrinatio academica* while still a student. The text states that Hager had sedulously assisted his teacher Johannes Faber (a German physician) for three years in his *praxis chirurgica* in patients' homes as well as in the hospitals of San Giovanni and Santa Maria della Consolazione; that he had also substituted for Faber in several cases; and that therefore he should be deemed entirely worthy to be entrusted with public functions (*publicae functiones*).[34] Interestingly, Hager was attested with *surgical* skills, although as a physician back home he would be expected to avoid doing any work conceded to the surgeons' guilds. Apparently, it was important to have had one's hand on the patients, as a testimony from 1608 confirms, certifying that Heinrich Valentin Knorr from Forchheim always "handled" his patients successfully (*manus feliciter admodum adimplevisse*).[35]

Thus application letters show how one-sided is our usual focus on physicians as writers of erudite books and how our standard notion of "learned physician" is a product of university culture.[36] To explain the growing emphasis on *experientia* in those erudite medical books in the sixteenth and seventeenth centuries (through the rise of *observationes, consilia,* and so on) primarily as a reorientation toward methods found in the Hippocratic corpus and natural philosophy ignores the rise of the importance of experience in many physicians' working lives in this golden age of civic medical office.[37] Historians of medicine have long focused on early modern physicians' claims that their education made them better healers than their unlearned competitors. Yet physicians' eagerness to prove their practical experience, so evident in their applications, shows that this claim is far from the whole picture: even the physicians often did not represent academic knowledge as superior to non-academic knowledge and leading to superior treatment. On the contrary, although physicians used academic education to differentiate themselves from competing healer groups in the medical market, the importance of academic knowledge was accepted by civic communities and their leadership only when physicians were able to prove their practical and even hands-on experience.

Finally, applicants claimed to have *specific* practical knowledge. This claim was advanced by those physicians who were able to report that they already had held the same public office in another town or had temporarily stood in for another town physician (usually because he was ill or deceased). To have accompanied a town physician in his work for a longer period (one's own father in the example above) came close to the value of having served as one. Experience as an officeholder or as an assistant to one indicated to city authorities that a candidate was already familiar with the duties and able to fulfill them. Philipp Höchstetter therefore stressed in his letter of application that—by standing in for an appointed town physician 18 years ago—he had "seen elsewhere and learned back then what is necessary for this Offici[um]."[38] This focus on prior experience explains why many physicians did not try to begin their civic careers by applying for a "first physician" civic post (*physicus primarius*),[39] but for lesser offices, like that of "plague physician" on a temporary contract or town physician's assistant. These lesser offices offered the same advantage of regular pay and the opportunity to enhance one's chances with future applications. Accordingly, many physicians claimed in their letters that they had already given their share of medical support to a local health care system by holding minor offices.[40] Slightly weaker in argument, but still making a point, were those applicants who had not yet worked by civic appointment to provide medical care to citizens but had successfully completed single tasks assigned to them by town authorities, like visitation of pharmacies or inspections for leprosy (*Siechenschau*).[41]

Social Relations

Though mandatory, academic education and practical experience were not the only qualifications. Applicants often intensified their plea by declaring that they had been born in the territory or town to which they were applying (their parents thus being local subjects or citizens) or were married to a citizen. Such applicants usually stated their urgent wish to serve their *Vatterland*.[42] This implied a claim to deserve civic office over equally qualified foreign applicants. It suggests that families with citizenship expected on principle to be appreciated by town authorities as useful building blocks of civic structure. Some of the letters confirm this notion, as their writers spell out the family's past usefulness to the city.[43] Ideally, an applicant could remind the city council that it had employed his late father or another relative as town physician.[44] Other services counted as well: Karl Widemann time and again invoked the memory of his father-in-law (long dead before his daughter's marriage to Widemann), who had served the city of Augsburg as a lawyer.[45] Conditions that had tested an applicant's loyalty, like long-term service at low pay or in a capacity different from the desired one of physician, were cited to exert moral pressure: medically educated Georg Henisch underlined that he had worked for the city of Augsburg as a schoolmaster for 22 years and therefore now wished to be made town physician, as he longed finally to put to use what he had once studied for nine long years.[46]

Experience of providing medical services to a town, however, was doubtless valued more highly by its authorities. Applicants who had not had the opportunity temporarily to fill a vacancy or to hold minor medical office tried at least to depict their service to the town to best advantage. Aside from assuring that they had won the confidence of many patients through successful treatment, physicians cited services to the community at their own expense; treating soldiers or the poor without payment either at home or in hospital; or standing firm and facing danger in times of epidemic and civic medical crisis.[47] If devotion to the community had led to personal harm or loss, the claim of *do ut des* carried even more weight: Johann Christoph Steeb reported that he had lost his wife when taking care of infected patients in the *pestilenzhaus* of Frankfurt on the Main in times of "contagion."[48]   Other   physicians   reported   having   fallen   ill   as a consequence of their duties in the hospital. Wendelin Hock von Bracke-nau begged to become town physician, as his weakened condition would soon prevent him from continuing his municipal hospital service:

> even if God gave me his special help and mercy, it would be impossible for me to stand this stench: the poisoned air, or work; as it has occurred within a short time that this stench of the hospital has brought deadly disease upon me.[49]

Administrative Practices and Obligations

Urban administration in early modern Germany was characterized to a large extent by formalized acts of communication and decision-making. To participate in or influence those decisions therefore required being familiar with established administrative practices. As we can see from their letters, physicians applying for office knew well how to argue according to such practices: they regularly reminded the authorities of assurances given or decisions made and their consequences.[50] First of all, they wrote as insurance they would not be forgotten after having been turned down: even if there was no official waiting list, any candidate who had already been passed over once or several times could claim priority the next time he applied. When Karl Widemann wrote to the privy council and city managers (*Stadtpfleger*) of Augsburg to support the renewed application of his son, Marcus Widemann, he recalled that after his son's failed first application, Marcus had been told that the members of the city council would "remember him, if a similar situation arises, before all others" and that this had been confirmed orally by the two *Stadtpfleger* several times over some years.[51] In this way, a city council could keep a number of applicants in competition for office through several elections over an extended period, and unsuccessful applicants could strengthen their claims each time around.

When reapplying, physicians usually added fresh information or pointed to their growing seniority with respect to competitors or to the fact that a previously successful colleague had moved on, in some cases "to eternal peace and bliss."[52] From time to time we notice a reproachful tone, when applicants point out that they have been passed over several times although it had been their turn. This was apparently considered an administrative failure, and so Marcus Banzer could hope to move authorities by complaining that they had passed him over several times.[53] Losing track of how long an applicant had been waiting also figured as a common failure of the authorities. Thus, Johann Ulrich Oeler, in his application for the vacant post of town physician of Lindau, informed the city council that he had now been working for 20 years as their plague physician and had always been content—because he had expected to be promoted in due time (that is, now).[54]

Some physicians tried to hasten decisions in their favor by reporting that they had declined offers from other towns or noblemen, reserving their knowledge and ability for their own town.[55] This information could be interpreted as an implicit warning: the authorities risked losing a useful citizen. Every town had to be interested in having a supply of capable men, especially academics, to run the administration and fulfill tasks linked to it. For this reason, some councils even gave study grants to the sons of citizens. Some of the applying physicians who had been funded in this way, or who had been able to study because their fathers had been employed by the town, hoped that they would therefore be supported further on. It seemed reasonable, in any case, to remind authorities that they had already regarded the applicant as trustworthy and invested in his education, from which they now could profit. For Johann Ludwig Witzel, it proved helpful to remind the council that it had paid not only for his studies in Germany, but also for his *peregrinatio* and that he, therefore, felt obliged to give something in return. Soon after, he became town physician in Frankfurt on the Main.[56]

Finally, by reporting that many of their patients, including important citizens, had pressed them to apply for office, physicians signaled that their applications were not only in their own interest but responded to the voice of citizen demand.[57] The applicant's *petitio* was thus multiplied, and for the council to decline it would have meant not only to turn down a single man, but to ignore the wishes of the community.

Thinking Ahead

Many applicants had clear ideas about their future duties as a town physician and the problems that might occur in the relationship between the authorities and the officeholder. Some had observed conflicts; others had learned about difficult situations from other physicians; and certainly, they used this knowledge in making their case. It is striking how often the physicians adopt the perspective of the authorities. In their letters, they anticipate problems *they* might cause and indicate solutions. Thus, they showed not only awareness of potential conflicts, but also how such conflicts could be avoided.

Many physicians assured authorities that no complaints would ever be heard about their behavior.[58] What kinds of misbehavior or negligence could cause complaints can be seen in physicians' promises of what they reliably would do: be available at all times,[59] give advice and medication to the poor for free (both promises anticipating the town physician's oath),[60] swear the same oath as their predecessors,[61] work as a plague physician, or support others in times of crisis.[62] One can easily recognize the kinds of past conflict that underlay these pledges, mostly concerning duties defined by town physicians' contracts.[63] Naturally, misbehavior on the part of the authorities was never mentioned, although such stories must have circulated among physicians. In their letters of application, they displayed only anticipatory obedience and thus seem implicitly to assure that, if ever conflicts arose, their colleagues would be to blame.

To show eagerness to serve, doctors tended to downplay the cost of employing them.[64] We often find the suggestion that the authorities should feel absolutely free to decide on the amount of payment as they saw fit. Christopherus Germanus, who applied to become *physicus* of Salzwedel in 1567, happened to be without predecessor, because the town had only just decided to establish the office. So, on request, he suggested a mode of payment: 60 Taler per year, ten loads (*Fuder*) of wood and one of coal, and accommodation.[65] Ten days later, when the council had still not answered, he evidently grew nervous that his suggestions might have made him a nuisance and might cost him the job. So he sat down to write in a second letter that for now he would be content with *any* amount of money (*qualicumq[ue] stipendio (...) contentus ero*) and, for accommodation, suggested a certain house that could be refurbished at low cost (*sumptu parvi*).[66] Other applicants developed more creative ideas for selling themselves to the authorities, including even that they could save the town money: Hieronymus Henninger offered to serve also by preaching the word of God[67]; Matthias Zacharias Pilling reminded the council of Altenburg that his late predecessor "had left a poor widow and many mostly still-to-be-raised orphans with little funds." He made

> the offer to leave an entire year's salary to this poor and very saddened widow for her benefit, voluntarily and of my free will, and nonetheless fulfill the duties of office and the tasks connected with it with the highest untiring industriousness and due obedience.[68]

It is likely that the penniless widow addressed the council with a supplication for help; and, unsurprisingly, Pilling soon became town physician of Altenburg.[69]

Beyond the City Walls

Whereas applying was an act of subordination, appeal to external referees could raise applicants' status. Usually referees were men of standing able to communicate with town authorities on an equal or higher footing.[70] Pursuing this strategy, some physicians confined themselves to a hint that a certain person of standing (usually named) figured as their patron.[71] More often, they asked supporters for direct help. We know this from applications in which we find formal support from co-signatories[72] or even letters of recommendation, either attached or sent under separate cover.

One entry in the city records (*Ratsprotokolle*) of Würzburg shows how such an intercession worked. In 1676, there were two competitors for the office of Würzburg town physician: Michael Werlein and Hieronymus Virdung.[73] An intercession for Virdung by the prince-bishop of Würzburg was made orally by Privy Counsellor Pfenning to the Elder Mayor of Würzburg, who was meant to recommend Virdung to the city council. The bishop requested that the Catholic convert Virdung, to whom he had already given a professorship, be made town physician

> for one reason or another, especially as he was recommended to Him [the bishop] *specialiter* by noble men, to whom he [Virdung] had, as He [the bishop] had heard, applied such cure that they had high hopes concerning [the value of] his experience.

The bishop stated that he wished the council's right of election (*ius eligendi*) to remain unaffected and that he certainly did not wish to impinge upon its traditional and free rights; nevertheless, he continued, he hoped that his wish to see Virdung in office would be granted, as this was the first time he had ever directed a request to the council. That this "most gracious will," as the scribe phrased it, was received as a command can be deduced from the prompt decision for Virdung. The record of the decision illustrates the combination of written and face-to-face communication that characterizes early modern politics: Dr. Virdung was "accepted for a *Stattphysicus*, immediately appointed, and the letter of appointment read to him, especially his obligation for [attendance during] mortal disease [*sterbensläufften*] and that he, when prescribing medicine, should not be too extravagant."[74] Interestingly, the city authorities also made note of reasons for choosing the other applicant, Werlein: that he was the son of a citizen and that he had risked his life serving in a local hospital during dangerous times. These arguments may have been copied from Werlein's letter of application and seem to have been kept in case the council someday had the opportunity to decide for Werlein.

The decisions of town authorities unfolded in broader, extramural context when applicants brought their religious confession to bear. When in 1584 Petrus Scipio wrote from the Catholic city of Würzburg to apply for office in the Protestant town of Kitzingen, he emphasized his wish to serve solely in a place where "the Pure True and Undoubted word of God prevails" and "the Holy Sacraments are established and celebrated according to our dear Lord Jesus Christ's installation."[75] He thereby appealed to the members of the council of Kitzingen to save a brother-in-faith from having to live in the nearby Catholic city and bishopric and to enable him to live in an environment of the right faith.[76] That this was a sound expectation is confirmed by an earlier letter of the council to the physician Johannes Posthius in Würzburg: the council informed Posthius that they knew him to be a follower of the "true" religion (*liebhaber der wahren christlichen Religion*), and as they obeyed Margrave Georg Friedrich of Brandenburg and his wish for a true preaching, Posthius surely would be glad to come to Kitzingen where he could practice his faith freely.[77] Laurentius Phronto, too, went beyond local reasons to hire him and reminded the burgomaster and council of their image beyond the walls: he outlined how the outside world highly regarded establishing a good "policy regarding the noble art of medicine" (*policei mit der Edlen kunst der Ertznei*) and described his future services to the sick as "support" (*fürderung*) of church and government.[78] Applicants had to vary such confessional arguments when applying to cities like Augsburg, which required equal numbers of Catholics and Protestants among its officeholders and even equal total pay to each group. Johann Henisius, for example, had studied the Augsburg officeholding situation in 1649 well enough to be able to argue that his appointment would laudably maintain confessional parity with regard to both numbers of persons and salaries.[79]

Profession, rather than confession, was the core of Johann Ulrich Oeler's argument. He wrote to the council of Lindau that physicians were facing such fierce competition with "idiots [that is, lay healers], barbers, nurses, pharmacists, hangmen and old wives" that they could survive only through civic appointments as *physici ordinarii*.[80] This claim to professional superiority seems also to have been an appeal to university-trained council members (mainly jurists) to support their fellow academics (physicians). Oeler's is the only example of this argument I have found so far. Johann Friedrich Graff made no such general plea to support academic physicians but a related (and flattering) appeal to a city's academic values and excellence when he stated that he would like to become town physician of Worms because he wished to send his children to a good school.[81]

Times of Hardship

The arguments discussed so far include academic education and practical experience, local family background and service record, familiarity with administrative practice, recommendations from supporters, and reference to confession and status. Besides these, some letters also reveal the personal situation of the applicant. Here we read about hardships like displacement due to war, responsibilities for large families, old age, poverty and illness.

Alone among these problems, poverty called for an explanation: a poor physician could be suspected of being a bad one. Thus, applicants who mentioned their financial problems usually described how these came about through no fault of their own and despite the large number of patients they had treated. Christian duty explained Bernhard Schludin's poverty: he had devoted his hard work to many patients—some for pay and some for free, but in the end more poor than rich ones.[82] Georg Laub, on the other hand, explained that he had treated many patients with the means to pay who had, however, not paid "because of [their] burdensome forgetfulness" (*aus beschwerlicher Vergessenheit*).[83] Authorities would certainly have put more trust in the experience of a candidate like Laub ("poor," but reporting a large number of well-to-do patients) than in a practitioner like Ulrich Kieffer who wrote that for lack of "required clientele" (*notwendiger Kundschafft*) his "*res domestica* will become deficient."[84]

Besides poverty, some physicians reported being themselves ill or infirm. It is unsurprising that physicians could fall ill, especially when working under the dangerous circumstances to which we have seen them refer, but surprising that personal ailment could be used as an argument for being appointed and not only for being rewarded for service. Evidently physicians did not expect town authorities to see their illness or old age as a hindrance. This may be because the usual case load of an early modern learned physician was only one to three patients a day.[85]

By revealing hardship, physicians came closer to being like most other supplicants. The wish to better one's situation can be seen as a characteristic element of all supplications.[86] When questions of survival were raised, however, the supplicant's wish became urgent need. Poor and ill (competent) physicians did not only apply for office: they called upon authorities' Christian duty of care.

Conclusion

To recognize the supplicatory character of physicians' letters of application and explore their arguments helps relocate the town and state physician beyond historiographical clichés, old and new, a desideratum articulated by Mary Lindemann:

> Today, few historians will argue that seventeenth- and eighteenth-century physici (and physicians) were knights of hygiene and science who sallied forth under the banners of enlightenment and medical science to battle ignorance and confound superstition. Now we are far more likely to encounter analyses that pin the physici in the jaws of a vice composed of local interests on the one hand and the aspirations of central territorial government on the other; or to view them as the protégés and creatures of territorial governments that ran on patronage and clientage relationships. Yet the experiences of the physici as a group, in particular the lives of those who never scaled the ladder to become body-physicians or to sit on a territorial collegium medicum, who never attained a professorship or authored a significant piece of medical literature, have not been examined in detail.[87]

Nearly all of the applicants discussed in this chapter meet this description of ordinary *physici*.[88] Through their letters, they communicated with town authorities as with a sovereign, offering their services and promising perfect fulfillment of duty in exchange for basic financial security and incorporation into civic life and structure. As we can learn from their letters, they knew well that civic authorities were not interested in the learned *habitus* that physicians also cultivated. This brings us to a final question and insight: why, then, did towns and cities recruit academic physicians at all instead of craft-trained practitioners, especially given that learned doctors were not primarily distinguished by their experience in everyday medical practice? One answer may be the moral standards an academic diploma was meant to assure. Another may lie in the importance of practical skills other than medical ones. All physicians had undergone the basic academic training involved in studying the liberal arts. This meant that they were highly experienced in written communication—everything from the use of language in persuasive writing to appropriate composition and layout of texts in different genres for different purposes. Students of the arts did not, of course, learn to write official documents, but they were trained—over many years—to recognize and imitate the structures and styles of classical texts. This capacity could translate directly into what physicians had to do when writing as town physicians: certify, report, indeed plea, and generally interact in writing, which entailed reproducing the styles and structures of official documents and adapting them to medical purposes, sometimes even developing new forms.[89] A letter of application itself—as a standardized and highly formalized text related to an existing genre (the supplication)—bore witness to this ability. Adapting Marshall McLuhan's famous phrase, the form was the message: signaling an understanding of the ways of public writing as well as an awareness of the topics and conventions of communication in and for the polity, thereby "producing trust" and displaying competence.[90] This was also the aim of the thoughtfulness some applicants showed concerning the everyday duties and financial aspects of civic medical office. On the other hand, applications conspicuously lack concrete comments or general statements on civic health care systems—for example, a promise to pursue possible improvements or an offer to share knowledge acquired in other towns. This may be because promoting oneself as an innovator implied future insubordination.

To know one's position and place was certainly important in early modern communities. This applied to council members themselves, as can be seen, for example, in "sophisticated seating arrangements" in meetings, which corresponded with the right to speak at certain times.[91] Among the many decisions made in these meetings were decisions among applicants for the office of town physician. Further research could be done on how such decisions were reached.[92] Council meeting records (*Ratsprotokolle*) often include not only the content of discussions—here we might see which arguments of the applying physicians worked and which did not—but also the *way* in which discussion and decision took place. In Hamburg, for example, we find the combination of written and oral communication that turns out to be characteristic of early modern politics: council members usually voted for a candidate via slips of paper and the winner's name was read aloud in front of the council.[93] This example also shows that, at least in Hamburg, physicians were *elected* to office by council. The records of such an election in Helmstedt in 1731 provide insight into how council members assessed candidates.[94] From among the six candidates who had applied and promoted themselves using the standard arguments—above all, reports on their practical experience—the council chose the physician who could prove the longest stretch of practice (20 years), a *licentiatus* named Siegesbeck. In the records, we read that the whole council, chaired by the burgomaster Cellarius, discussed the matter thoroughly. Cellarius argued for Siegesbeck on the basis of "certain messages that he [i.e., Siegesbeck] was a skillful *Medicus Practicus* and had written one or two treatises."[95] In Helmstedt unlike Hamburg, decisions had to be unanimous, and this one was not reached until all agreed Senator Schieckelmann's proposal that the new town physician treat members of the senate (that is, the council and the burgomaster) free of charge and Senator Haenichen's stipulation that the town physician always "concede the senators their rank" (*als Stadt-Physicus denen Senatoribus den Rang geben möchte*). Giving precedence at public events enacted hierarchy before citizens' eyes.[96] Town physicians, it seems, were not meant even to mingle with those of their learned peers, the jurists, who were members of council or to walk with them in processions. Civic ceremony was thus supposed to display not the physician's translocal academic status, but his position in a local system of administration. Heightened attention to local rank in ceremony, as in Helmstedt in 1731, suggests that the singularity and importance of civic medical office and its holders' academic qualifications had come to pose an implicit challenge to civic hierarchy, at least by the eighteenth century.

Picturing the town physician walking near but decently behind the councilors, while knowing very well how to gain the council's attention by writing, helps us to understand the place and experience of physicians as members of early modern communities and, by the same token, the nature of those communities in so far as they enlisted and depended on the services of physicians—learned and competent, in ways both medical and political.

Notes

1 On the development of this office, see Wolfram Kaiser and Arina Völker, *Universität und Physikat in der Frühgeschichte des Amtsarztwesens* (Halle/Saale, 1980), pp. 9–11; Manfred Stürzbecher, "The Physici in German Speaking Countries from the Middle Ages to the Enlightment," in Andrew W. Russell (ed.), *The Town and State Physician from the Middle Ages to the Enlightment* (Wolfenbüttel, 1981): 123–29, pp. 124–25; Mary Lindemann, *Health and Healing in Eighteenth-Century Germany* (Baltimore, London, 1996), p. 77. See

also Dross, "'De Officiis'," Chapter 4 of this volume; Kinzelbach, "Negotiating on Paper," Chapter 6 of this volume; and Pomata, "A Sense of Place," Chapter 8 of this volume.

2 See Dross, "'De Officiis'," Chapter 4 of this volume. On town physicians' benefits in Frankfurt on the Main, see Thomas Bauer, "'der stede arzt': Stadt und Gesundheit in Frankfurt am Main vom Mittelalter bis zur Neuzeit," in Thomas Bauer, Heike Drummer and Leoni Krämer (eds), *Vom "stede arzt" zum Stadtgesundheitsamt: Die Geschichte des öffentlichen Gesundheitswesens in Frankfurt am Main* (Frankfurt a. Main, 1992): 11–50, p. 11.

3 See the case of Jörg Chümerlin: Stadtarchiv Esslingen, Bestand Reichsstadt, Faszikel 81, Nr. 61, Jörg Chümerlin to the mayor and council of Esslingen, n.p., 1545; see also Georg Naber, "Der Arzt als städtischer Amtsträger im alten Amberg" (Med. dent. diss., University of Erlangen-Nürnberg, 1967), p. 22.

4 On the structure of supplications, see Alexandra-Kathrin Stanislaw-Kemenah, "Zwischen Anspruch und Wirklichkeit: Supplikationen des 16. und 17. Jahrhunderts zur Aufnahme in das Dresdner Jakobshospital – eine linguistische Analyse," in Philipp Osten (ed.), *Patientendokumente: Krankheit in Selbstzeugnissen* (Stuttgart, 2010): 81–97, p. 83. Ulbricht points out that academics wrote supplications for illiterate people, but does not mention physicians: Otto Ulbricht, "Supplikationen als Ego-Dokumente: Bittschriften von Leibeigenen aus der ersten Hälfte des 17. Jahrhunderts als Beispiel," in Winfried Schulze (ed.), *Ego-Dokumente: Annäherung an den Menschen in der Geschichte* (Berlin, 1996): 149–74, p. 153.

5 On the *supplicatio* as a characteristic genre in the administration of the Holy Roman Empire of the sixteenth and seventeenth centuries, see Helmut Neuhaus, *Reichstag und Supplikationsausschuß: Ein Beitrag zur Reichsverfassungsgeschichte der ersten Hälfte des 16. Jahrhunderts* (Berlin, 1977), pp. 87–88; see also Ulbricht, "Supplikationen," p. 152.

6 See Ulbricht, "Supplikationen," p. 150; Neuhaus, *Reichstag*, p. 88.

7 Koziol defines this as a language "that communicated two facts: the petitioner's humility and the benefactor's graciousness": Geoffrey Koziol, *Begging Pardon and Favor: Ritual and Political Order in Early Modern France* (Ithaca and London, 1992), p. 8; on the religious dimension of supplications and especially the notion that secular authorities are installed by God, pp. 8–9.

8 On such elements and their origin in medieval court ceremonies, see Koziol's chapter on "The Language of Petition": Koziol, *Begging*, pp. 25–58, on forms of address, esp. p. 38.

9 See Stanislaw-Kemenah, "Anspruch," pp. 88–89.

10 Stadtarchiv Lindau, A III: 49/6, s.p.: letter of application by Wolfgang Ringler, Lindau, 22.11.1652: "E[dlen] v[esten] e[hrsamen] f[ürsichtigen] und Weisen darmit der allegeweltigen hohen hand Gottes zum allem gesegneten wol ergehen, glücklicher Regierung, denenselben aber mich zu beharrlicher Obrigkeittlicher großgünstigkeit und wolgewogenheit underthänig und gehorsamlich empfehlend als E[euer] v[ester] e[hrsamer] f[ürsichtiger] underthänig gehorsamer Bürger Wolfgang Rincklerus dr." Thanks to Sebastian Felten for help with translating this passage. For a similar example, see Stanislaw-Kemenah, "Anspruch," pp. 86–87.

11 See Stanislaw-Kemenah, "Anspruch," pp. 94–95.

12 On the difference between supplications for mercy and those for justice (which required an opponent), see the synopsis by Alexandra-Kathrin Stanislaw-Kemenah, *Spitäler in Dresden: vom Wandel einer Institution (13. bis 16. Jahrhundert)* (Göttingen, 2008), p. 334.

13 Stadtarchiv Lindau, A III: 49/6, s.p.: letter of application by Johann Ulrich Oeler, Lindau, 7.9.1666. On typical phrasing like this in German supplications, see Stanislaw-Kemenah, "Anspruch," p. 88.
14 Stadtarchiv Augsburg, Reichsstadt, Rat, Deputatio ad Collegium Medicum und die Apothekerordnung, CM VIII 85 (2): letter of report by Dr. Johannes Henisius, representing the Collegium Medicum of Augsburg, Augsburg, 30.3.1638.
15 The sample analyzed in this article is comprised of letters preserved in the archives of Altenburg, Augsburg, Esslingen, Frankfurt (Main), Freiburg, Lindau, Oldenburg, Strasbourg, Weißenburg (Bavaria), Worms, Würzburg, and Uppsala (Waller Collection: records of Kitzingen). It draws on a long-term database project of the Bavarian Academy of Sciences collecting the correspondence of physicians in the German-speaking territories from 1500–1700, accessible online at www.aerztebriefe.de. I would like to thank Michael Stolberg and Ulrich Schlegelmilch for providing me with photos of unpublished manuscripts from the archives of Lindau and Würzburg and Tilmann Walter for references to database content.
16 Lindemann notes "themes … endlessly repeated in almost all the petitions" of applying physicians (p. 98) but focuses mainly on interaction between the Collegium Medicum and the privy council of Braunschweig-Wolfenbüttel and their decision-making in the eighteenth century (Lindemann, *Health*, pp. 95–107). The bounds of her excellent study are extended here to the previous two centuries, across many towns and polities, and by survey of arguments used with respect to how successful they were.
17 See Stürzbecher, "Physici," p. 123. A well-studied exception is the non-academic "Stadtschnittarzt" (town surgeon) Jacob Ruf, who was promoted to the office of town physician: see Hubert Steinke, "Medizinische Karriere im städtischen Dienst," in Hildegard Elisabeth Keller (ed.), *Jakob Ruf: ein Zürcher Stadtchirurg und Theatermacher im 16. Jahrhundert* (Zurich, 2006), pp. 87–88. For further examples, see Dross, "'De Officiis'," Chapter 4 of this volume; Kinzelbach, "Negotiating on Paper," Chapter 6 of this volume.
18 Husanus defined his academic status as "defectu[s] gradus Doctorei" and described in detail what he would present: his "gradum oder vitae ac eruditionis testimonium publicum, sonderlich will ich der örter, da ich meine studia medica continuieret, occasiones und competitiones angeben": Stadtarchiv Altenburg, VIIIb, 15, Nr. 2, Bl. 3r–4v: letter of application by Johannes Husanus, n.p., 30.1.1612
19 See Ulrich Rasche, "Die deutschen Universitäten und die ständische Gesellschaft: Über institutionengeschichtliche und sozioökonomische Dimensionen von Zeugnissen, Dissertationen und Promotionen in der Frühen Neuzeit," in Rainer A. Müller (ed.), *Bilder, Daten, Promotionen: Studien zum Promotionswesen an deutschen Universitäten der Frühen Neuzeit* (Stuttgart, 2007): 150–273, p. 165.
20 See Rasche, "Deutsche Universitäten," p. 165 (with references).
21 See Rasche, "Deutsche Universitäten," p. 230.
22 As quoted by Rasche, "Deutsche Universitäten," p. 231: "auch die herrschaften jederzeit wissen mögen, wie ein jeder seine geschicklichkeit halben bei kirchen und schuelen, auch in der regierung oder sonst dem gemeinen nutz zum besten zu gebrauchen."
23 See Stolberg, "The Many Uses of Writing," Chapter 2 of this volume; Włodzimierz Kaczorowski, "Elias Kuntschius und sein Sohn Elias – zwei Oppelner Ärzte und Dichter," in Gerhard Kosellek (ed.), *Oberschlesische Dichter und Gelehrte vom Humanismus bis zum Barock* (Bielefeld, 2000): 329–38; Walther

Ludwig, "Die Sammlung der *Epistolae ac Epigrammata* des Ulmer Stadtarztes Wolfgang Reichart von 1534 als Dokument humanistischer Selbstdarstellung," in Klaus Arnold (ed.), *Das dargestellte Ich: Studien zu Selbstzeugnissen des späteren Mittelalters und der frühen Neuzeit* (Bochum, 1999): 117–38.

24 Hohenlohe-Zentralarchiv Neuenstein, Sf 160 Bü 127 [Nr. 4]: letter of application by Johann Christoph Spieß [Öhringen], 5.7.1697.

25 "ohn Ruhm zu vermelden, nit allein in Teutschlandt, zu Strasburg, zu Wittenberg, zu Basel: sondern auch in fremdten Landen mit großen umbkosten, mühe undt arbeit in Louen zu Brabandt, zu Douai in Artesia, zu Paris, zu Orleans undt letzlich zu Padova, Bononia"; Universitetsbibliotek Uppsala: Waller Collection, Waller Ms de-00248, 1r–2v: letter of application by Petrus Scipio, Würzburg, 26.12.1584.

26 See Vivian Nutton, "Medicine at the German Universities 1348–1500," *Würzburger Medizinhistorische Mitteilungen*, 16 (1997): 173–90, p. 179.

27 Nutton, "Medicine," p. 178.

28 Staatsarchiv Oldenburg, Best. 20–7, 446: letter of application by Wilhelm Günther Brügge [Zerbst], 23.3.1694.

29 Institut für Stadtgeschichte Frankfurt (Main), Sanitätsamt: Akten des Rats (Medicinalia) 138: letter of application by Eucharius Rößlin d.J., Frankfurt (Main), 11.2.1528.

30 "Non est mihi dubium, quin Ampliss[imus] Senatus non exspectabit in me inanem titulum, nihilominus tamen, ubi rediero, ex patria testimonium scholae philosophicae Marpurgensis et studii medici iudicium de me perlegendum exhibebo, atq[ue] operam dabo, quo magis me conversatio et vita quam litterae commendent": Kirchenbibliothek St. Katharinen Salzwedel, Ms. Elias Hoppe: Soltquellensien, vol. 2, p. 264: Christopherus Germanus to Jacobus Praetorius, n.p., 30.6.1567 (transcription by the Salzwedel city archives).

31 One applicant referred to his service to the Duke of Saxony-Lauenburg as a physician to the princely army: Institut für Stadtgeschichte Frankfurt (Main), Ratssupplikationen 1.686, pp. 63 and 65: letter of application by Johann Jakob Rasor, Frankfurt (Main), 20. 4.1686; another listed his services to three bishops and the local cathedral chapter: Stadtarchiv Augsburg, Reichsstadt, Rat, Deputatio ad Collegium Medicum und die Apothekerordnung, CM VIII 96: letter of application by Andreas Bischof, Augsburg, 25.8.1649. Besides members of the princely houses and the Church, various members of the lower nobility or "noblemen" of the town are also named.

32 By stressing that he had gathered experience while working in different hospitals during his medical travels abroad (*DurchReisung frembder Länder*), Johann Sparr reveals that he considered his *peregrinatio academica* worth mentioning, but useful only as an argument if combined with information on his practical work: Institut für Stadtgeschichte Frankfurt (Main), Ratssupplikationen 1.686, Bl. 63–64: letter of application by Johann Caspar Sparr, n.p., 20. 4.1686.

33 See, for example, the letter of application by Georg Abraham Mercklin, who offered such testimony from his hometown, Weisheim: Stadtarchiv Weißenburg (Bayern) 7243, Weißenburg, 13.7.1640.

34 Fondo Faber, Biblioteca dell'Accademia dei Lincei e Corsiniana, Rome, Vol. 420, fol. 471; see Silvia De Renzi, "Medical Competence, Anatomy and the Polity in Seventeenth-Century Rome," *Renaissance Studies*, 21/4 (2007): 551–67, p. 563. I thank the author very much for sending me her transcription of the original text of this testimony and the following one.

35 See ASR, S. Spirito, Atti di Decreti e Spedizioni, busta 130, anni 1606–1614.

36 See the quotation from Mary Lindemann cited in the conclusion of this article.

37 On *ratio* and *experientia* as criteria for reliable knowledge in the sixteenth and seventeenth centuries, see Michael Stolberg, "Formen und Strategien der Autorisierung in der frühneuzeitlichen Medizin," in Wulf Oesterreicher, Gerhard Regn and Winfried Schulze (eds), *Autorität der Form – Autorisierungen – institutionelle Autorität* (Münster, 2003): 205–18, pp. 207–08. On the interdependency between everyday practice and the development of certain genres of medical writing, see Gianna Pomata, "Sharing Cases: The *Observationes* in Early Modern Medicine," *Early Science and Medicine*, 15 (2010): 193–236, pp. 208–09.

38 Stadtarchiv Augsburg, Reichsstadt, Rat, Deputatio ad Collegium Medicum und die Apothekerordnung: CM VIII 63: letter of application by Philipp Höchstetter, Augsburg [9.12.1627].

39 Cities often hired more than one physician and split their duties. Frankfurt on the Main, for example, had four town physicians: a *physicus primarius*, two subordinate *physici ordinarii*, and one *physicus extraordinarius* for paperwork only: see Bauer, "stede arzt," p. 17; see also Annemarie Kinzelbach, "Heilkundige und Gesellschaft in der frühneuzeitlichen Reichsstadt Überlingen," *Medizin, Geschichte und Gesellschaft*, 8 (1989): 119–49, p. 136.

40 See below. Especially in Augsburg, an Imperial city with a sophisticated health care system, applicants often tried to be promoted from lower civic medical offices such as physician to a pox house (*Blatterhaus*) or infirmary (*Brechenhaus*) to the higher post of regular town physician. On the often confusing variety in name and structure of such institutions in German towns and cities, see Annemarie Kinzelbach, "Hospitals, Medicine, and Society: Southern German Imperial Towns in the Sixteenth Century," *Renaissance Studies*, 15/2 (2001): 217–28, p. 219.

41 One applying physicians described his former involvement in the *Sondersiechenschau* in another town (*anderer orten*) as an *officium*: Stadtarchiv Augsburg, Reichsstadt, Rat, Deputatio ad Collegium Medicum und die Apothekerordnung: CM VIII 45: letter of application by Maximilian Merman, Augsburg, 18.5.1621. On the *Sondersiechenschau*, an examination for leprosy, see Fritz Dross, "Vom zuverlässigen Urteilen: Ärztliche Autorität, reichsstädtische Ordnung und der Verlust 'armer Glieder Christi' in der Nürnberger Sondersiechenschau," in *Medizin, Geschichte und Gesellschaft*, 29 (2010): 9–46. On examinations performed by the medical officers of Nördlingen, see Kinzelbach, "Negotiating on Paper," Chapter 6 of this volume.

42 Institut für Stadtgeschichte Frankfurt (Main), Ratssupplikationen 1.688, vol. I, pp. 275–76: letter of application by Johannes Hieronymus Niemand [Frankfurt (Main)], 20.11.1688.

43 On referring to former services as a typical line of argument, see Stanislaw-Kemenah, "Anspruch," pp. 85, 91; Ulbricht, "Supplikationen," p. 151.

44 On the preference for sons of well-established families, see Werner Piechocki, "Die Anfänge des halleschen Stadtphysikats," *Acta Historica Leopoldina*, 2 (1965): 5–28, p. 8 on the example of Halle. Patscheider suggests that the sons of local physicians were preferred because they were assumed to have a better knowledge of citizens' health: see Hubert Patscheider, "Die Stadtärzte im alten St. Gallen," *Schriften des Vereins für Geschichte des Bodensees und seiner Umgebung*, 115 (1997): 89–132, p. 131.

45 Stadtarchiv Augsburg, Reichsstadt, Rat, Deputatio ad Collegium Medicum und die Apothekerordnung: CM VIII 25: letter to the *Stadtpfleger* and the privy council by Karl Widemann, concerning the application of his son Marcus, Augsburg, 22.2.1614; see also note 51.

46　Stadtarchiv Augsburg, Reichsstadt, Rat, Deputatio ad Collegium Medicum und die Apothekerordnung: CM V 8 (1): letter of application by Georg Henisch, Augsburg, 23.7.1596.

47　Johann Ulrich Rumler claimed he had faced mortal danger: "bey jungst sterble-uffen, aus damals eingerissener unordnung, auch nit wenig Gefahr erstanden": Stadtarchiv Augsburg, Reichsstadt, Rat, Deputatio ad Collegium Medicum und die Apothekerordnung: CM V 10: letter of application by Johann Ulrich Rumler, Augsburg, 27.11.1597.

48　Institut für Stadtgeschichte Frankfurt (Main), Ratssupplikationen 1.674, Bl. 2–3: letter of application by Johann Christoph Steeb, Frankfurt (Main), 8. 1.1674.

49　Archives de la Ville et de la Communauté Urbaine de Strasbourg, VI, 368, 6: letter of application by Wendelinus Hock von Brackenau, n.p., 19.3.1516: "wo got der almechdig sin besündare hilff und genod mir gebe, wer unmüglich miar semlich geschmack: vergift luft, odar arbayt [zu] liden, als sich auch in kurzar zyt hat beschwer, das mich der geschmack des spitals in dotliche krankhayt bracht hat."

50　This applies as well to supplications for a place in a hospital: see Stanislaw-Kemenah, "Anspruch," p. 90.

51　Stadtarchiv Augsburg, StadtAA, Reichsstadt, Rat, Deputatio ad Collegium Medicum und die Apothekerordnung: CM VIII 46: letter to the *Stadtpfleger* and the privy council by Karl Widemann, concerning the application of his son Marcus, Augsburg, 22.5.1621: "uff begebenden weitteren fall seiner vor alle ander eingedenck zu sein"; on the use of verbatim quotations in the letters of supplications, see Stanislaw-Kemenah, "Anspruch," p. 91.

52　Institut für Stadtgeschichte Frankfurt (Main), Ratssupplikationen 1.688, Bd. I, pp. 281–82: letter of application by Conrad Hieronymus Eberhardt, Frankfurt (Main), 20.11.1688. Another typical example is the plea of Jeremias Erhard: "mich als ein hiesig bürgerskind und under den unbedienten in Medico nostro collegio ex senioribus vor anderen competitorn [...] zue bedenken": Stadtarchiv Augsburg, Reichsstadt, St. Martinsstiftung, Nr. 50 (7): letter of application by Jeremias Erhard, Augsburg, 6.4.1623.

53　Stadtarchiv Augsburg, StadtAA, Reichsstadt, Rat, Deputatio ad Collegium Medicum und die Apothekerordnung: CM VIII 62: letter of application by Marcus Banzer [December 1627]: "obwohlen dieser zeit als ich hier bin, zu unterscheidlichen mhalen vacierende stellen sich begeben, bin ich doch allzeit biß dato übergangen worden."

54　Stadtarchiv Lindau, A III: 49/6: letter of application by Johann Peter Oeler, Lindau, 7.12.1686.

55　The more rival towns one named, the better, as can be seen in the letter of the physician Allmacher: Institut für Stadtgeschichte Frankfurt (Main), Ratssupplikationen 1.686, 66–8: letter of application by Johann Friedrich Allmacher, n. p., 20.04.1686.

56　Institut für Stadtgeschichte Frankfurt (Main), Ratssupplikationen 1.655, Bd. I, 139–40: letter of application by Johann Ludwig Witzel, Frankfurt (Main), 15.5.1655.

57　Eucharius Rößlin confidently reported that he visited Frankfurt only on request of his patients but would be willing to stay if he were offered civic office: Institut für Stadtgeschichte Frankfurt (Main), Sanitätsamt: Akten des Rats (Medicinalia) 125: letter of application by Eucharius Rösslin, n.p., 7.5.1517; see also Karl Baas, "Eucharius Rösslins Lebensgang," *Archiv für Geschichte der Medizin*, 1 (1908): 429–41, p. 436; Oswald Feis, "Unbekannte Briefe von Eucharius Rößlin (Vater und Sohn)," *Sudhoffs Archiv*, 22 (1929): 102–04, p. 103.

58 Stadtarchiv Augsburg, Reichsstadt, Rat, Deputatio ad Collegium Medicum und die Apothekerordnung: CM XIX 78: letter of application by Jeremias Kneulin, Augsburg, 29.8.1628: "dass kein Mangel noch Klag sich befinden solle."

59 Karl Wideman stressed that he lived in the city center, where he could easily be found also at night, and that he never travelled: Stadtarchiv Augsburg, StadtAA, Reichsstadt, Rat, Deputatio ad Collegium Medicum und die Apothekerordnung: CM XIX 81: letter of application by Karl Wideman, Augsburg, s.d. On the obligation of being resident as a clause of the appointment contracts, see Martin Kintzinger, "Status Medicorum: Mediziner in der städtischen Gesellschaft des 14.–16. Jahrhunderts," in Peter Johanek (ed.), *Städtisches Gesundheits- und Fürsorgewesen vor 1800* (Cologne, 2000): 63–91, p. 73; on the town physicans' oath, see Dross, "'De Officiis'," Chapter 4 of this volume.

60 Typical phrasing: "Ich verspreche in solchen [!] ambte also mich zu verhaltten, damit denen Patienten ... ohne underschied so arm als reichen und zwar der armuth ohn endgeld undt bezahlung der müh noch der arzney ohnverdrossen auffwarthung und beyhülffe nach bester müglichkeit geleistet werde" – "I promise to behave in this office such that the patients ... will be given untiring attention and aid at [my] utmost capacity, without discriminating between the poor and the rich and, for those in poverty, without charge or fee for labor or remedies": Stadtarchiv Altenburg, VIIIb, 15, Nr. 2, 10r–11v: letter of application by Matthias Zacharias Pilling, Altenburg, 8.2.1669. On the physicians Pilling, see Gustav Wolf, "Matthias Zacharias Pilling und seine Söhne – eine fast vergessene Altenburger Arztfamilie," *Altenburger Geschichts- und Hauskalender*, 16 (2006): 143–49.

61 The physician Höchstetter combined this promise with the a promise not to cause complaints: Stadtarchiv Augsburg, StadtAA, Reichsstadt, Rat, Deputatio ad Collegium Medicum und die Apothekerordnung: CM XIX 52: letter of application by Philipp Höchstetter, Augsburg, 9.11.1609.

62 Several applicants argued that during epidemics the number of physicians was always too low: see for example, Stadtarchiv Augsburg, Reichsstadt, Rat, Deputatio ad Collegium Medicum und die Apothekerordnung: CM VIII 34: letter of application by Raymund Minderer, Augsburg, 20.8.1616.

63 See Dross, "'De Officiis,'" Chapter 4 of this volume; Pomata, "A Sense of Place," Chapter 8 of this volume.

64 See Lindemann, *Health*, p. 103, who states that "the questions of salary constituted the most frequent stumbling block to the appointment of the physicus."

65 Kirchenbibliothek St. Katharinen Salzwedel, Ms. Elias Hoppe: Soltquellensien, vol. 2, pp. 260–63: letter of application by Christopherus Germanus, n.p., 20.6.1567.

66 See note 30.

67 Stadtarchiv Esslingen, Bestand Reichsstadt, Faszikel 81, Nr. 48: letter of application by Hieronymus Henninger [Bern], 30.04.1532.

68 Stadtarchiv Altenburg, VIIIb, 15, Nr. 2, Bl. 10r–11v: letter of application by Matthias Zacharias Pilling; Altenburg, 8.2.1669: "ein arme wittibe undt viele meist noch ohnerzogene kinder als waisen, darneben ein weniges an mitteln hinderlaßen"/"ahnerbohtig, bemeldeder Ehlender undt hochst bedriebeder wittiben zum besten ahn der besoldung ein gantzes jahr aus eigener bewegniß freywillig zu überlaßen nichts minder jedoch dem Physikat und was dem anhengig mit hochstem unverdrossenen fleiß undt schuldiger observanz vorzustehen."

69 On the contract of appointment, see Wolf, "Pilling," p. 145.

70 See Lindemann, *Health*, pp. 79–80, on "pulling strings."

71 See the example of Hans Zehler: Stanislaw-Kemenah, "Anspruch," p. 91.

72 On this court practice of having men of rank speak as intermediators for the supplicant, see Koziol, *Begging*, pp. 70–76, esp. p. 70.

73 Universitätsbibliothek Würzburg, M.ch.f. 660/14, p. 510v: "und umb ein und anderer ursach wegen, sonderlich weilen Ihro derselbe von vornehmen herren specialiter recommendiret worden, und wie Sie vernehmen, der Zeit solche curam gethan, das an seiner experienz gute Hoffnung zu machen, mögen Sie gerne sehen, daß ihm das Stattphysicat zu gleich conferirt würde, das Sie zwar E.E. Rath das ius eligendi nit benehmen, oder dem alten herkommen und raths freyheiten was präiudiciern wollten, Sie wollten aber verhoffen, weilen dies das erste begehren sey, das Sie ahn E.E. Rath thäten, mann würde Ihro diesfalls nit zu widersetzen."

74 *Ibid.*; see Philipp Hoffmann-Rehnitz, "Discontinuities: Political Transformation, Media Change, and the City in the Holy Roman Empire from the Fifteenth to Seventeenth Centuries," in Jason Philipp Coy, Benjamin Marschke and David Warren Sabean (eds), *The Holy Roman Empire, Reconsidered* (New York and Oxford, 2010): 11–24, p. 16, 24; for the interweaving of oral and written parts within the appointments, see Dross, "'De Officiis'," Chapter 4 of this volume.

75 "ich an keinem andern Ort solches zu thun willens gewesen, dann eben an dem, do das Reine, Wahre undt Ungezweiffelte Gottes Wort seinen gang hatt, undt die heilige Sacramenta nach unseres lieben herrn Jesu Christi einsatzung gerichtet und genossen werden": see note 25 above.

76 One physician combined the arguments "influential aquaintances," "rivalry among competitors," and "right faith" cleverly by reporting that he had been offered positions by the Archbishop of Salzburg, the Bishop of Bamberg, and the Provost of Ellwangen but had declined all of these because of his religion: Stadtarchiv Weißenburg (Bayern), 1050: letter of application by Nicolaus Eberhard Winckler, Feuchtwangen, 5.11.1612.

77 Universitätsbibliothek Würzburg, M. ch. f. 660/14, 77r–v: letter from the burgomaster and the council of Kitzingen to Johannes Posthius, Kitzingen, 28.4.1577.

78 Germanisches Nationalmuseum Nürnberg: Historisches Archiv, Papierurkunden 1560 Juli 8: letter of application by Laurentius Phronto, Kitzingen, 8.7.1560.

79 Stadtarchiv Augsburg, Reichsstadt, Rat, Deputatio ad Collegium Medicum und die Apothekerordnung: CM II 5: letter of application by Johannes Henisius, n.p., 1649: "were die paritet sowol ratione personarum als salarii lobwürdig erhalten."

80 Stadtarchiv Lindau, A III: 49/6: letter of application by Johann Ulrich Oeler, Lindau, 7.12.1686.

81 Stadtarchiv Worms, Abt. 1B (Reichsstädtisches Archiv), Mappe 1, Bl. 9–10: letter of application by Johann Friedrich Graff, n.p., c. 1704.

82 Stadtarchiv Augsburg, Reichsstadt, Rat, Deputatio ad Collegium Medicum und die Apothekerordnung: CM IV 24: letter of application by Bernhard Schludin, Augsburg, before 30.10.1546: "reichen und arme[n] min vermugliche[n] vleyß mittgetailt, als umb zimliche[n] lon als och umb sunst, dermaßen als das ich ob schon gleich wol vil krancke hab gehabt, doch merren thail arme[n] den reichem [!]."

83 Stadtarchiv Augsburg, Reichsstadt, Rat, Deputatio ad Collegium Medicum und die Apothekerordnung: CM III 5: letter of application by Georg Lauber, Augsburg, 19.12.1595.

84 Stadtarchiv Augsburg, Reichsstadt, St. Martinsstiftung, Nr. 50 (8): letter of application Ulrich Kieffer, Augsburg, 26.11.1630.

85 See Philipp Klaas, Hubert Steinke and Alois Unterkircher, "Daily Business: The Organisation and Finances of Doctors' Practices," in Martin Dinges et al. (eds), *Medical Practice, 1600–1900: Physicians and Their Patients* (Leiden, 2016).

86 See Stanislaw-Kemenah, "Anspruch," p. 82.

87 See Lindemann, *Health*, p. 75; I extend Lindemann's observation back to the the mid sixteenth century.

88 Today Johannes Posthius is better known as a Neo-Latin poet; some town physicians became personal physicians to higher clergy or nobility.

89 See Di Giammatteo and Mendelsohn, "Reporting for Action," Chapter 5 of this volume. Writing certainly came to the fore of official communication in the sixteenth century, which was when cities and towns established the *Physikat*.

90 See Hoffmann-Rehnitz, "Discontinuities," p. 24.

91 See Alexander Schlaak, "Overloaded Interaction: Writing in German Imperial Cities, 1500–1800," in Jason Philipp Coy, Benjamin Marschke and David Warren Sabean (eds), *The Holy Roman Empire, Reconsidered* (New York and Oxford, 2010): 35–47, pp. 17–18.

92 See note 16 above.

93 The record of this meeting highlights an irregularity in this procedure: Staatsarchiv Hamburg, Best. 111–1, Cl. VII, Lit. Mb, Nr. 1, Vol. 1a1, Fasz. 1, Extractus protocollorum: 1660, fol. 307: "Dr. Garmers clara voce zum Sub-Physico erwehlet, doch ohne praejudicio der gewohnten Wahl per schedulas."

94 See Robert Schaper, "Arzt und Apotheker – Das Physikat in Helmstedt," *Aus der Heimat – für die Heimat*, Supplement to *Helmstedter Kreisblatt*, 10 September 1966 (unpag.). Discussions like this one may not have been different in the sixteenth and seventeenth centuries. For the exact wording of the following in German, see *ibid.*; see also Lindemann, *Health*, pp. 95–107.

95 Given that Siegesbeck held only the degree of a *licentiatus*, these "treatises" probably are not learned medical publications, but the typical short manuals on the handling of plague, bloody flux, and so on that town physicians were obliged to provide.

96 See Schaper, "Arzt und Apotheker."

4 De officiis

Doctors' Oaths and Appointments in Early Modern Nuremberg

Fritz Dross

When, in December 1459, Sebastian Mulner was appointed a Nuremberg town physician, the municipal authorities issued a short decree stating that his appointment should stand for five years, that he would receive 100 florins per year paid quarterly, and that he must not refuse to serve the burghers of the city when requested.[1] The decree ended by stating that Mulner had sworn the physicians' oath exactly as it was written on page nine of the official "book of the city." This short notice provides insight into what it meant to be a physician in an urban polity and, vice versa, how such polities looked after their health. There was nothing exceptional in Mulner's appointment. *Every* physician in early modern Nuremberg had to be officially appointed—and in this elaborate and precisely specified way, with its mix of oral and written forms of authentication. To be a physician in Nuremberg was also to be a physician of and for Nuremberg.

This chapter thus provides one in-depth answer to the question "town physician or physician in a town?"[2] More than previous studies in this area, I take the perspective of urban administration and its paperwork. Complementing the analysis of physicians' letters of application by Sabine Schlegelmilch in this volume, this chapter focuses on the oral and written process of the appointments that those applications aimed to secure. Town physicians' oaths and contracts show both the procedure of obligation and the obligations themselves, such as holding or assessing examinations and awarding certificates.[3] How did early modern urban authorities obligate physicians? What did urban councils and administrations expect physicians to do? These questions have a wider historiographical context. Relations between physicians and patients in late medieval and early modern Europe could be highly contractual and subject to juridical procedure, as we know from Gianna Pomata's work on "contracting a cure" in Bologna.[4] Refocusing from physician–patient relations to those between physicians and urban authorities, what did "contracting a doctor" mean? Pomata showed slow erosion of what constituted a fair patient–physician relationship and its proper regulation. How, I ask, did the polity–physician relationship change over time?

DOI: 10.4324/9781315554693-6

Answering these questions entails analyzing appointment procedures. My opening example of Sebastian Mulner in Nuremberg shows an appointment procedure that mixed oral and written forms of authentication: at the center of the appointment procedure we find the oath that had to be sworn but which became valid only by an official decree stating that it had been sworn, as well as naming the exact source of the oath's precise text. Certainly by 1459 the oath itself had already become a written tradition; only the procedure of swearing remained an oral practice, which, at the same time, needed to be confirmed by a written decree. Since medieval times, the entitlement to practice healing in Nuremberg required swearing an oath as well as signing an appointment contract—which at the least means that sixteenth-century doctors should by no means be regarded as constituting a liberal profession. Consequently, a first step is devoted to the Nuremberg physicians' oath and swearing, which continued to be at the core of the relationship between the town and its physicians. In a second step, I will look at appointment contracts that individualized and enhanced the concept of one general oath to be sworn by every doctor permitted to practice in Nuremberg. How was the collective practice of swearing amended (but definitely not replaced) by individually contracting the doctors? In the third part of this chapter, I will show that in the late sixteenth century doctors attempted to turn around their subjection to the authorities by claiming their superiority in affairs of health, which eventually meant subjecting the urban administration to the physicians' professional concerns. Why, when, and how did the Nuremberg physicians aim to develop their official role by promoting the establishment of an institution like the Collegium Medicorum? How did the doctors conceptualize their collective relationship to the municipal administration?

This analysis concentrates on the Imperial City of Nuremberg in the sixteenth and seventeenth centuries. The (Free and) Imperial Cities within the Holy Roman Empire acted as Imperial States, and their authorities thus held a juridical status comparable to that of the territorial princes. In historiography, they are considered to have developed the early forms of bureaucratic administration in the German territories since the sixteenth century.[5] Nuremberg had gained special importance since the fourteenth century and is known for being one of the centers of the German Renaissance in the fifteenth and sixteenth centuries. Around 1500, Nuremberg was inhabited by about 30,000 people *intra muros* and, together with Augsburg, was the second largest city of the Holy Roman Empire after Cologne.[6] At the same time, Nuremberg possessed a huge domain, which, beyond urban administration in the narrow sense, means that the urban authorities and their administration were effectively in charge of ruling this territory.

Regarding the sources, this article analyses the administrative paperwork of the sixteenth-century Nuremberg authorities and suggests that, in the mid-fifteenth century, municipal administration in German Imperial cities modernized and established bureaucratic procedures by issuing and keeping records of their administrative practices—instead of just documenting their legal outcome by issuing charters. Studying the collections of official oaths of the urban officeholders as well as the small annual booklets recording who had sworn the oaths and contrasting this survey by an analysis of several individual appointment contracts, I hope to paint a differentiated and subtle picture of what "town physician" meant.

Swearing the Physicians' Oath

Whenever a physician was allowed to practice in Nuremberg for a period of several years, he had to swear the official oath and be admitted as a sworn town physician.[7] The Nuremberg physicians' oath goes back at least to the mid-fourteenth century[8] and was expanded in the sixteenth.[9] The physicians' oath was nothing special in Nuremberg's personnel administration. Annually swearing an oath was demanded of every officeholder, beginning with the councilors themselves, dozens of scribes and registrars, and ultimately amounting to more than 100 oaths of office or of fulfilling special functions for the authorities. The Nuremberg City Archive holds 16 huge volumes containing oaths sworn by members of professional guilds whose duties to the authorities were thus fixed explicitly; several more such volumes are preserved in the Nuremberg State Archive.[10] In contrast with the oaths of healing professionals, oaths sworn by persons responsible for security, criminal justice, and criminal prosecution, for example, have been analyzed much more comprehensively for Nuremberg and other cities.[11] Generally, in-depth study of officeholders remains a desideratum for cultural history of early modern urban administration, at least regarding the German territories.[12] Nuremberg doctors' oaths had nothing to do with the Hippocratic Oath (which is not even mentioned in my sources), as they did not confirm a professional ethic but instead were clearly aimed at controlling the physicians and securing the *personal* responsibility of each doctor to the authorities.[13] Finally, being accepted and sworn as a learned town physician did not mean that either the authorities or other healing practitioners accepted doctors as a superior profession, as Annemarie Kinzelbach demonstrates in Chapter 6 of this volume.[14] In short, using the case of Nuremberg to look closely at physicians' oaths alerts us to ways in which it may be entirely misleading to consider early modern doctors as comprising a liberal profession.

What exactly did Nuremberg physicians swear to do? In its sixteenth- and seventeenth-century form,[15] the oath obliged doctors

1 to be willing to take care of every individual living legally in the city and
2 to charge moderate prices. These are no more than standard stipulations meant to legitimate the rule of authorities over their subjects. The oath

becomes more precise as it moves on to the relation between physicians and apothecaries. The doctors had to swear

3 to order remedies only from the city's legally admitted apothecaries and

4 not to favor one apothecary over another or to negotiate special contracts.

5 If a doctor received a special license to prepare and sell drugs, he had to use the weights prescribed for the apothecaries.

6 If a sick person called two, three, or more doctors, the physicians were obliged to visit the patient together as well as to deliberate and arrive at an agreement concerning the prescription in a cordial manner.

Finally, several phrases state the ways in which physicians had to be at the authorities' disposal:

7 When requested by the authorities, the physicians had to inspect pharmacies and evaluate their stores of medicines and medical ingredients.

8 In the Holy Week before Easter, they had to serve in an extensive annual inspection for leprosy ("Sondersiechenalmosen").

9 Above all, physicians were forbidden to leave town overnight and to accept foreign clients (that is, non-Nuremberg patients) without permission from the authorities.

10 Physicians were obliged to remain in town during epidemics or times of plague. The seventeenth-century version of the oath added that

10a physicians had to notify the authorities if they suspected a person of being infected.[16]

11 Finally, doctors had to swear to pay their taxes (*gemeine losung*).

Trying to understand the rationale for these duties, one could wonder how swearing to pay taxes could be part of the city's efforts in health care provision. Equally instructive is what the oath lacks from our perspective. It does not mention hospitals and their maintenance, organization of medical care, or access to it for the poor and ill. Omissions could, on the other hand, be covered elsewhere: behavior in times of pestilence is ignored in the oath (beyond the rule to stay in town and, later, to report suspected cases) but treated in detail by special ordinances (*Sterbsordungen*) in the sixteenth century and thereafter. Finally, the oath does not include points we would expect from a more specifically medical ethic—how to behave toward patients, their families, and one's peers in cases of uncertain diagnosis or prognosis, and so on.

Yet these are all clues on how to understand the oath in the terms of its time and place. Taking the perspective of early modern municipal administration, the physicians' oath can be regarded as belonging to trade policy and regulation (*Gewerbepolizei*). The oath's instructions concerning doctors' behavior among themselves are much the same as the well-known instructions concerning craft guilds, which aimed at preventing rivalry and competition.[17]

From the authorities' point of view and in terms of the administrative logic of sixteenth-century Nuremberg, the duties and rules listed in the physicians' oath follow the rationale of policing trade and commerce in an early modern urban "republic." Far from an element of health care policy, the physicians' oath regulated a professional group that, unlike the barber-surgeons and the apothecaries, was not constituted as a corporation or guild.

The picture becomes more intriguing if we compare the Nuremberg physicians' oath to oaths sworn by members of the other healer and body-care groups. Nuremberg's midwives swore an oath,[18] as did the "Honorable Women" ("Ehrbare Frauen")[19] who aided the midwives at births. The midwives' oath dates from 1562 and was expanded in 1579, 1660, 1682, and 1704. In the eyes of the Nuremberg authorities, midwifery was the most delicate health-related business to manage, necessitating the most comprehensive of all of the oaths examined here. Turning to pharmacy, we find an apothecaries' oath,[20] which was old enough to have already been expanded in 1555; a journeymen's oath[21]; and a separate oath for journeymen in the hospital.[22] Nuremberg had three different oaths for its barber-surgeons. First, the oath of the "sworn masters"[23] was taken by the three masters of the "Barbiere" (Barbers) and the three masters of the "Bader" (Bathers), which were separate but collectively governed guilds with overlapping functions. Second, there was the oath taken by all *Barbiere* and *Bader* as healers ("Aller Wundttärtzt Ayd"—*Wundarzt*, literally "wound healer," usually translated as "barber-surgeon" in English),[24] and finally there was an oath for the barber-surgeons of the city hospital.[25] The six masters were in charge of examining candidates for membership in the guilds and for admitting those who passed. These new members then had to be presented to the authorities, as was the case for all other Nuremberg guilds.[26] Thus, in effect, the masters were responsible for ensuring that no barber-surgeon practiced in town without permission. This was a responsibility to the authorities. Furthermore, the six barber-surgeon masters were officially obliged to deliver their professional opinion when requested, especially on wounds. Like the physicians' oath, the oaths of the barber-surgeons as well as those of the apothecaries should be understood as part of trade regulation, defining the privileges and duties of different crafts and trades. Unlike the physicians, the barber-surgeons did not have to swear that they would pay their taxes: as members of guilds, they were already fully integrated into the corporatively organized world of early modern urban society.

The texts of these oaths and dozens of others are extant in two large and costly made volumes from the first half of the seventeenth century, called "Oath and Duty" books ("Eid- und Pflichtbücher"), spanning 330 folios and 570 folios respectively, and showing signs of wear.[27] (See Figure 4.1) The physicians' oath appears in the first volume, which covers the more powerful and eminent offices; oaths of the other health-related professions appear in the second volume. Another large volume, Nuremberg's Book of Offices ("Ämterbuch"), lists dozens of offices and

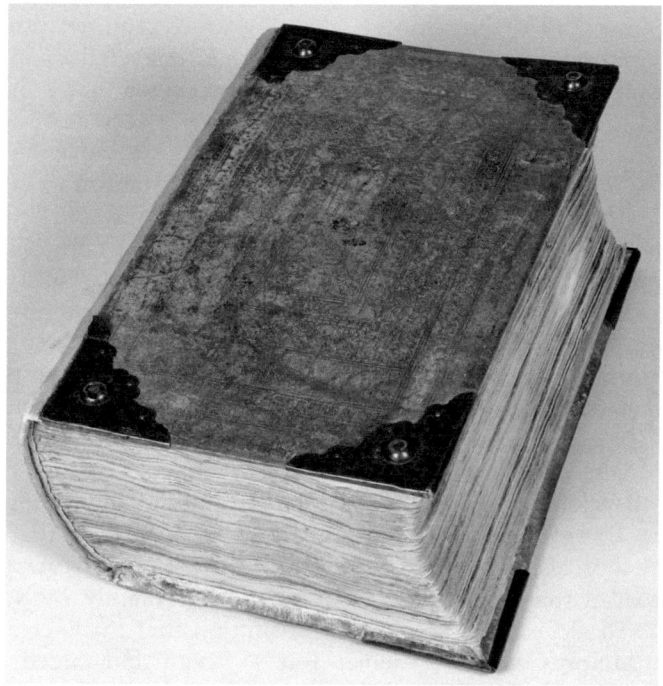

Figure 4.1 Volume II of the Oath and Duty Books of the Imperial City of Nuremberg, seventeenth century. Courtesy of Stadtarchiv Nürnberg: B 11 Eid-
und Pflichtbücher der Reichsstadt Nürnberg, No. 146.

their associated oaths from medieval times through the eighteenth
century.[28] This shows that swearing oaths remained an irreplaceable
ritual for offices both great and small. The page that starts the list of
the Nuremberg sworn physicians from 1475 to 1795, states that each of
the listed doctors was accepted by the Nuremberg authorities and had to
swear the oath every year, after the council's election at Easter, in the
town hall.[29]

Swearing oaths is an ancient oral practice. Yet the Nuremberg example
shows that, at least since the fifteenth century, oaths and their swearing
also comprised a complex of practices of reading and writing, which were,
moreover, bound up in the paper technology of public administration. Following recent historiography, this could be at least partly explained by the
idea that early modern legal acts had to be performed through some kind
of physical action, which would then be documented—and perhaps in
some sense further performed—on paper.[30] Let us see how extensive, elaborate, and precise this activity actually was.

When in 1553, for example, Heinrich Wolff became a sworn physician of the Imperial City of Nuremberg, the magistrate required three written decrees to confirm the procedure. The first one, delivered on August 30, states that Dr. Heinrich Wolff should be accepted as a Nuremberg physician and receive 100 florins per year; the second decree of September 7 states that the doctor was summoned by the authorities; and the third one of September 8 states that he had sworn the oath.[31] Returning to my opening example of Sebald Mulner, the decree concerning his civic appointment in 1459 states not only that he swore the physicians' oath, but that he swore the oath written down in a city register ("statbuch") on folio nine.[32] Notwithstanding that no contemporary reading or hearing the decree would have gone to the town hall to look in the *statbuch* to verify the words Sebastian Mulner had spoken when he swore the physicians' oath, and even though the decree was kept succinct, its writers found it important enough to refer to the official volume containing the oath and even to the folio number.

Though they had to be spoken, oaths were bound up with paperwork not only by being fixed in writing and decreed in writing that they had been sworn, but also through official recording of the swearing itself—a ritual procedure that, moreover, was carried out mainly by scribes and registrars.[33] The legislative year of the institution that made civic appointments, the Minor Council ("Kleiner Rat"), began and ended at Easter. Councilors were (re-)elected, and then every municipal officeholder had to renew his duty by swearing. These proceedings were both organized and recorded using a handy Booklet of Offices ("Ämterbüchlein"), still extant in a run from 1396 to 1806.[34] Compared to the large, expensively made volumes in which the oaths themselves were preserved in writing, these booklets belonged to routine paperwork of administration. Beginning in 1481, there was one for each year. The number of offices grew. In 1568, for example, the sworn physicians ("Geschworne Doctores der Arznei") appeared in position 104, after the officers competent in assessing coinage, out of 125 total offices; by 1588, the physicians had moved back to position 135 out of still more offices. Each new year's booklet listed the sworn officeholders, amended by adding names between or below the lines of the original list and by crossing out the names of those who left Nuremberg, annotated with symbols such as circles and crosses whose meaning is not yet clear. When in 1569 the Dutch physician and anatomist Volcher Coiter came to Nuremberg, the scribes added his name three times to the same list. (See Figure 4.2.) Adding new names either did not always happen attentively or had to be repeated for some reason (perhaps failure to attend). Either way, the handwriting shows that the new year's booklet was copied from the previous one at the end of the legislative period. Having this list when the swearing ceremony began after Easter, a scribe could mark off who attended, amending and notating as needed throughout the year.

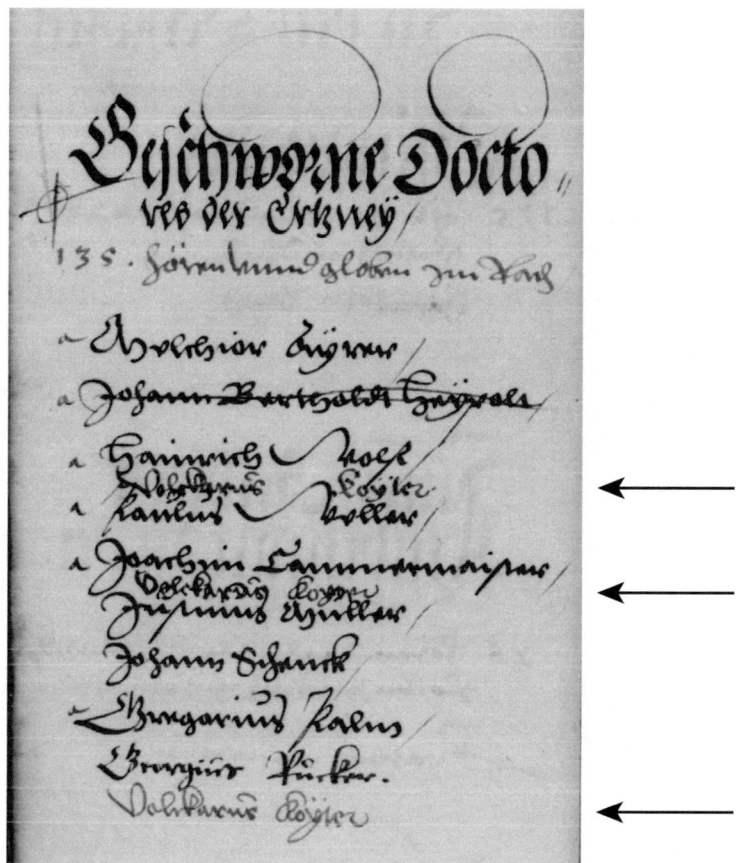

Figure 4.2 Booklet of Offices, Nuremberg, 1569: page for the Sworn Doctors of Medicine, showing Volcher Coiter listed thrice. Courtesy of Staatsarchiv Nürnberg: Rep. 62, Reichsstadt Nürnberg, Ämterbüchlein, No. 88 (1569): Geschworene Doctores der Artznei.

Booklets of Offices listed the sworn physicians, followed by two magistrates (not physicians!) in charge of overseeing drugs and raw materials in pharmacies, and then the midwives. (See Figure 4.3) The barber-surgeons do not appear; the apothecaries appear from the second half of the sixteenth century. Typically, these groups numbered nine sworn doctors, six apothecaries plus one in the hospital; 14 to 18 midwives in the city and two additional ones in the suburbs. In addition to the midwives, the booklets include lists of the "Sworn Women" in charge of supervising the midwives and the "Honorable Women" helping the midwives.[35]

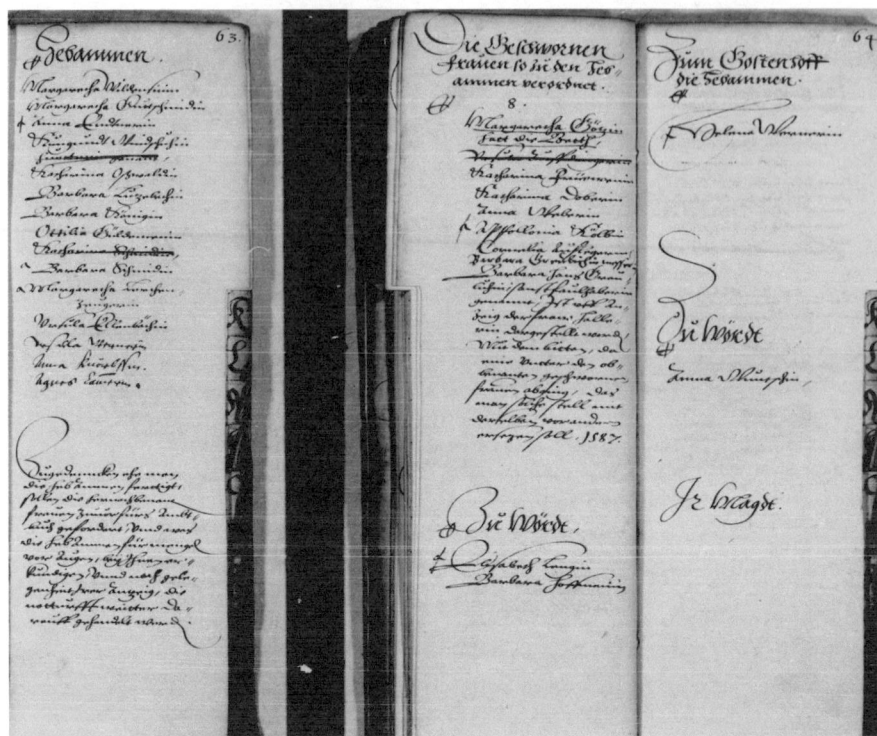

Figure 4.3 Booklet of Offices, Nuremberg, 1588: page for Midwives and for Sworn Women in charge of supervising the midwives. Courtesy of Staatsarchiv Nürnberg: Rep. 62, Reichsstadt Nürnberg, Ämterbüchlein, No. 107 (1588): Hebammen, Geschworne Frauen.

Beginning in the 1560s, these booklets recorded where and how the officeholders swore their oaths. They first had to "listen to their duty" ("die Pflicht hören") spoken aloud to them, and then they had to swear the oath aloud. Officers charged with assessing coinage[36] heard their duty in the chancellery and swore before the council.[37] The doctors' swearing ritual comprised both acts in the same place—in the town hall *coram consilio*.

Historians have elucidated the function of oaths in early modern social and political order.[38] Looking closely at practice in Nuremberg shows the written as well as oral dimension of this function. This combination makes sense if we regard swearing as a communicative practice of face-to-face society using different media: the oral ritual as well as the written paper.[39] Both lasted a long time together. On the one hand, the premodern performative ritual did not fade over time. When the jurist Veit Guggenberger published *Oath Book* in 1699,[40] two engravings at the start of the volume

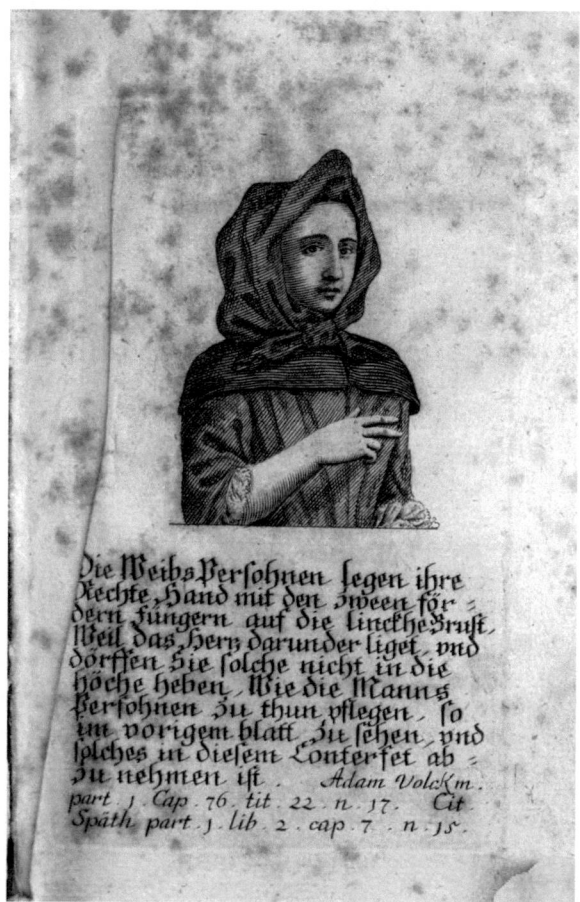

Figure 4.4 Illustration showing proper positioning of the hand and fingers for women in swearing oaths: Veyt Guggenberger, *Ayd Buech* (Munich, 1699). Courtesy of Bayerische Staatsbibliothek.

illustrated proper positioning of the hand and fingers when swearing: one position for men and one for women. (See Figure 4.4.) In the late eighteenth century, Krünitz's encyclopedia, which criticized some oaths as superfluous, still instructed how to move one's hand and fingers into proper position for swearing.[41] On the other hand, as we have seen, already in the fifteenth century in Nuremberg, oaths were valid only after an official decree had declared that an oath had been sworn, designating the volume and page where the written wording of the oath was to be found in the town hall. By the seventeenth century, the city's hundreds of oaths and ongoing record of their swearing had been brought together systematically into large books.

These were not necessarily closed to the public. Their location in the town hall was well known. In 1641, a Lutheran Pastor named Johann Sauber went into the town hall to negate having sworn to observe certain dogmatic rules of religious confession introduced by the city after the Reformation. He was not dismissed for this action.[42] The performative act of swearing could be renounced after the fact. How? By pen on paper. Sauber crossed out his name.

Contracting with the City

Beyond the oath, physicians were sometimes appointed in early modern Nuremberg by written contract with the city. These belonged to the tradition and institution of the charter. In the archive today, Nuremberg's chronological series of charters runs for 115 shelf meters.[43] Among these thousands of documents are 37 appointment contracts involving 21 medical practitioners between 1524 and 1625. Sixteen of these concern university-educated practitioners designated by their academic title of doctor. The oldest of these documents is in fact a termination of contract (of a barber-surgeon), suggesting that the extant series is fragmentary and that the practice of civic contracts with medical practitioners began earlier than 1524. To gain a more complete picture of the conditions of civic medical appointments, one would have to study the records of the "Losungsamt" (tax office), which include protocols of when, how, to whom, and for what reason the authorities promised remuneration. Still, had the physicians' oath and its decree (which stated remuneration) defined their relationships to the municipal administration entirely and in all cases, there would have been no need for contracts. Clearly the authorities deemed these necessary for at least some appointments to medical office. Why?

Hans Gaugenrieder's appointment as barber-surgeon ("Schneidarzt") was terminated in writing in September 1524.[44] As this is the oldest surviving medical contractual document in the Nuremberg charter series, we do not know whether the appointment had begun by contract. By 1526, Gaugenrieder had signed a new contract for appointment for eight years at 36 florins annually.[45] At the end of this time, in 1534 and again in 1545, his service continued under new contracts and higher salaries.[46] Gaugenrieder's son Ciriacus, appointed "Schneydartzt" in 1538, achieved such follow-up contracts and salary raises four times.[47] His son did the same, tripling his salary to 60 florins over the course of three contracts between 1567 and 1576. On the one hand, appointment contracts were clearly being used for changing remuneration, whereas the oath remained unchanged. On the other hand, the contracts did more, by almost literally repeating points from the physicians' oath, such as the promise to care for both the rich and the poor, the young and the old, and to charge patients moderately (when not treating them without charge within the framework of annual remuneration for service to the city).

Comparing such contracts with the names in the oath lists reveals that sworn town physicians could be appointed without contract and, more importantly, that doctors could be contracted without being listed as sworn town physicians.[48] This discrepancy shows change in what a "sworn physician" was. Every doctor allowed to practice in Nuremberg had to swear the physicians' oath. Yet the contracts show that not every doctor who had taken the oath thereby became a "sworn physician" of the city. And doctors with contracts who were not, however, listed as sworn physicians of the city were special cases, to which we now turn.

The most intricate of these were the cases of practitioners already under appointment of service to another polity. Ulrich von Anngelburg was a town physician of Munich, about 170 kilometers from Nuremberg, when he contracted with the Nuremberg authorities as a learned physician, surgeon, and oculist.[49] In Munich, he was under contract from 1548 to 1564. This position allowed for other appointments at the Munich authorities' discretion. They allowed Anngelburg to serve simultaneously as personal physician to Bavarian Duke Wilhelm IV, who resided in Munich. When the duke died in 1550, the Munich authorities allowed Anngelburg to sign with Nuremberg, which he did for four years at 50 florins annually. As he lived in Munich, Anngelburg's contract stipulated that he would travel to Nuremberg whenever the Nuremberg authorities ordered and the Munich authorities allowed. He promised to care for a horse in order to make the journey immediately upon request.[50]

This case suggests that the Nuremberg authorities engaged in head-hunting for medical practitioners renowned for special skills. The urban administration clearly felt able to offer extraordinary appointment conditions to those who met special requirements. Anngelburg was contracted for his expertise as an oculist, not for being a learned physician, and so did not have to be put at the city's constant disposition. Anngelburg's was one of several such cases. In 1575, the physician Anton Fuchs was contracted for a lifetime appointment, explicitly highlighting his expertise—"seiner kunst," literally "his art"—with respect to cancer and leprosy.[51] In 1564, physician and surgeon ("Leib- und Schneidarzt") Benedict Fröschel signed a contract with Nuremberg while under contract with another Imperial city, Augsburg.[52] His father, Benedict Fröschel the Elder, had been town physician in Augsburg since 1508 (without having been academically trained); the younger Fröschel, since 1537, from which he was allowed to travel to treat the Archbishop of Salzburg as well as the Bavarian duke, an exalted clientele that probably helped bring him to Nuremberg's attention. Signed in 1564, his contract with Nuremberg was, unlike most other such contracts, unlimited in duration and stated that he would serve there as a surgeon twice a year for one to four weeks.[53] As with Anngelburg, Fröschel also promised to care for a horse so that he could come as quickly as possible to Nuremberg when needed.[54] At 200 florins annually, Fröschel was well paid for attending only twice a year for a couple of weeks.[55] Unlike the oath, an appointment contract enabled both parties to make special arrangements for special purposes. When in 1553 Heinrich Wolff became a Nuremberg physician, the decree stipulated remuneration of 100 florins per annum but also a gift of 25 florins to assist him in becoming comfortably established.[56] The gift was to be kept secret.[57] Contract periods ranged from three years (six cases), four years (four cases), five years (five cases), to lifetime ("per integrum vitae meae curriculum"). Annual salaries ranged from 40 florins to 200 florins, paid two or four times a year. The four physicians who were contracted twice obtained better conditions with their second contract.[58]

As there was no contemporary label for municipal officeholders as a group, they were called "faithful servants" ("getreuwe diener")—from the lowest ranks of workmen ("Stadtknecht") to the highest judges and finance administrators.[59] Thus it should not surprise us that physicians' contracts include lengthy passages of subjection to the authorities, in language the doctors' matched in their letters of application.[60] All of the contracts gave the authorities the right of immediate termination at any time. Thus, it seems plausible that the authorities were also entitled to do the contrary, namely, to renew a contract without executing a new instrument. So, it is conceivable that Dr. Johannes Neudörffer simply stayed a town physician in Nuremberg after his three-year 1603 contract ended, before signing a new one in 1611. Contracts made doctors subject to the Nuremberg authorities and legal courts in the event of disagreement with Nuremberg burghers concerning fees. Usually they were obliged to live in the city, not to leave without permission, and to serve on military campaigns. Altogether, contracts bound physicians to the authorities and thus reflected the role of those authorities as representatives of both territorial power and sovereign autonomy within the empire. Their power was expressed in their capacity to make contracts tailored according to what they held to be the city's special needs and priorities.

Lack of rules for appointment contracts made them tools for expanding the scope and nature of publicly funded medical services, usually by attracting doctors from outside. Volcher Coiter from Groningen and Steffan Holtmann from Hamburg were lured with contracts that included exemption from taxation, apart from the "Ungeld," a special consumption tax.[61] The strategy of attracting physicians from elsewhere by offering tax exemptions can be found in other cities such as Frankfurt am Main.[62] Using appointment contracts to settle physicians in Nuremberg who were not, or did not become, burghers of the city entailed special arrangements with respect to juridical status, such as agreeing to be subject to the city's legislation and to accept the decisions of its council and courts. Not being obliged to become a burgher and enter completely into the political community of the city (which would have meant paying municipal taxes) could thus be regarded as a special privilege.[63] Accepting physicians without charging them municipal taxes and contracting surgeons who did not come to live in Nuremberg allowed the authorities to recruit experts who could not have been hired otherwise.

Lack of rules for appointment contracts also made them tools of negotiation by both sides. Some physicians signed contracts that excluded remuneration, such as Erasmus Flock in 1545 and Georg Palma in 1568.[64] More frequently, doctors showed success in improving their financial conditions through renewals. Melchior Ayrer, for example, was hired for three years at a rate of 40 florins per annum in 1549, which was extended for an additional three years in 1552. In 1555, he was contracted for six years for 52 florins, and this was extended for another six years. In 1567, he was dismissed.[65] Renewing a contract could also include expanding a physician's duties without changing his pay. When, in 1585, the authorities embarked on contracting a physician specially for times of pestilence, they began negotiations with three resident doctors already in the city's service and pay. Paul Weller claimed to be too feeble for the additional duties. Johann Schenk declined, citing the burden of his appointment as hospital physician and his assignment to the patients with the "French disease." Anton Fuchs agreed—under the condition that the authorities sign a special appointment securing him sufficient income ("damit er auskomme") and granting him a horse for reaching patients.[66] The authorities accepted Schenk's reasons for declining but declared that Weller's refusal was grounds for reconsidering the pay he already received. Contracting a doctor could play off one physician against another and entail negotiative gamble by the authorities and the physicians—at some risk to both.

Becoming Incorporated

What has been shown here is that the doctors of Nuremberg were not a collective, even though they all swore the same oath and had the same basic civic duties and constraints. Some were more successful, some less so, in cutting deals with the administration, and the contracts of the minority of practitioners who had them varied widely. Either way, the authorities did not negotiate or even communicate with the physicians as a group. In the corporatively organized world of an early modern urban republic, the doctors lacked a corporation of their own.

Oaths, contracts, and their own letters of application cast physicians as "faithful servants" of the Nuremberg authorities. In the late sixteenth century, the physicians began to reverse this obligation. The reverse idea that the authorities were responsible for the doctors came to the fore after 1571 in a physicians' initiative for a Collegium Medicum. The following focuses on the nature of this argument—in the context of oaths, contracts, and appointments as pictured in this chapter—rather than on the establishment of the Collegium in 1592 and its early history.[67]

On December 27, 1571, the Nuremberg physician and scholar Joachim Kammermeister, known as Camerarius the Younger , presented a memorandum on why and how to establish a Collegium Medicum. The medical arts, he lamented, were badly treated in his times.[68] Political and administrative confusion led many people to disdain doctors who were in fact kind-hearted, honest, and law-abiding. It was up to the authorities to change this situation for the good of all. Accordingly, the memorandum was dedicated to the Nuremberg authorities and began with a letter to the council praising them.[69] The next folio presents article 134 of the Holy Roman Empire's Constitutio Criminalis Carolina of 1532, which prescribed severe punishment of healers who caused death by their medical practice, especially those who practiced without proper medical education.[70] The memorandum continued in four main parts, on (1) the office of a physician ("Von dem ambt eines artzts"); (2) the office of an apothecary ("Vom ambt eines erfarnen apoteckers"); (3) surgeons, barbers, midwives and other healers; and (4) examination for leprosy and inspection of the municipal hospitals.

The first part begins by proposing a doctors' ethic. The son of one of the most famous classicists of sixteenth-century Germany, Camerarius had the erudition to do this from classical sources. Physicians had responsibility for their patients; yet more generally, as Camerarius emphasized with reference to Galen, the physician was supposed to be nature's servant and to help mankind preserve its health. It seems strange that Camerarius did not mention the Hippocratic Oath, which would have complemented his argument, but which was little used until later times, mainly as a rationale against outside regulation: physicians are bound by their own ethic and thus cannot submit to any other authority.[71] Camerarius was one of the first German physicians to stake out such a position. After his introductory letter praising the civic authorities, he ceases to refer to them, even when outlining doctors' duties. On the contrary, as the authorities were responsible for the health of their subjects, the learned Nuremberg doctor asserted they were also responsible for caring for their physicians. The memorandum and its proposed Collegium were a strategy for ending domination of doctors by cities' authorities and administrations: doctors, following their own ethic of service to others, did not need control but protection—against other healing trades (which lacked such an ethic) and against patients' misguided belief that they were best served by choosing whichever healer they wished. Camerarius thus proposed breaking with that which—since late medieval times—had been commonly considered the free and fair relationship between patients and healers. He thereby proposed reshaping health regulation around the primacy of the physician. Thus, the proposed Collegium Medicum would be in fact a Collegium Medicorum, a college of physicians with a collective professional role in the city.

The city deliberated on this for 20 years. In 1592, the Nuremberg authorities finally accepted Camerarius's proposal by enacting a medical constitution or comprehensive ordinance ("Medizinalordnung").[72] The title page bears the Nuremberg city arms and the motto "AEgrotorum salus svprema Lex esto." This echoed the logic of Camerarius's memorandum by recapitulating a major rule of the Hippocratic Oath.[73] As doctors exclusively served their patients' benefit (in the abstract, while concretely setting rules and norms of patient compliance with doctors), the authorities must serve the doctors and not vice versa. Nevertheless, the new, professional logic accommodated the old civic one: swearing the civic oath is mentioned prominently where the ordinance states that every physician who was licensed to practice in the city and who swore the physicians' oath every year would be made a member of the Collegium.[74] Further along in the text, however, the ordinance extends Collegium membership to physicians who had finished their academic training and been allowed to practice—without mentioning any additional obligation toward the authorities. Moreover, the Collegium was also comprised of the medical professors at Nuremberg's university in nearby Altdorf, who were not sworn town physicians of Nuremberg. Apothecaries, surgeons, barbers, and midwives were obliged to be examined by the Collegium. The "Medizinalordnung" forbade any other inhabitant from practicing as a healer or hosting any such person, imposing a penalty for this of 10 florins. The authorities nonetheless reserved the right to entitle any person they wanted to practice as a special healer in certain situations—as we know they had long been doing through special contracts. Whereas the physicians' oath specified only that they treat rich and poor and charge accordingly, the "Medizinalordnung" fixed a flat rate: 1 florin for the first visit and a quarter of this sum (1 Orth) for every further visit. This effectively removed the doctors' burden of having to "contract a cure" with patients and removed the safeguards of such contracts for patients. Special higher prices would have to be paid, especially by the wealthy, in times of pestilence and serious epidemics.[75] Collegium members, on the other hand, were not allowed to evade a call to session, even in times of plague.[76] In short, the medical ordinance of 1592 and the Collegium it established provided the rules and institutions for turning the physicians of Nuremberg into a professional body, analogous to the corporations and guilds of trades and crafts.

Conclusion

The initial question of "town physician or physician in a town?" has been answered: both. At least in Nuremberg. Often the same person was both. Oral and written forms and forces of community—oaths, contracts—pulled in both directions. And, finally, both were subsumed in a shift over time toward collectivity through incorporation.

On the one hand, the annual oath of the town physician is overwhelmingly significant. Its specified duties comprised no public health program yet defined physicians and their activities as public benefit under public regulation. The oath connected every doctor to the authorities and did so in the same way: as a sworn town physician in its service. On the other hand, the contracts differentiated doctors into unrelated physicians in a town—differently specialized, differently salaried for different periods, some with special functions, and so on. Yet, at the same time, these strongly differentiating contracts were all city contracts of service to the citizens and inhabitants. Oaths unified, contracts differentiated (and unified because they were all with the city and for serving it), pulling physicians in contrary directions and in one direction at the same time. In these manifold ways, as we can now see, the city was a complex medical polis and not just an urban medical marketplace.

Already as applicants to cities and towns, physicians were diverse in academic training and practical experience, social and economic background, and confessional affiliation, as their letters of application and their contracts show.[77] Once appointed, their function as sworn physician and urban officeholder remained only part of their working lives. Neither oath nor contract defined a position and a salary commensurate with a physician's whole livelihood; his economic existence had to remain differentiated and multisided.[78] And, finally, there was a tension in being a town physician. At bottom, an early modern urban republic can be understood as the confraternity of all who swore its oath. The annual ritual performance of swearing produced community. Yet physicians had a strong continuing outside affiliation, which many of them practiced in writing all the time. Being part of the learned world, the wider Latin community of the universities (from which their qualifications came) and the *res publica litterarium*, physicians could not easily or fully be integrated into the early modern municipal community. To appoint a doctor as a sworn town physician was to bring together two spheres of the early modern world: (1) that of scholarship and the early modern academic and scientific community, and (2) that of the rise of the modern administrative polity in its early urban form, which, moreover, was arranged as much as possible according to corporations—which the Nuremberg doctors were not until after 1592.

The Collegium Medicum established by Nuremberg's medical ordinance of 1592 acted as a Collegium Medicorum—a general assembly of the learned medical doctors. This made the physicians more like all the other corporative groups of which the city was in many ways composed. At the same time, however, in creating the Collegium, the city in effect accepted and institutionalized a reversal of obligation argued by the doctors led by Camerarius. Though individual doctors continued to swear obligation to the authorities, the authorities now obligated themselves to support the doctors. This can be understood as one beginning of a political process of authorization of university-educated physicians and thus of that which distinguished them from other healers: their universal academic knowledge.

If Nuremberg thus provides one important story of the creation and development of civic medicine, it was inconceivable without pen and paper and indeed specific forms of written record and written communication. Far from sparing themselves and their busy scribes the trouble, the authorities made innovative use and combination of existing forms of administrative and legal paperwork. By the mid-fifteenth century, Nuremberg's oaths were being written down in a register—the "city book." Hence swearing came to involve reading. The oaths became written tradition and were kept in impressive volumes that did not gather dust on the shelf but showed the signs of regular use. Writing and reading did not replace speaking but made it precisely repeatable. Though necessary, swearing aloud was insufficient, becoming a legally binding act only when confirmed by written decree. Moreover, the authorities began registering each annual act of swearing in lists in booklets that were carefully preserved in series for centuries and that came, by the 1560s, to include a brief protocol of the performance. Thus, in addition to its oral performance, the physician's bond to the community and his place in the polity came to be enacted, validated, and perpetuated by four kinds of paperwork: (1) the written oath, (2) the decree confirming it had been sworn, (3) the listing of those who had sworn, and (4) the swearing protocol. On top of all this came, in the sixteenth century, written contracts. These, in turn, were preserved and managed over time through the administrative paper technology of the municipal tax office in charge of paying the doctors. Finally, in 1593, the Nuremberg doctors' position in relation to the authorities and the municipal administration as well as within urban society generally became organized on a corporative basis and fixed on paper by a printed "Medizinalordnung," which still relied on the medieval oath.

Notes

Acknowledgments: I thank Andrew Mendelsohn for his patience and diligence in shaping this chapter.

1 Nicolas Damm, "Der Nürnberger Stadtarzt Sebald Mulner (†1495): Eine Biographische Skizze," *Mitteilungen des Vereins für die Geschichte der Stadt Nürnberg*, 88 (2001): 139–70, p. 151: "Zu wissen, daz doctor Sebolt Mullner ist bestelt worden, daz er der stat phisicus und artzt sein sol fünff jare die nehsten nacheinander volgende, und man gibt im yedes jars C gulden in landswerung an müncz, ungeverlich nemlich alle quatemper XXV guldin an müncz. Und er hat den burgern des diensts in derselben zeite nit abzusagen, sunder wenn er in nit füglich oder eben wer, so mugen sie im den dienste wol absagen, wenn sie wollen. Und er hat der ertzt aide gesworen, der im statbuch folio IX geschriben steet, und tritt mit seinem solarium an auff Invocavit schirst."

2 Ruth Schilling, Sabine Schlegelmilch, and Susan Splinter, "Stadtarzt oder Arzt in der Stadt? Drei Ärzte der Frühen Neuzeit und ihr Verständnis des städtischen Amtes," *Medizinhistorisches Journal*, 46 (2011): 99–132. "Town physician" in some cases meant no more than allowance to practice; in other cases, it meant the duty to fulfil specified tasks. On the German *Stadtarzt*, see Schlegelmilch, "Promoting a Good Physician," Chapter 3 of this volume; and Kinzelbach, "Negotiating on Paper," Chapter 6 of this volume. For town physicians in a context close to Nuremberg, see Annemarie Kinzelbach, "Heilkundige und Gesellschaft in der frühneuzeitlichen Reichsstadt Überlingen," *Medizin, Gesellschaft und Geschichte*, 8 (1989): 119–49.

3 See Kinzelbach, "Negotiating on Paper," Chapter 6 of this volume.

4 Gianna Pomata, *Contracting a Cure: Patients, Healers, and the Law in Early Modern Bologna* (Baltimore, 1998); see also Michael Stolberg, "Formen und Strategien der Autorisierung in der frühneuzeitlichen Medizin," in Wulf Oesterreicher (ed.), *Autorität der Form – Autorisierung – institutionelle Autorität* (Münster, 2003): 205–18.

5 Robert Brandt, "Reichsstadt," in Friedrich Jaeger (ed.), *Enzyklopädie der Neuzeit*, vol. 10: *Physiologie – Religiöses Epos* (Stuttgart, 2009): cols. 945–48.

6 Michael Diefenbacher, "Nürnberg, Reichsstadt: Politische und soziale Entwicklung," in *Historisches Lexikon Bayerns*, URL: www.historisches-lexikon-bayerns.de/artikel/artikel_45427 (consulted 2 February 2015); Rudolf Endres, "Zur Einwohnerzahl und Bevölkerungsstruktur Nürnbergs im 15./16. Jahrhundert," *Mitteilungen des Vereins für die Geschichte der Stadt Nürnberg*, 57 (1970): 242–71.

7 The contemporary terms in Nuremberg were "geschworne Leibärzte" or "bestelte Leibärzte."

8 Werner Schultheiß, *Satzungsbücher und Satzungen der Reichsstadt Nürnberg aus dem 14. Jahrhundert: Einleitung (1. Teil): Abdruck der Texte, Personen- und Ortsregister*, Nürnberger Rechtsquellen vol. 3 (Nürnberg, 1965); August Jegel, "Aus dem Altnürnberger Ärzteleben vor 1500," *Münchner medizinische Wochenschrift*, 81 (1934): 1091–93.

9 Stadtbibliothek Nürnberg (StadtBibN), Ms. Cent V 42, fols. 1r–2v, also published in: Klaus G. König, *Der Nürnberger Stadtarzt Dr. Georg Palma (1543–1591)* (Stuttgart, 1961); Universitätsbibliothek Erlangen (UBE), Ms. 1143, fols. 2r–3r.

10 Stadtarchiv Nürnberg (hereafter: StadtAN), B 11, Eid- und Pflichtbücher der Reichsstadt Nürnberg, Nos. 145–160; Staatsarchiv Nürnberg (hereafter: StaatsAN), Rep. 52b, Reichsstadt Nürnberg, Amts – und Standbücher, Nos. 100–106.

11 Andrea Bendlage, *Henkers Hetzbruder: das Strafverfolgungspersonal der Reichsstadt Nürnberg im 15. und 16. Jahrhundert*, Konflikte und Kultur: Historische Perspektiven, vol. 8 (Konstanz, 2003); Peter Schuster, *Der gelobte Frieden: Täter, Opfer und Herrschaft im spätmittelalterlichen Konstanz* (Konstanz, 1995).

12 As an exception, see Kirill A. Levinson, *Beamte in Städten des Reiches im 16. und 17. Jahrhundert* (Halle, 2004).

13 For other cities' regulations that did reflect the so-called Hippocratic Oath, see Thomas Rütten, "Hippokrateskommentare im 16. Jahrhundert: Peter Memms Eidkommentar als Paradigma eines gegenwartsbezogenen Genres," in Brooke Holmes (ed.), *The Frontiers of Ancient Science: Essays in Honor of Heinrich von Staden* (Berlin, 2015): 557–609.

14 See also Annemarie Kinzelbach, "Erudite and Honoured Artisans? Performers of Body Care and Surgery in Early Modern German Towns," *Social History of Medicine*, 27 (2014): 668–88.

15 StadtBibN, Ms. Cent V 42, fols. 1r–2v, also published in: König, *Nürnberger Stadtarzt*, p. 29f.; UBE, Ms. 1143, fols. 2r–3r; in a seventeenth-century version: StadtAN, B 11, No. 145, Eid- und Pflichtbuch der Reichsstadt Nürnberg, fols. 243r–245r.

16 StadtAN, B 11, No. 145, Eid- und Pflichtbuch der Reichsstadt Nürnberg, fols. 243r–245r.

17 Johann Heinrich Zedler, *Großes vollständiges Universal-Lexicon*, vol. 12 (Halle and Leipzig, 1735), "Hand-Wercker," col. 455; Michael Stürmer, *Herbst des alten Handwerks: Quellen zur Sozialgeschichte des 18. Jahrhunderts* (Munich, 1979). On the surgeons' guild in eighteenth-century Düsseldorf, see

Fritz Dross, *Krankenhaus und lokale Politik, 1770–1850: Das Beispiel Düsseldorf*, Düsseldorfer Schriften zur Neueren Landesgeschichte und zur Geschichte Nordrhein-Westfalens, vol. 67 (Essen, 2004), pp. 139–42.

18 StadtAN, B 11, No. 146, fols. 254r–255v.

19 StadtAN, B 11, No. 146, fols. 256r–264v.

20 StadtBibN, Ms. Cent. V 42, fols. 3r–6r; also published in Egon Philipp, *Das Medizinal- und Apothekenrecht in Nürnberg: Zu seiner Kenntnis von den Anfängen bis zur Gründung des Collegium pharmazeuticum (1632)* (Frankfurt a.M., 1962); StadtAN B 19, No. 134; StadtAN B 11, No. 146, fols. 1r–4r.; "Der Apotheker Aydt vnd Ordnung."

21 StadtAN, B 11, No. 146, fols. 4v–5v.

22 StadtAN, B 11, No. 146, fols. 363r–363v.

23 StadtBibN, Ms. Cent. V 42, fol. 7r–7v, "Der Geschwornen Mayster Aydtt."

24 StadtBibN, Ms. Cent. V 42, fols. 8r–9v, "Wundtärtzt Ordnung. Aller Wundtärtztt Aydtt"; followed by "eines E Raths Warnung den Barbierern vnnd Bader beschehen, jn Anhang einer Straff," fols. 9v–11r. See also StadtAN B19–150 "Ordnung der Bader gesellen Knecht und Jungen alhir zu Nurenberg."

25 StadtAN B 11, No. 146, fols. 395r–396r.

26 StadtBibN, Ms. Cent V 42, fol. 7: "wie auff andern handtwercken gewohnheitt ist."

27 StadtAN, B 11, Nos. 145 and 146.

28 StadtAN, B 11 Ratskanzlei, No. 140a.

29 StadtAN, B 11 Ratskanzlei, No. 140a, fol. 50r.: "Volgen hernach dießer Statt woll verordtnete Herrn Doctores Medicinae, Welche von Einem E.E. Rath, Angenommen vnd Jederzeit auch Ihre Pflicht, nach gehaltener Österlichen Wahl, der gebühr nach, Jn der Rath Stuben laisten, vnd ablegen müßen."

30 Barbara Stollberg-Rilinger, "Einleitung," in Stollberg-Rilinger (ed.), *Vormoderne politische Verfahren*, Zeitschrift für historische Forschung, Beiheft 25 (Berlin, 2001): 9–24.

31 The three decrees are quoted in Wolfram Brechtold, *Dr. Heinrich Wolff, 1520–1581* (Würzburg, 1959), p. 245: "Herr Hainrich Wolffen/der artzney doctor/umb die begerten 100 gulden järlicher dienstbesoldung annehmen"; "Herr Hainrich Wolffen/der artzney doctor/zu der pflicht zu erfordern"; "Herr doctor Hainrich Wolff medicus/hat seine pflicht im rathe gehört und mit dem eide verstattet."

32 Damm, "Nürnberger Stadtarzt Sebald Mulner," p. 151: "Und er hat der ertzt aide gesworen, der im statbuch folio IX geschriben steet."

33 Compare for Augsburg Levinson, *Beamte*, pp. 271–75.

34 StaatsAN, Rep. 62, Reichsstadt Nürnberg, Ämterbüchlein, Nos. 1 (1396) to 325 (1806). See Peter Fleischmann: "Die Nürnberger Ämterbüchlein," in *Das Nürnberger Buchgewerbe: Buch- und Zeitungsdrucker, Verleger und Druckhändler vom 16. bis zum 18. Jahrhundert* (Nürnberg, 2003), pp. 560–69.

35 StaatsAN, Rep. 62, Reichsstadt Nürnberg, Ämterbüchlein, No. 107 (1588): "Die Geschwornen Frauen so zu den Hebammen verordnet"; "Die Erbaren Frauen so zu den Hebammen und geberennden weibern gebeten werden."

36 For instance: "Gewardein oder Probirer der Müntz," "Eisengraber," "Ambtman jn der Schau," "Ambtmann in der Wexel."

37 "Hören jnn der Canzley vnnd globen jm Rath."

38 Paolo Prodi, *Das Sakrament der Herrschaft: Der politische Eid in der Verfassungsgeschichte des Okzidents*, Schriften des Italienisch-Deutschen Historischen Instituts in Trient, vol. 11 (Berlin, 1997); André Holenstein, "Seelenheil und Untertanenpflicht: Zur gesellschaftlichen Funktion und theoretischen Begründung des Eides in der ständischen Gesellschaft," in Peter Blickle (ed.), *Der*

Fluch und der Eid: Die metaphysische Begründung gesellschaftlichen Zusammenlebens und politischer Ordnung in der ständischen Gesellschaft (Berlin, 1993): 11–63.

39 Rudolf Schlögl, "Vergesellschaftung unter Anwesenden: Zur kommunikativen Form des Politischen in der vormodernen Stadt," in Schlögl (ed.), *Interaktion und Herrschaft: Die Politik der frühneuzeitlichen Stadt*, Historische Kulturwissenschaft 5 (Konstanz, 2004): 9–30, p. 25: "habituell gebrauchte Schriftlichkeit."

40 Veit Guggenberger, *Ayd-Buech: Warinnen findig, Was Ayd, vnd Aydschwur seyen, wie manicherley derselben gefunden, wie vnd welchermassen sie sowol am Kayserlichen Cammer-Gericht, als sonsten im Römischen Reich: in Specie aber in Chur-Bayrn gebraucht werden* (Munich, 1699), www.mdz-nbn-resolving.de/urn/resolver.pl?urn=urn:nbn:de:bvb:12-bsb10554157-6 (consulted 2 February 2015).

41 Johann Georg Krünitz, *Oeconomische Encyclopädie, oder allgemeines System der Staats- Stadt- Haus- u. Landwirthschaft*, vol. 10: E–Einguß (Berlin, 1777), col. 318: "Mannspersonen verrichten ihn mit Aufhebung der beyden vordersten Finger, auch wohl dazu des Daumens, an der rechten Hand, welche sie vor sich einwärts (nach dem Leibe zu) in die Höhe halten; Frauensleute aber mit Auflegung solcher Finger auf die linke Brust, nachdem vorher eine scharfe Vermahnung und Warnung, vor einem Meineide sich zu hüten, an diejenigen, die schwören sollen, ergangen ist."

42 Ernst Riegg: "Eigenwille und Pragmatismus: Der Konflikt um die Norma Doctrinae in der Reichsstadt Nürnberg," in Rudolf Schlögl (ed.), *Interaktion und Herrschaft: Die Politik der frühneuzeitlichen Stadt* (Konstanz, 2004): 237–68, p. 241.

43 StadtAN A1 (Urkundenreihe).

44 StadtAN A1 1524.09.26 (Gaugenreider, Han[n]s).

45 StadtAN A1 1526.05.02_1 (Gaugenrieder, Hans).

46 StadtAN A1 1534.04.24_1 (Gaugenrieder, Hans); A1 1545.11.01_1 (Gaugenrieder, Hans).

47 StadtAN A1 1543.08.23_1, A1 1547.09.26_1, A1 1552.09.26_1, A1 1557.02.01_1 (Gaugenrieder, Ciriacus); StaatsAN, Rep. 60c, Reichsstadt Nürnberg, Verlässe zum Losungsamt, 1 (1526–1600), V 22, fol. 30.

48 StadtAN, B 11 Ratskanzlei, No. 140a, fols. 50r–52v, for example.

49 StadtAN A1 (Urkundenreihe) 1550.11.01, Anngelburg: "doctor der Ertzney auch Schneid vnd augenartzt ytzund zu münchen"; StaatsAN, Rep. 60c, Reichsstadt Nürnberg, Verlässe zum Losungsamt, 1 (1526–1600), V 22, fol. 51.

50 Ibid.: "So sol vnnd wil ich mich allweg auff erlanngte erlaubdtnus vnuerhindert rechter erhaffter leibs not doch auff Jrer Erberkait oder der Jren, denen ich also zu gutem hieher geuordert wurde gepürlichen rossen und Zerung, darzu ich mich aber selbs beritten machen soll, on verzug vnnd widerrede, alher gein Nürmberg oder wohin mich Jr Erbere Weyshait in Jrem gepiet beschayden werden, verfügen."

51 StaatsAN, Rep. 60c, Reichsstadt Nürnberg, Verlässe zum Losungsamt, 1 (1526–1600), V 22, fol. 93; StadtAN A1 (Urkundenreihe) 1575.02.16_2 (Fuchs, Anton); "merertails von wegen seiner kunst fur den krebs vnd zum Taill fur den Aussatz."

52 StadtAN A1 (Urkundenreihe) 1564.11.01_III-Fröschel; Stadtlexikon Augsburg: Fröschel https://www.wissner.com/stadtlexikon-augsburg/artikel/stadtlexikon/froeschel/3827 (consulted 2 February 2015).

53 StadtAN A1 (Urkundenreihe) 1564.11.01_III-Fröschel: "yedes mals ein wochen drey oder vier oder wie lanng es die notturfft erfoderen wurde, alda verharren"; "von dato ditz briefe an so lang es Iren Erberkaiten gefellig."

54 StadtAN A1 (Urkundenreihe) 1564.11.01_III-Fröschel: "So soll vnnd will Jch mich allweg doch Jmselben fall auf Jrer Erbarn weißhait oder der ienen denen Jch also zu gutem hieher geforderet wurde, geburlichen vnnd zimlichen costen vnnd Zerung auf mein Person auch ainen knecht vnnd zwey pferdt, mit denen ich mich selber beritten machen soll."

55 StadtAN A1 (Urkundenreihe) 1564.11.01_III-Fröschel: "ain yedes Jar zweymal, als vngeuerlich vmb walburgis vnnd Egidij. Daselbsthin gein Nurmberg verfuegen. Yedes mals ein wochen drey oder vier oder wie lanng es die notturfft erfoderen wurde, alda verharren vnnd mich als ein Schneid Artzt Auch mit meiner Kunst der leib Artzney souil mir zu meinem thun, des Stain vnnd Bruchschneydens gebürt vnnd von nöten ist vnnd sunst Jnn allem dem, das Jch aus Gottes gnaden kan, willig vnnd gern geprauchen lassen."

56 Brechtold, *Wolff*, p. 245: "damit er sich desto besser allhir einrichten möge."

57 Ibid.: "doch daß solches der anderen doctoren wegen im stillen und gehaim gehalten werden."

58 StadtAN A1 1564.11.01_II_1-Weller, Paulus Dr (second contract of 1568 noted in the bottom space oft he instrument); StadtAN A1 1602.02.2_II_1-Herden, Balthasar Dr; A1 1611.08.10_1-Herden, Balthasar Dr.; StadtAN A1 1603.05.01_III_1-Neudorffer, Johannes Dr; A1 1611.11.1_II_1-Neudorffer, Johann Dr.; StadtAN A1 1622.09.12_1-Kirchberger, Johann Heinrich Dr; A1 1625.07.04_1-Kirchberger, Johann Heinrich Dr.

59 Levinson, *Beamte*, pp. 99–100.

60 For example, "wie mir als ainem getreuwen diener schuldigklich zu thun gebürt," "Ir Erbare weißheit aber sollen gut macht vnnd gewalt haben," and so forth. For application letters, see Schlegelmilch, "Promoting a Good Physician," Chapter 3 of this volume.

61 StadtAN A1 1569.10.06_1-Coiter, Volkherus Dr ("das ich in der stadt Nurenberg mit aigenen rauch ohne alle burgerliche beschwerden außerhalb des vngelts das ich gleich anderen zu raichen vnnd zu geben schuldig sein soll heußlich wohnen vnd sitzen mog"); similar wording in StadtAN A1 1560.11.01_1-Holtmann, Steffen Dr, also published in Robert Herrlinger, *Volcher Coiter, 1534–1576* (Nürnberg, 1952), pp. 60–62; see Fritz Dross, "Gelehrte mit Migrationshintergrund – Volcher Coiter und die Nürnberger Ärzte des 16. Jahrhunderts," in Brigitte Korn, Michael Diefenbacher, and Steven M. Zahlaus (eds), *Von nah und fern: Zuwanderer in die Reichsstadt Nürnberg* (Petersberg, 2014), 141–44.

62 See the introduction to Schlegelmilch, "Promoting a Good Physician," Chapter 3 of this volume.

63 Compare the Amberg case: Gerhard Naber, *Der Arzt als städtischer Amtsträger im alten Amberg* (Erlangen, 1967).

64 Otto Clemen, "Erasmus Flock, ein Nürnberger Arzt und Mathematiker," *Zeitschrift für Bayerische Kirchengeschichte*, 14 (1939): 195–202; Klaus G. König, *Der Nürnberger Stadtarzt Dr. Georg Palma, 1543–1591* (Stuttgart, 1961).

65 Doris Wolfangel, *Dr. Melchior Ayrer (1520–1579)* (Würzburg, 1957), p. 77.

66 E[rnst] Solger, "Aus dem Sanitätswesen der Reichsstadt Nürnberg im 16. Jahrhundert," *Deutsche Vierteljahrsschrift für öffentliche Gesundheitspflege*, 2 (1870): 67–90.

67 StadtBibN, Ms. Cent V 42; Karl Gröschel, *Des Camerarius Entwurf einer Nürnberger Medizinalordnung "Kurtzes und ordentliches Bedencken" 1571* (Munich, 1977).

68　StadtBibN, Ms. Cent V 42, fol. 90r: "Heu male nunc artes medicas haec secula tractant"; see Fritz Dross: "Vom zuverlässigen Urteilen: Ärztliche Autorität, reichsstädtische Ordnung und der Verlust 'armer Glieder Christi' in der Nürnberger Sondersiechenschau," *Medizin, Gesellschaft und Geschichte*, 29 (2010): 9–46.

69　StadtBibN, Ms. Cent V 42, fol. 90r.: "Den Ernhaften, fürsichtigen, Erbarn und weißen Herrn Burgermeister und Rath der Stadt Nürnberg meinen großgünstigen und gebiettenden Herrn."

70　"…auff leichtuertige leut/die sich ärtzenei vnderstehn/vnd der mit keynem grundt gelernet haben."

71　Karl-Heinz Leven, "Der Hippokratische Eid: Tradition, Mythos, Fiktion," *Imago Hominis*, 18 (2011): 307–16.

72　*Gesetz Ordnung vnd Tax Von einem E. Raht der Statt Nuermberg dem Collegio Medico, den Apotheckern vnd andern angehœrigen daselbsten gegeben. (Folget der verneuert Apothecken Tax wie er forthin allhie zu Nuermberg gehalten soll werden)* (Nürnberg, 1593).

73　Rütten, "Hippokrateskommentare."

74　*Gesetz Ordnung vnd Tax*: "So vil nun erstlichen die anstellung solches Collegij Medici belangt/sollen demselben alle von einem Erbarn Raht angenommene Doctores der Artzney (welche järlichen ihren Erbarkeiten die gewonliche Pflicht leisten) incorporirt und eingeschriben werden."

75　*Gesetz Ordnung vnd Tax*: "…inn gefehrlichen contagios Kranckheiten als in Pestilentzischen Fiebern vnnd sonderlichen da die Pestis regiert"; "in gantz gefehrlichen Seuchen vnd Kranckheiten."

76　In contrast with collegia medica in eighteenth-century German territorial states, the Nuremberg Collegium was not in charge of public health administration; see Ole Peter Grell, Andrew Cunningham, and Robert Jütte (eds), *Health Care and Poor Relief in 18th and 19th Century Northern Europe* (Aldershot, 2002); Dross, *Krankenhaus*, pp. 147–56; Mary Lindemann, *Health and Healing in Eighteenth Century Germany* (Baltimore, 1996). Public health administration in Nuremberg was carried out by special commissions ("Ratsdeputationen") of the magistrate, which, like most early modern Italian health boards, did not include physicians; see Di Giammatteo and Mendelsohn, "Reporting for Action," Chapter 5 of this volume.

77　See Schlegelmilch, "Promoting a Good Physician," Chapter 3 of this volume.

78　Tilmann Walter, "Ärztehaushalte im 16. Jahrhundert: Einkünfte, Status und Praktiken der Repräsentation," *Medizin, Gesellschaft und Geschichte*, 27 (2008): 31–73.

Part II
Evaluating, Reporting

5 Reporting for Action

Forms of Writing between Medicine and Polity in Milan, 1580–1650

Laura Di Giammatteo and J. Andrew Mendelsohn

"Bad news about the plague" greeted Giovanni Battista Arconato on 28 October 1629. Arconato was a nobleman and senator of Milan, then serving as president of its Tribunale di Sanità, the city's board of health during the period of Spanish rule, 1535 to 1706. He read on:

> When we arrived in Olginate, the countrymen told us that the region of Chiù had been infected because of the passage of German soldiers [...] We were also informed through notifications by the vicar of Galbiate that in two days 23 persons died with pestilential signs [...] We ascertained the same and have given a reliable notification to the Tribunal [...]. The Tribunal must now issue provision plans concerning surgeons, *monatti* [i.e., persons charged with transporting the sick and the dead in times of plague], the cleansing of houses and wares, and we will issue instructions to the commissioner for the territories, Daniel Herba, whom we have appointed [...]. We have already issued public health provision plans concerning the soldiers at the borders, we have also barred streets and isolated villages, we have issued provision plans for the sick and also for the healthy, in order to prevent the spread of the contagion [...][1]

To the casual eye, there is nothing remarkable in this snippet from the records of a city's response to plague. To the eye alerted by hours in the Milan archives, however, certain words leap from the page: notifications, provision plans, instructions, and the title given to this document itself: report. In the Italian of the Milanese archives, these were specific terms of art—*avvisi, provvisione, istruzione, ragguaglio*—and there were many more of them. Any document of significance usually bears one or another of these labels as its title.

This grammar seems to have been strictly observed. Woe to one who used the wrong heading, the wrong kind of paperwork for his purpose or addressee, the wrong form for a given function. Or for his own status and

DOI: 10.4324/9781315554693-8

role: few were entitled to write and receive such papers, for they had consequences. Each was a node for the interconversion of information and action in the Milanese polity. The *ragguaglio* quoted here was not written by a peer of Arconato's in the senate or by an administrator. It was written by a physician, together with a jurist. And that introduces the research problem we wish to define and explore in this chapter.

Recent work has highlighted the kinds of writing used by physicians. *Consilia, consultationes, regimina, curationes, observationes, loci communes* were the most important learned yet practical and empirically based of these kinds of writing in the early modern period, often intersecting with vernacular forms such as the recipe.[2] But there is also the question of how physicians wrote in their other roles. No such variety of writing has hitherto been highlighted for physicians as holders of public office or participants in government. This is a different point from the well-known fact that jurists and physicians shared ways of writing, such as the advisory genre of *consilium*.[3] When the physician Alessandro Tadino (1580–1661), member of Milan's health Tribunale and holder of its highest medical office, addressed a *ragguaglio* on the plague to Tribunale president and Milan Senator Arconato, he did not use the term lightly. Nor did he normally write *ragguagli*—reports—when he reported on cases to his medical colleagues, or *istruzioni* when he instructed patients or students. For *istruzioni* and *ragguagli* belonged to neither academic nor healing practice. They designated specific forms of communication within and around government. This chapter is about such forms. Its primary aim is to demonstrate the existence of a range of specific kinds of writing that flourished as two rising learned groups, physicians and jurists, became increasingly involved in government and as European government leaped in size, functions, and organizational complexity in the sixteenth and seventeenth centuries. The same questions of specificity, genesis, use, and implications for the development of knowledge and practice apply here as they do in current historical work on *consilia, observationes*, patient histories, recipes, and other kinds of learned and vernacular writing. This chapter can hardly answer those questions; it aims to make a case for asking them. A case that does this well is that of Milan.

Milan and Its Tribunale di Sanità

Milan's health system was distinctive but not unique in the Italian and wider European context. It had a health board, the Tribunale di Sanità, with executive, juridical, and legislative powers, unlike health commissions in most of early modern Europe but like the health boards of other Italian cities. Yet unlike the other Italian boards, whose directorate was typically non-medical and whose medical membership was advisory rather than executive and administrative, the Milan Tribunale included physicians as full members of its directorate, two of whom held the top positions beneath the board's president and were, moreover, endowed with powers of decree.[4] This peculiarity makes Milan an experiment in what happens, under early modern conditions, to physician and polity—and the practice of informed governance—when doctors are so empowered and when those powers are collaborative with non-physicians rather than singular to public medical office.

Health boards emerged in the sixteenth century in northern Italian city-states such as Florence, Venice, Genoa, Lucca, and Milan. These "special magistracies" combined "legislative, judicial, and executive powers."[5] Thus they were much more than advisory and supervisory bodies, like medical *collegia*, faculties, and guilds of doctors or barber-surgeons. And they were collectives, unlike offices such as that of town physician (*medico condotto, Stadtarzt* in German-speaking Europe) or that of civic or state chief physician (*protomedico*) in Spain and Italy.[6] Closest to the Italian health boards were the health councils of Swiss cantons, such as the Zurich *Wundgschau*, which included administrators and members of the city council alongside physicians and barber-surgeons, and its *Sanitätsrat*, which consisted mainly of city councilmen and included a secretary from the chancery.[7]

That said, the functions of an Italian health board were hardly unknown to urban government elsewhere in Europe. Like a ruling city council advised by its official doctors, a permanent health board had to legislate in matters of health, organize and run a health system, and prevent and respond to epidemic disease through administrative delegation of measures within and beyond city walls. Preserving the health of Milan also meant inspecting and regulating trades and industries such as soap production, a function shared with the Tribunale di Provvisione, overseeing cleanliness of water supply and canalization of waste water, keeping vital statistics, certifying merchandise through *bollette* or *attestati di sanità*, and negotiating with neighboring foreign governments over quarantine and trade. Milan's Tribunale had the power to confiscate merchandise and to order corporal punishment of people disobeying its orders, particularly during epidemics.[8] Many cities of late medieval and early modern Europe developed a similar range of functions, partly through laws and procedures of *police* or *Policey*.[9] These functions were, however, those of the ruling body—as in the German *Rat* or council—and of a number of separate offices, rather than concentrated in the activity and power of a single agency of mixed membership.

The Milanese peculiarity of empowering physicians as co-magistrates went back to the Magistratura di Sanità introduced in 1534 by the Sforza duke Francesco II to integrate medical functions. When Milan became a Spanish Habsburg territory in 1535, the Holy Roman Emperor and King of Spain, Charles V, confirmed the Sforza statute and, in 1541, promulgated a sanitary constitution based on this statute and adding new rules.[10] The Tribunale di Sanità was composed of seven members: a president elected by the Milanese Senate from one its number; a secretary chosen from among those of the senate; two doctors of law, called *questori*, whose role included that of police commissioner; the *protophysicus* elected by the senate with approval from the King of Spain; and two further doctors of medicine, called *conservatori di sanità*, or health preservers. The two *questori* were elected to the health board by the senate from the Milanese collegium of noble jurists. The two *conservatori* were elected to the board from the Milanese medical collegium, also composed of local nobility.[11] The *conservatori* were the most magistrate-like physicians in Milan—and therefore in Europe. And they were the European physicians whose public functions were most collaborative. Indeed, when the senator and president, the *conservatori di sanità*, the jurist *questori*, the *segretario*, and the *protophysicus* met, which they did weekly, they referred to themselves not in a language of bureaucratic procedure but using the usual term for deliberating in council: *congregati*.[12]

But what did this mean in practice? On paper, the powers of the *conservatori di sanità* were breathtaking:

> The officers of public health have absolute and complete authority and power in matters pertaining to their office and in any way regarding them. Let them be granted the right to give orders to any subject of this state, to impose fines, to confiscate goods, to inflict any form of corporal punishment short of the penalty of death [...].[13]

This heady job description in the city's *Novae Constitutiones* (1541) was fulfilled in practice: the Milanese archives boast a mass of Tribunale files filled with reports, provisions, instructions, orders, notifications, cautions, and decrees written by the health preservers. Their roles and powers of informed and informing governance existed not only on paper, but through it.

System of Information, Deliberation, and Action for Health

Instead of focusing on one or two forms of writing by physicians or jurists or administrators, as most previous work has done, this chapter reconstructs all of the writing of the healthy polis and aims to show it comprised a system.[14] Table 5.1 identifies different kinds of paperwork and their range of authorship as represented in the files of the Tribunale, mainly from 1550 to 1650. The files contain papers written by the *conservatori di sanità*, by the tribunal's provincial commissioners, by the *protophysicus*, by the president and by the *questori*. Of course, the table does not cover all paperwork of the Milanese polity, but that used in carrying out—indeed in creating or developing—informed governance, especially when this involved representatives of the two main learned groups, physicians and jurists. These kinds of paperwork were common to the Tribunale di

Table 5.1 Analysis of forms and functions of official and unofficial writing by physicians, jurists, and others around health in Milan in the sixteenth and seventeenth centuries.

Writing Agents/Genres		Medical and Juridical Professionals			Tribunale di Sanità (Board of Health)					Other
		Civic Doctors/ Town Physicians	Jurists	Physici Collegiati (College of Physicians)	Jurists as Questori	Protophysicus	Conservatori di Sanità	President of the Tribunale	Commissioners and Deputies	Diplomats, Vicars, Church Elders
Writing as Professional	Case	▨								
	Consilium	▨								
	Parere	▨								
	Observatio	▨								
Writing as Office Holder	Avviso	▨	▨		▨	▨	▨		▨	▨
	Ragguaglio/ Relazione				▨	▨	▨		▨	▨
	Avvertenza					▨	▨	▨		
	Istruzione/ Ordine					▨	▨	▨		
	Provvisione					▨	▨	▨		
	Avvertimento					▨	▨	▨		
	Bolletta di Sanità					▨	▨	▨		
	Grida						▨	▨		

Sources: Archivio Storico Civico e Biblioteca Trivulaziana and Archivio di Stato, Milan.

Sanità and other organs of Milanese state and civic government, such as its supreme judicial body, the senate; its highest civic authority, the Tribunale di Provvisione; and the Consiglio Segreto, privy council to the governor.[15] Each paper was usually distinguished by the heading put above the text and by designation of office of sender and addressee. These not only demarcated forms of writing. They articulated functions and linked institutions. Yet the functions and files of the Tribunale di Sanità are such that the survey also naturally takes in more widely used kinds of writing. These stretch from the most inclusive to the most exclusive, from writing by members of the public who submitted *avvisi* or *lettere* to writing by Tribunale members who had the rare authority to issue official reports and decrees. Thus, this chapter also explores the polity-building effect of both official and unofficial public communication as well as what this meant for the knowing activity of the physicians who used these genres—or who were, in effect, used *by* them, for they guided as much as empowered.

First of the office-holder forms listed in Table 5.1 is the *avviso*. *Avviso*, or notice, warning, advice, eventually "news," was a fundamental form of early modern manuscript communication. The *avviso* form had long been used by merchants, diplomats, and militaries, while city governments in northern Italy and in the Holy Roman Empire communicated as often as daily about unfolding events, including spread of disease.[16] In the sixteenth century, *avvisi* became the major public form of circulating information, through the growth of a whole business of newsletters called *avvisi*, for which reporter-like *menanti* or *gazzettieri* gathered and wrote information for postal dissemination, for which a new consumer public paid to receive.[17] Yet, at the same time, anyone literate could write "avvisi" to others in a city or its authorities—or indeed to doctors and other widely networked scholars—to apprise them of events that had occured or warn of events that might occur and that could be relevant to the "good of all the city."[18] *Avvisi* were addressed to the Milanese health board to inform it of dangerous health situations in the hope of activating the administration to issue orders or provisions or both. The passage with which this chapter began, with its medical *avvisi* from a vicar, exemplifies how news informed and activated planning and intervention.

Second in Table 5.1 is *ragguaglio* or *relazione*: a report in the form of a longer letter usually including information from, or indeed copies of, multiple received *avvisi* as well as provisions and orders issued by the board or its physician members. *Ragguaglio* was thus a macro-genre into which flew other genres, procedures, pieces of an unfolding story. A form of communication specifically between offices, reports could be sent only by Tribunale deputies or commissioners and by its core members, the *conservatori*, the *questori* or the *president*.[19] Whereas *avvisi* linked public office and public sphere, a report was made on the basis of "received *avvisi*" and "verified *avvisi*"—that is, *avvisi* confirmed through inspections conducted by officeholders. In these ways, the *ragguaglio* was the key synthetic writing form of public office and the basis for decisions.

Third, *avvertenza*, or caution, consisted of non-binding suggestions for how to deal prudently with difficult situations. *Avvertenze* were thus predictive or anticipatory. They were issued by the healthcare preservers to Tribunale deputies, such as the urban commissioners (*commissari urbani*) and the *commissari foranei* appointed in the territory around the city.[20]

Fourth, *istruzione* or *ordine*, instructions or orders, were usually handwritten. Particularly important instructions to more than one addressee could be printed, as in the following two examples:

> Instructions to the Territorial Commissioners
> for Quarantine of Travelers ...
> [from]
> The President and Health Preservers of the State of Milan

Passengers [...] in quarantine at the Ponte della Tresa and other locations of this State who are in good and continuing health 21 days from the day of their arrival will be dismissed to continue their travel, but first having all of their clothing and other belongings disinfected with all diligence [...]. 12 July 1628.

* * *

> Instructions to the Captain & to the Soldiers
> of the Guard of the City of Milan,
> Regarding Dangers of the Plague
> [from]
> The President and the Health Preservers of the State of Milan

1. You soldiers must stay day and night, live, and sleep at the gates of this City [...]. And as we are obliged occasionally to allow a license to stay overnight at home, it is up to your captain to allow this, but he must first write a deposition to our President [of the health board].
[...]
11. No one is to be admitted without a certificate [*bolletta*] under the pretext that he is a citizen [*del Borgo*] or that he is well known to the soldiers [...]. 18 January 1632.[21]

Such instructions were binding on those who received them. They were often issued by the health preservers to commissioners or mayors in the towns, instructing them in how to deal with disease prevention, treating the sick, or passage of foreigners across the borders. As early as the 1580s, we find the *conservatori* writing instructions to the *anciani*, or elders in the churches throughout the Milanese territory, on how to carry out inspections with assistance from the collegium of barber-surgeons.[22] Instructions legitimated as well as guided their recipients in new functions, expanding what their responsibilities and interactions with inhabitants meant. Instructed *commissari*, *anciani*, and others acted as the arm of the *conservatori di sanità* throughout city and

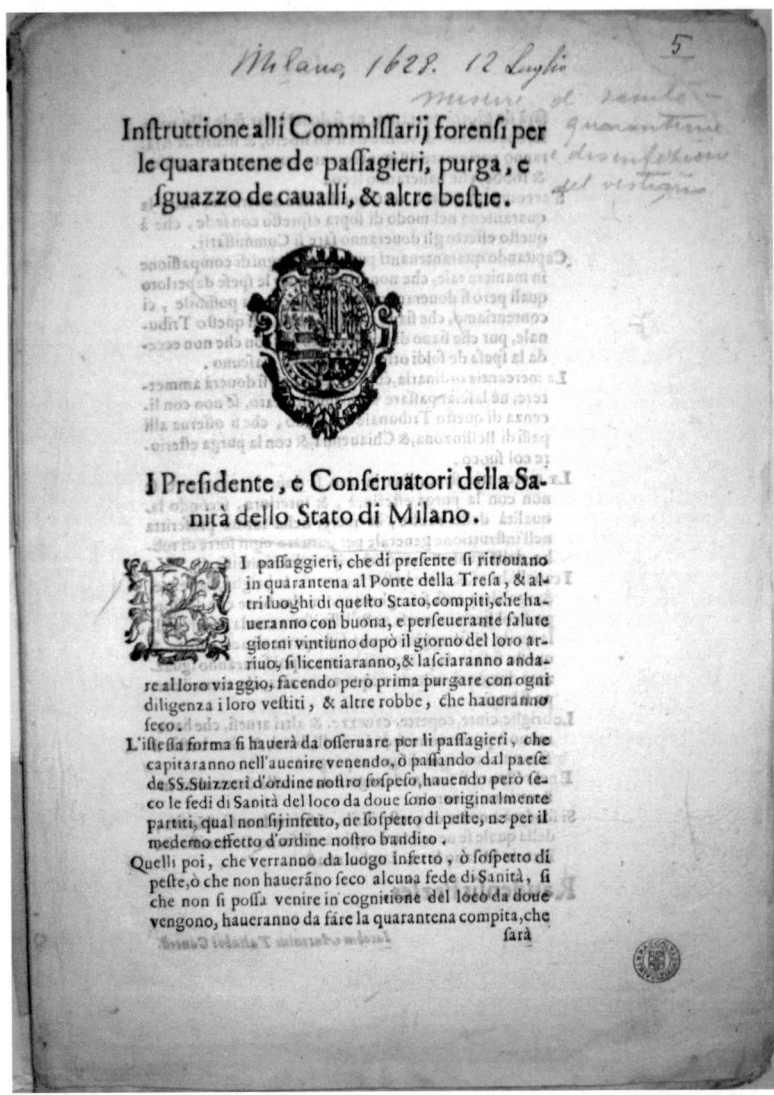

Figure 5.1 Example of seventeenth-century Milanese public health instructions. Instruttione, 12 July 1628, by President and Health Preservers of the State of Milan. Courtesy of Archivio Storico Civico e Biblioteca Trivulaziana, Milan: Gride, Carton 6, Fasc. 106. © Comune di Milano.

territory, yet also as their eyes: recipients were supposed to report on the effects of what the instructions prescribed, thus producing observations and information for further rounds of judgment, planning, and decision-making. If, as historians have shown, official instructions could create "order through ink and quill," they could also open order to the creation of new capacities beyond what the instructors already saw, knew, and wanted done.[23]

Fifth, *provvisione*, or providing plan, was a higher and more generalized form of instruction. It could be issued only by the two health preservers or the president of the Tribunale. This was not only a matter of authority. The greater generality of a *provvisione* required synthesis of wide-ranging notifications and observations as well as reasoned justification of multiple interventions in an overall course of action. Physicians as *conservatori di sanità* could recommend provisions not only to their president, but also to the Governor, Senate, or other Milanese tribunals. "The City of Milan is being destroyed," the Governor was avized on 4 July 1630 by Conservatore Tadino and Questore Visconti, "not only because of the mortality of 450 or 500 persons each day, but also because of the lack of the necessary *provisioni*." The two noble *doctores*, one of medicine, one of law, reported in detail on the epidemic and on provisions they had distributed to the sick and the healthy in a village they had visited and to soldiers guarding the border. Therefore we pray Your Excellency, they continued,

> to ponder these problems and the riots occurring in Milan and to carry out provisions needed to bring the aristocracy and the heads of houses back to Milan and to return the people to the concern of the senators [...] Through *provvisioni* we have ordered all women and children under the age of 12 to be sequestered in their homes [...] and we consider our order justified because of the growing number of infected persons in the city of Milan. Considering all these aspects, we pray Your Excellency to issue provisions for food to be given to the poor women and children sequestered in their homes.[24]

Providing food was within the competence of the Tribunale di Provvisione and the governor. Thus, in a single document of their synthetic activity, the physicians and jurists of the health board can be found reporting on *provvisioni* they have issued and outlining higher *provvisioni* beyond their authority, evaluating and justifying along the way. Altogether, *provvisioni* and the reporting and justifying activity around them integrated physicians into complex government action. This complexity was reflexive. The actors themselves conceived a *provvisione* as an interdependent "plan" to be formulated, implemented, and evaluated in practice through collaboration among different offices for the benefit of the collective.[25] This also helps make clear that, much more than a board, the Tribunale di Sanità comprised a system of interdependent offices and rules and a procedural hierarchy of competences, duties, employees, and other participants.

Sixth, *avvertimento*, or caution for government,[26] was to *avvertenza* what *provvisione* was to *istruzione*: that is, a higher form of caution with systemic scope of information input, reasoning, and potential application. *Avvertimenti* were addressed to directing members of the tribunal, not to its employees and deputies, who received *avvertenza*. *Avvertimenti* were generally written by the health preservers to the president, but also to the tribunal of provision, to the senate, or to the governor. They not only anticipated and warned, but also gave *prudenti consilii*: strongly recommended prudent counsel.

Seventh, *bolletta di sanità* was a health certificate for wares or persons, certifying that they had been disinfected before entering the State of Milan.[27] The decision to introduce requirements for *bollette* in a certain time and place was made by the preservers, or the *protophysicus*, or the tribunal as a whole, yet always in communication with the supreme civic authority, the Tribunale di Provvisione, responsible for supplies and administering the budget.

Eighth, *grida*, a law declared aloud in public, was a form sometimes used by the President of the Tribunale di Sanità or in extraordinary situations (hence *grida straordinaria*) by the physician health preservers.[28] Whereas *istruzioni* and *provvisioni* were issued for the benefit of all yet addressed only to those with government functions, a *grida* was addressed to all members of the community. In the *grida* of 25 November 1630 pictured in Figure 5.2, for instance, the president of the health board ordered all who carried out functions for the board yet also ordinary citizens and inhabitants—*alberghieri, osti* (innkeepers, publicans)—to watch for "suspicious" travelers and help prevent those with no *bolletta di sanità* from entering Milan. The generality of a *grida* was such that, in effect, the whole polis was supposed to collaborate with the Tribunale in such an effort, with the promise of monetary reward for informing and the threat of fines for failing to do so.

Thus, in their observations, evaluations, reports, recommendations, orders and so on, physicians as health preservers of Milan acted within a system of forms of writing. They also acted through that system on a world of health and disease, interaction and separation, behavior and environment. Even their actions on the material and human world were acts of communication on paper—a *provvisione*, an *istruzione*, an *avvertenza*, a *grida*. Each was far from interchangeable in form with the others. And each depended on the system as a whole for its meaning and operation. System concepts from sociology have helped historians explore processes of social and especially functional differentiation.[29] We make a different point here. Milan's system of action by writing preceded physicians' (and others') uses of its elements in the same way that, applying the distinction introduced by the founder of structural linguistics Ferdinand de Saussure, language (*langue*) precedes utterances (*parole*) of its users.[30] Elements of the *langue* of political papers such as certificates (*bolleta*) and decrees about certificates (*grida*) were hardly meaningful without each other. The function of each paper resulted from its position in relation to other forms, a relationship that was not classificatory or only procedural, but logical (you could hardly have *provvisioni* without *ragguagli* and *ragguagli* without *avvisi* and so on), enchaining interactants, defining their capacities and dependencies and the nature of their

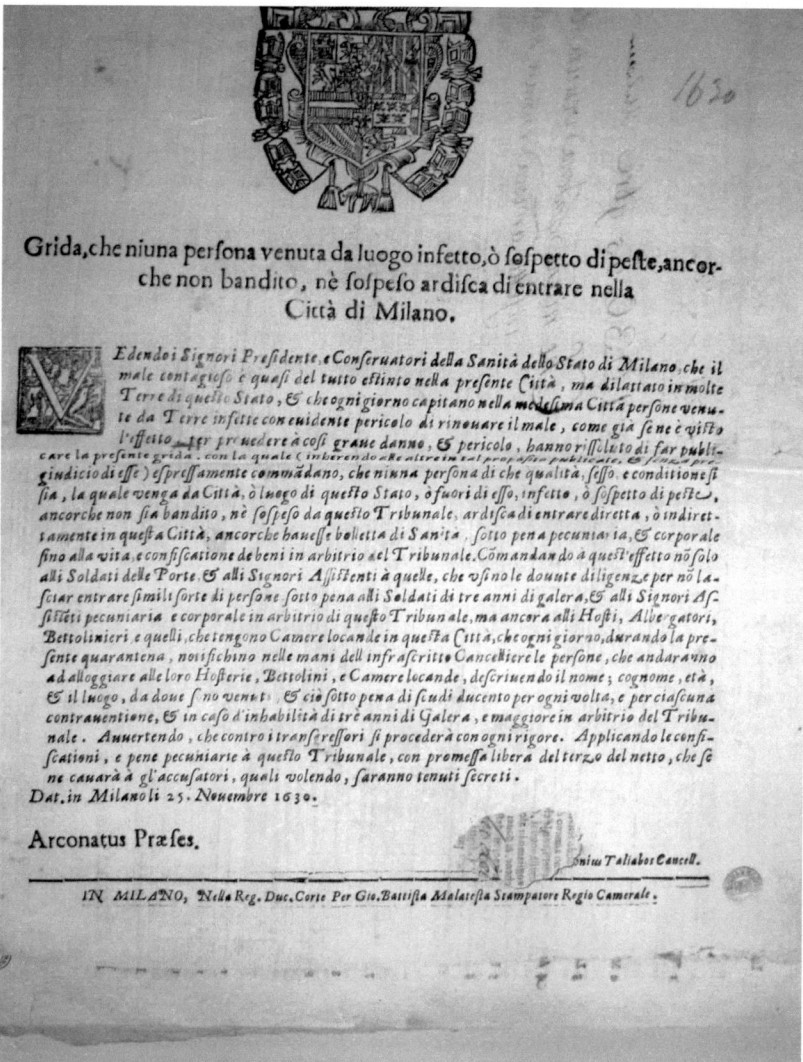

Figure 5.2 Example of seventeenth-century Milanese public health decree. Grida, 25 November 1630, by Tribunale di Sanità. Courtesy of Archivio Storico Civico e Biblioteca Trivulziana, Milan: Gride, Carton 6, Fasc. 106. © Comune di Milano.

actions. Chains of observance were also meant to be chains of observation and thus an empirical foundation for policy. At any point in these chains, a link could fail, papers could be ignored (and were, as we shall see), but the grammar remained.

Unlike words in languages, the polity's forms of writing typically came labeled with their grammar, as though "noun," "verb," "conditional," "imperative," and so on were to be written above the words in a sentence. The heading on a *folio di comunicazione* and its corresponding form and content (*ragguaglio, provvisione*) not only activated—or was supposed to activate—a network of specific interlocutors, but also their understanding of their place in the system. Papers with their headings repeatedly instantiated to readers how empirically informed government was supposed to work. Each form of writing was therefore instrumental yet also descriptive and prescriptive of itself, continually constituting government as tool, account, and norm of informed action. This system of writing was not just a means of government. It *was* government, no less than was deliberation in the senate or the Consiglio Segreto or accounting in the fiscal Magistrati.

Polis by Papers?

Milan's system of papers for health looks like bureaucracy and was. It was equally society, or an aspect thereof. For it was participation in governance—by officeholders who were citizens elected to service rather than career civil servants, by the groups from which they were elected, and by members of the public who contributed information "from below" to the empirical basis of policy and intervention. Only research on sources beyond those of the health board archive could find ways of measuring whether such participation actually built political community (and health in each other's image), but a frame for this question can be sketched here.

Consider more closely the physicians of Milan and their subgroups: the city physicians, the noble medical collegium members, and the three of these who belonged to the health board. The city physicians or *medici cittadini* of Milan, though university graduates, were not eligible to serve on the Tribunale since they were not noble and therefore could not belong to the College of Physicians, from which the *conservatori* and *protophysicus* were elected. This was not just social hierarchy translated into political privilege. It was a difference between the old model of civic doctors recruited often from outside (*condotto* meant hired by the community) and civic doctors homegrown from a city's old leading families.[31] Thus noble here meant local and is not to be confused with nobility of lordship or nobility granted by a king. So important was this "nobility" that College rules even prohibited members, on pain of explusion, from teaming with so-called *exteri* to handle difficult cases and co-author consultations—yet another shaping via forms of writing.[32] The evidently different ways in which these two models—outsider and insider—fulfilled or shaped or failed to fulfill political and epistemic desiderata of impartiality, efficacy, and the public interest would bear further examination.

And yet the analysis in Table 5.1 reveals that belonging to the locally well-born few got you only so far. Noble collegiati could contribute to *consilia* and *pareri* (expert opinions) on request from the senate. But nothing higher. The College as corporation and nobility could conceivably have wielded higher genres of knowledgeable governance but was excluded from them. Thus, forms of writing distinguished government from the rank and power of those from whom its officeholders were nonetheless drawn. Forms of writing thereby defined—if not secured—office as a tool of public rather than group interest. This was to grow the knowledgeable state out of corporation and class yet, at the same time, to create the civic beyond them.

Writing and reading structured participation on a scale of access and competence beginning with the widely accessible genre of *avvisi* and narrowing through *ragguaglio* to the exclusive *grida*. Most forms of writing used in and around the Tribunale were not written to or read by members of the public. Yet these relatively closed circuits of communication were nevertheless open, for they were based on information, *avvisi* and *lettere*, "from below" or simply outside. Anyone could contribute in this way to the wellbeing of the community and the functioning of its government, and some indeed were required to do so, as we saw for innkeepers and publicans, a requirement that made visible the dependence of government, and the health board in particular, on public participation.[33]

The news/instruction nexus bound together governors and the governed in a common interest and fate: the wellbeing of the city. It also thereby had the potential to bind together the disparate groups, classes, and sectors of society whose interests diverged or conflicted, whose degree of medical security or insecurity varied widely, as did their costs and benefits in relation to regulation for health. More than an ideal, health was a buzz of talk and writing, of communicating observations and drawing implications from them, animated and gathered into a focus by the Tribunale di Sanità. How similar yet different this was from the much looser world of urban politics by information exchange, which, as has been shown for Venice, unfolded not least through the health world of a city's everyday life and via those circulating communicators, the doctors, and those very newsy places, the shops of apothecaries and of barber-surgeons.[34] Communication around the board of health both fits and defies standard categories. It is well described neither as *arcana imperii* (though access and genre use were restricted) nor as public sphere (though public participation was essential). Its written exchanges lack the spontaneity of the public sphere yet also the secrecy of state. These forms had recently grown from the single notebook carried around by a late medieval lord and his secretary (from "secret"), through times of exploding organization and documentation to a resulting emphasis, exemplified by Venice, on oral as opposed to written reporting, prohibition on note-taking during speeches and deliberations in council, and strict control of access to written versions deposited in the Venetian archive appropriately named *Secreto*, however leaky its secrecy actually was.[35] Though usually the subject of separate histories, handwritten government and handwritten news were in fact twin non-Gutenberg phenomena, exploding in the early modern period.[36] Milan shows how these two could form a system encompassing state and civil society—even in a time well on its way to leaving behind the less differentiated world of *vivere civile* and despite radically sharpening distinctions between what those in office and those not in office could read and write and thereby do.

Milanese thus had their place in the polity not only by social stratification and group membership, but as potential contributors to the whole, the common good, and as potential beneficiaries of action for the whole. Or as potential losers by such action: the merchant whose shipments were held up, the soap manufacturer whose operations had to be moved, the families quarantined, being too poor to flee.[37] If such participation, benefit, and loss —potential or actual—helped create political community (in conflict as well as consensus), it did so differently from other forms of political participation, such as voting, supplication, petition, and denunciation.[38] Milan invites us to think less in terms of participation than in terms of (1) dependency of institutions like the Tribunale di Sanità on an informed citizenry capable of acting for the public good, and (2) constraint on what such institutions and their leadership could do, or decide not to do, with information they received. Constraint is another lesson of the analysis in Table 5.1: the most authorized writers were the least authorial. Least free, they inhabited the world according to the table more than anyone else did. For what made (or at least was supposed to make) such government something other than insiders doing what they wished, or what someone paid them under the table to do or not do, or doing nothing at all, was the Tribunale's system of writing and—recalling the heterogeneity of its members—its institutionalized mix.

Physicians in the Mix

What did civic office, its purpose, and its system of writing mean for the present and future of knowing disease and intervening for health? Tackling this question requires a switch from surveying forms of writing in context to following the writers through their roles and fields of action and interaction. These were more various than one would expect from standard concepts of medical practice, medical marketplace, learned medicine, court medicine, or even public health. Perusing the Milan archives, we can follow Conservatore Tadino and his senior colleague Lodovico Settala,[39] elected *protophysicus* in 1628, visiting the *Ospedale Maggiore* or the leper house or patients in their homes, writing *consilia* whether for a patient or the polity (a whole sheaf of these survives),[40] stopping at the house of the Tribunale president to attend the weekly meeting of its leadership, the *congregati*, and on such occasions reading *avvisi* aloud, discussing *avvertenze* and *provvisioni*.[41] We can see Tadino taking charge of the archive of the College of Physicians of Milan, reorganizing its *decreta* and other papers according to an index of actions, such as *protestationes* against Cardinal Carlo Borromeo's meddling in the health care of the city.[42] We can see Tadino calling a session of the College to formulate *pareri* or *responsi* (expert opinions) to *quaestiones* put by the Milanese Senate,[43] whether on a suspicious death or the properties of a plant or other natural material. We can follow Tadino attending meetings of the Tribunale di Provvisione as one of its "Twelve," or directorate, discussing questions of drug taxation or the introduction of wares from infected areas. Not least, we can see Tadino the indefatigable, visiting villages and towns around Milan during the plague of 1629–1630, sending back *lettere, ragguagli*, and *avvisi* to the Tribunale di Sanità, or drafting *provvisioni* and *ordini*.[44]

Tadino's itineraries and activities suggest that the effects of office and its written ways on its holders and perhaps also their peers unfolded along three main lines, each following from the previous: collectivity, heterogeneity, and interdependence, all via mechanisms of transfer or merger of ends and means between medicine, government, and publics. Altogether the effect of these was to open up new possibilities as to what medicine was. And perhaps government too.

First, collectivity of object and action. Serving in *ufficio di sanità* meant seeking to know and act on a collective in addition to individuals, as physicians did in their practice as healers, which in Milan as elsewhere was itself an office (*ufficio del medicare*). Some genres were shared across this difference. Tadino and colleagues might write a *consilium* for a patient or a *consilium* for the polity. Tomasso Rangone, Venetian doctor and patron of the arts, published a regimen for Venice.[45] Being tied to town and serving a community, as Gianna Pomata shows in Chapter 8 of this volume, could habituate civic doctors to see health and disease as part of a complex local whole rather than individualize illness as the doctor–patient dyad encouraged them to do. Civic doctors' case histories could become disease histories yet remain *observationes*. What difference might the size and complexity of larger cities and city-states like Milan have made? These distributed knowing and intervening beyond the confines of a single-authored *observatio* (with its recipes and regimen) through a web of written forms. These comprised coordinated action, unlike the prescription of one doctor for a whole community as though it were a single patient, as in Rangone's regimen for Venice. They also comprised coordinated empiricism, with division of functions among different and unequal contributors, unlike the collective empiricism of sharing cases and generalizing from lots of them, as communities of physicians learned to do through redactive paper-and-ink practices different from those displayed in Table 5.1 for Milan.[46]

Second, heterogeneity, or writing for (and with) diverse non-medical readers. When early modern physicians advised courts of law, they tended to cite authorities to help support their arguments, notably by analogy among cases or juridical situations. Chief physician of the Papal States Paolo

Zacchia, foremost representative of this activity in the time of Tadino and Settala, studded his *consilia* with references to the Latin literatures of medicine and law.[47] This practice contrasts strikingly with the kind of written governance exemplified by his Milanese counterparts. Tribunale papers by *conservatori* and *protophysici* contain few such references. This points up a difference between serving on a government board and serving a court of law. Physicians serving courts wrote for jurists, members of the other learned group with a literature of rules and cases analogous to that of medicine, whereas a physician on the health board, though working closely with jurists, wrote for its deputies and other lay administrators, senators and secretraries, and members of the public. We know much about the former activity, through the historiography of legal medicine, but less about the latter, as its history has been written mainly as history of the plague and public health. Did translating doctrine into use without doctrine change doctrine? Did reducing descriptive information to give government reports punch, as can be seen in the Tribunale archive, rather than maximizing information as physicians tended to do in their case reports or *observationes*, subtly or slowly change the practice of the latter? This is a question for research with an eye to difference between juridical and administrative activity and an open mind for what unknowns lurk behind such concepts as "administration." The Milan example suggests answers that lie not in Weberian or other characteristics of administrative office, "bureaucracy" affecting medicine, but rather in systems of governance like that of the Tribunale bringing together differently trained and experienced groups through communicative activity of inquiry, observation, evaluation, intervention, and cycles thereof.[48]

Third, interdependence. Interacting and working together through empirically informed writing was in itself nothing new to physicians, nor specific to their participation in governance. They were used to communicating far beyond the doctor–patient dyad or even its extension across patients' families and friends. As practitioners, physicians summarized cases to each other in requests for advice and answered such requests by writing *consultationes* or *consilia*. Those who participated still more actively in the medical republic of letters shared cases as *observationes* or less formally in their regular correspondence with one another.[49] Yet this was homogeneous interaction (physicians only), it was hardly necessary to medical practice (most patients did not become the subject of a *consultatio*), and only the albeit leading minority of learned physicians devoted much of their working lives to writing and sharing *observationes*. In health board deliberations, on the other hand, a physician could know and act *only* by interaction and *only* by interaction with non-physicians. More than collaboration, this was interdependence.

The Tribunale's mix prevented policy from unduly expressing the education, experience, and interests of any one group—jurists, senators, secretaries, physicians. So did the Tribunale's system of interdependent papers with their specified writers, readers, and functions, homogenizing the information and evaluation practices each participant brought from his background. In trials and consultations, by contrast, genres from those backgrounds, such as physicians' and jurists' *consilia*, flourished anew rather than being overriden. The interdependence among diverse *folii di comunicazione* within and around the health board entailed an interdependence among positions and offices and, therefore, also the groups and institutions that fed into them: collegia, senate, secretariat, patriciate, bourgeoisie. The self-designation *congregati* aptly captured this collaborative interdependence, which was certainly unlike being *peritus*, the virtuosic expert providing a *consilium* to answer questions put to him by a court as—drawing the contrast again—Zacchia did for the Roman Rota.[50]

This meant more than physicians, jurists, commissioners, senators, and so on interacting. It meant the creation of forms of intercollegiality, indeed transcollegiality. These ran contrary to the corporative system of collegia. On the one hand, this can be viewed as typical of the modernizing process by which state-building first drew upon and then eroded corporative institutions, a process completed in Milan after 1750 with reforms introduced by Maria Theresa of Austria dissolving the collegia system.[51] On the other hand and less teleologically, trans- or intercollegiality can be studied as itself an important historical form: integral to the creation of a civic common good, observable in paper-and-ink practice as outlined in this chapter, exemplified by, yet hardly unique to, Milan, lasting for two or three centuries, the golden age of the civic doctor.

Civic intercollegiality for health and security was not all harmony. Physicians and jurists were old rival groups. Senators could have their own points of view. Not everyone, including doctors, was equally devoted to the common good. Politics could prevent physicians from seeing their views realized in policy, as Tadino later claimed had happened in Milan during the plague of 1629–1630. Thus the heterogeneity of the Tribunale di Sanità represented both a potentiality for and a limitation on innovation in learned government and public medicine. The potentiality lay in the fact that a civic health system could hardly exist without aligning medical, juridical, social, economic, religious, corporative and other group perspectives. The limitation lay in the same structural challenge. The solution? In the short term, Tadino thought: rely on the system of writing. In the longer term, he found: go public.

Physicians like Tadino learned to speak and write in interdependent coordinated action on and for a collective body rather than individual ones, as well as between learned medicine and administration, senatorial government, lawmaking, trades and industries, neighborhoods and soldiers and church elders. Still, did the interdependence of physicians, jurists, senators, and secretaries as well as Tribunale deputies and informants and the imperative of coordinated action on and through a complex whole entail dialog, or translation, or indeed merger of competences and perspectives, or all three? This chapter shows that this is not just a bonus question if we happen to be interested in understanding communication, but a crucial question for understanding polity and knowledge. Whatever the answers, this interdependence and coordination suggest that what the diverse *congregati* were doing is not well characterized as either politics, or administration, or law, or medicine, or all of the above, and therefore that none of these, including medicine, is well understood as (what we think of as) itself. In so far as physicians' practice was public as well as private, medicine must be understood as the set of answers to these questions and not only as a healing practice or learned art and science or corporatively defined occupation.

Making Medicine Public

How might published medicine have expressed the breaking down of its corporative and learned identity through interdependent, coordinated empiricism and action on complex wholes? Signs of this process can be found in mixture of genre and in novel use of genres. Milan provides an instance of each.

Avertenze et osservationi appartenenti alla compositione de i medicamenti, published by Settala and Tadino in 1630 on the composition of drugs, seems a good example of mixture. *Avertenze*, as we have seen, was a specific form of vernacular written political and administrative communication, here especially recognizably so because it was from the pen of two holders of high public office. *Osservationi*, on the other hand, was the Italian for *observationes*, which in the late sixteenth century had become the major learned Latin genre of empirical case writing by jurists and physicians. *Avertenze et osservationi* was advertized as a translation by Tadino from a Latin work by Settala.[52] The bulk of this work, the first seven books of an eventual nine, had seen many editions since they first appeared in 1614. They had the character of a learned treatise of practical medicine, advising when to let blood and when not, brimming with references to Hippocrates and Galen as well as Settala's experience. In contrast, the eighth and ninth books struck out in a different direction. The eighth was about surgery, especially knowledge and treatment of wounds; the ninth about the composition of drugs.[53] These were the two major areas of medicine least specific to the tradition of the learned physician and most specific to his role in public office: surgery and pharmacy because civic doctors had become their regulators; wounds and drugs/poisons because of their centrality to juridical cases in which physicians acted as expert witnesses. Thus we can believe that these two books published almost simultaneously in Latin (under Settala's name) and Italian (under both names) in 1629–1630 came about "thanks to [the office of] Protophysicus of Sig. Settala" as Tadino wrote in a preface,[54] and that the processes of translation went beyond the linguistic to encompass collaboration on the health board as a center of evaluation and far-reaching communication and a forum of *congregati*.

Office demanded inspecting pharmacies and regulating materia medica according to civic pharmacopoeia and via *avvertenze* and like genres. Published, these became *avvertenze* not between offices—as the genre normally was used in seventeenth-century Milan—but beyond office. A genre of paperwork was not merely printed, but elevated into a book by two *doctores*. This, moreover, vernacularized the learned genre of *observationes* in amalgam with the paperwork of office. Amassing and articulating experience in the administrative form of *avvertenza* could better guide and develop the medical art, for instance, by making explicit and simplifying the training of surgeons through guidelines and by clarifying doubts about treatments.[55] How common such mixtures were, and how they were received and used, become worthy questions for further study. Fruits of office "offered to the world" in both vernacular and Latin, Tadino and Settala's joint work on therapeutics—the flashpoint between Galenism and the new chemical medicine—showed that neither of these, nor corporative medicine or the medical marketplace, but rather a civic medicine was the future. What makes this especially interesting is that Tadino and Settala were, at the same time, leaders of the medical old regime. It was thus becoming a new regime, via public office and public sphere, contrary to the story of decline and crisis or sellout to consumers characteristic of corporative medicine in London and Paris.[56]

And there was another way of publishing from public office and thereby opening up the scope of its possible effects. This is exemplified by the book on the plague published by Tadino in 1648. This was not the systematic scholarly plague treatise we might expect from a learned physician, like the densely referenced 300 pages of Latin his friend Settala had once dedicated to Cardinal Borromeo.[57] Nor was it a contribution to the burgeoning vernacular literature of treatment and prevention manuals, which we might expect to come from the pen of an experienced civic doctor in the plague years of Europe, as one did from Settala's pen in 1630, solicited by Tribunale president Senator Arconato and styled in the dedication "avertimenti compendiosi" easy to understand and useful "for every person."[58] Nor, finally, did Tadino's book fit the rising erudite empirical genre *historia epidemica*, or learned histories of particular epidemics, though it was written with considerable attention to particulars and titled *Report on the Origin and Daily Progression of the Great Contagious, Poisonous and Evil Plague that Befell the City of Milan and Its Duchy from the Year 1629 to the Year 1632.*[59]

The "great" plague of Milan came to be known as an indictment of the city for injustice—poison rumors resulting in trial and execution of alleged plague-spreaders—and for neglect, a symbol of Italian decline under Spanish rule.[60] This has overshadowed much of what one finds in the Tribunale archives: the system of information, evaluation, and prescription for action outlined in this chapter at work in high gear. Tadino published some of that paperwork in his 1648 *Report*, or *Raguaglio*, a book itself titled according to one of the governing genres. Had Tadino aimed to elevate vernacular into learned practice, he would have done as some other civic and state physicians did: publish juridical and administrative papers with Latin commentaries and introductions or indeed translate them into Latin.[61] Instead, the purpose affirmed in his *dedicatio* was to inform the public about how the plague had been investigated and managed,[62] or mismanaged, and through no fault of the Tribunale. Tadino aimed to show that policy and action had not reflected the *ragguagli* and *avvertimenti* submitted by the *conservatori di sanità* and the *protophysicus* until it was too late. Moreover, he charged officials high and low and even members of his own group, the physicians, with greed, corruption, and denial of danger, allowing disease to spread, neglecting the people, especially the poor, and thereby all but destroying the city.[63] To make this charge years after the fact was no longer quite the bold move it might have been. There is evidence that Tadino prepared long for it.

Lost in the archives of the Tribunale di Sanità is a curious piece of writing by which Tadino, we suggest, geared up for the *J'accuse* aspect of his *Raguaglio della gran peste* of 1648. Dated 1644, entitled "Raguaglio di Parnaso," it is a fictive report on a crisis of Milan, a report from Mount Parnassus where Apollo holds court, hears testimony, and pronounces wise justice and policy.[64] The Parnassus literary tradition had begun as poetry in the fourteenth century and developed into a genre of political satire in the fifteenth and sixteenth, culminating in the widely read and translated *Ragguagli di Parnaso*, published in Venice by Traiano Boccalini in 1612–1613.[65] In Tadino's never-published theatrical report from Parnassus, a string of medical witnesses starting with Asclepius, Hippocrates, and Galen blame newcomer "chemical" physicians for a decline of medicine. Then a surprise witness, a holder of public office who is not a physician, reveals that precisely the officeholding noble representatives of the old medicine have been corrupted by power and have used their positions for personal gain, compromising the city's physical as well as moral and political health in so doing.[66] To himself and perhaps a coterie of readers or listeners, Tadino thereby rehearsed accusations he would publish four years later.

The situation he dramatized was dire. Neither noble virtues nor Hippocratic or corporative ethos, neither political and religious ideals of the common good nor even public office as such could ensure health and good governance. For it turned out that none of these could resist corruption and the pursuit of individual or group interest at the expense of the public interest. There was only one thing left: the system of writing. Only its ways, if defended, could expose abuses and failures and ensure or restore the wellbeing of the polity. Tadino did not proclaim this. His text enacted it. Tadino's "Raguaglio di Parnaso" turned Apollo's tribunal into the Tribunale di Sanità: in the fictional trial on Parnassus penned by Tadino, *questori* receive *avvisi* of doctors' doings (including news heard in apothecary shops); Apollo hears *ragguagli* from Tribunale *delegati*, who are figured as the physicians Giulio Cesare della Scala (Julius Caesar Scaliger) and Giovanni Argenterio, representing conservative and reform medicine, respectively; the *delegati* hold inquiries and propose *provvisione* to Apollo; the *congregati* prepare *pareri*; and there are *resoconti* (accounts), *diligenze*, *ordini*, and of course Apollo's *sententia*. All would be well.

Down from the Mount though, in real Milan, no Apollo had held court. Only alleged plague-spreaders (*untori*) had been tried, no physicians and high officials. So Tadino undertook this himself, if rather long after the fact, by publishing *Raguaglio della gran peste*. Integrating examples of the forms of writing analyzed in this chapter into a chronological and explanatory account of the epidemic, Tadino guided the reading public behind the scenes of *grida* and *avvisi* and showed how the health board's system of observation, evaluation, and action was supposed to work and how it had been prevented from working as it should have. This act of publication made imaginable a history that had not taken place, that should have happened—not in Tadino's personal view but in archival view of what no one but himself, as the leading *conservatore* privy to all the papers, had seen: the would-be healthy polis of Milan on paper and by it. Tadino urged no reform. Human beings had failed; the system was sound. And its nature was clear: of the state yet also of civil society, expert yet collective and documented, corporative yet transcollegiate, learned yet vernacular, neglecting no sufferer too poor, as empirical and reasoned as *ragguagli* subject to discussion had to be, answerable as well as enabled by being public—in short, civic. This, Tadino wished Milan to show, is what medicine could be.

Notes

Acknowledgments: We thank Ruth Schilling, Annemarie Kinzelbach, Silvia De Renzi, Lars Behrisch, Volker Hess, and Maria Pia Donato for helpful comments and Josephine Fenger for help with formatting Table 5.1.

1 Alessandro Tadino, *Raguaglio dell'origine et giornali successi della gran peste contagiosa, venefica, & malefica seguita nella Città di Milano, & suo Ducato dall'anno 1629 sino all'anno 1632. Con le loro successiue prouisioni, et ordini* (Milan, 1648), pp. 26–27.

2 Studies on the more empirically related genres or forms of writing in early modern learned medicine include Jole Agrimi and Chiara Crisciani, *Les "consilia" médicaux*, Typologie des sources du moyen âge occidental, 69 (Turnhout, 1994); Chiara Crisciani, "Fatti, teorie, narratio e i malati a corte: Note su empirismo in medicina nel tardo medioevo," *Quaderni Storici*, 36/3 (2001): 695–718; Gianna Pomata, "Praxis Historialis: The Uses of *Historia* in Early Modern Medicine," in Pomata and Nancy G. Siraisi (eds), *Historia: Empiricism and Erudition in Early Modern Europe* (Cambridge, MA, 2005): 105–46; Michael Stolberg, "Formen und Funktionen medizinischer Fallberichte in der Frühen Neuzeit (1500–1800)," in Johannes Süßmann (ed.), *Fallstudien: Theorie—Geschichte—Methode* (Berlin, 2007): 81–95; Silvia De Renzi, "A Career in Manuscripts: Genres and Purposes of a Physician's Writing in Rome, 1600–1630," *Italian Studies*, 66/2 (2011): 234–48; Elaine Leong and Alisha

Rankin (eds), *Secrets and Knowledge in Medicine and Science, 1500–1800* (Aldershot, 2011); Michael Stolberg, "Medizinische Loci Communes: Formen und Funktionen einer ärztlichen Aufschreibepraxis im 16. und 17. Jahrhundert," *NTM: Zeitschrift für Geschichte der Wissenschaften, Technik und Medizin*, 21 (2013): 37–60; Gianna Pomata, "The Recipe and the Case: Epistemic Genres and the Dynamics of Cognitive Practices," in Kaspar von Greyerz, Silvia Flubacher, and Philipp Senn (eds), *Wissenschaftsgeschichte und Geschichte des Wissens im Dialog—Connecting Science and Knowledge* (Göttingen, 2013): 131–54; Nancy G. Siraisi, *Communities of Learned Experience: Epistolary Medicine in the Renaissance* (Baltimore, 2013).

3 See Carla Casagrande, Chiara Crisciani, and Silvana Vecchio (eds), *Consilium: Teorie e pratiche del consigliare nella cultura medievale* (Florence, 2004).

4 See generally Carlo Maria Cipolla, *Public Health and the Medical Profession in the Renaissance* (Cambridge, 1976), ch. 1, esp. pp. 20–22; and specifically Ann G. Carmichael, "Contagion Theory and Contagion Practice in Fifteenth-Century Milan," *Renaissance Quarterly*, 44 (1991): 213–56, esp. pp. 215–21, 251–54, on plague reporting and control in the previous, ducal period; and Leonida Besozzi, *Le magistrature cittadine milanesi e la peste del 1576–1577* (Padua, 1988). On Milan's administation in the "Spanish" period: Attilio Bricchi, *Medici milanesi in tempo di dominazione spagnola* (Milan, 1922); Alessandro Visconti, *La pubblica amministrazione nello stato milanese durante il predominio straniero (1541–1796): saggio di storia del diritto amministrativo* (Rome, 1913). On the Milan College of Physicians: Giovanni Battista Selvatico, *Collegii mediolanensium medicorum origo* (Milan, 1607); Alessandro Tadino, *Venerabilis Collegii Physicorum Mediolanensium antiquitas, privilegia, statuta, ordinationes in compendium redacta* (Milan, 1654).

5 Carlo Maria Cipolla, *Fighting the Plague in Seventeenth-Century Italy* (Madison, 1981), p. 4.

6 David Gentilcore, "All That Pertains to Medicine: Protomedici and Protomedicati in Early Modern Italy," *Medical History*, 38 (1994): 121–42; Andrew W. Russell (ed.), *The Town and State Physician in Europe from the Middle Ages to the Enlightenment* (Wolfenbüttel, 1981).

7 Gustav Adolf Wehrli, *Die Krankenanstalten und die öffentlich angestellten Ärzte und Wundärzte im alten Zürich* (Zurich, 1934), pp. 76–82, 88–91.

8 Archivio di Stato, Milan (hereafter: ASM), Sanità, Parte Antica (hereafter: P.A.), e.g., Carton 67 Protomedicati (e.g., Protofisico Giussano on water supply and legitimate industrial procedures, 1632); Carton 89 Acque; Carton 282 Peste, stranieri, svizzeri, e.g., documentation in 1629 of negotiating quarantine with the Swiss. Archivio Storico Civico e Biblioteca Trivulziana, Milan (hereafter: ASCM), Materie, Cartons 255 and 867, for soap industry.

9 See Mendelsohn, "Public Practice," Chapter 1 of this volume.

10 Visconti, *La pubblica amministrazione*, pp. 285–90; *Novae Constitutiones* (Milan, 1746), p. 76.

11 ASM, Sanità, P.A., Carton 47 Uffici, Provvidenze generali al 1746, Compendio cronologico-storico del Magistrato di Sanità; see Giulio Vismara, "Le istituzioni del patriziato," in Fondazione Treccani degli Alfieri (ed.), *Storio di Milano*, Vol. IX: *Il declino* spagnolo (Milan, 1958): 226–86; Cesare Mozzarelli and Pierangelo Schiera, *Patriziati e aristocrazie nobiliari: ceti dominanti e organizzazione del potere nell'Italia centro-settentrionale dal XVI al XVIII secolo* (Trento, 1978).

12 ASM, Sanità, P.A., Carton 291 Registri.

13 *Novae Constitutiones*, p. 78.

14 Studies focusing on one or more forms: see note 2 and note 17; Peter Becker and William Clark (eds), *Little Tools of Knowledge: Historical Essays on*

Academic and Bureaucratic Practices (Ann Arbor, 2001); Michael Niehaus and Hans-Walter Schmidt-Hannisa (eds), *Das Protokoll: Kulturelle Funktionen einer Textsorte* (Frankfurt am Main, 2005).

15 On these institutions and distinctions as well as blurring of state and civic authority among them, see Stefano D'Amico, *Spanish Milan: A City within the Empire, 1535–1706* (New York, 2012), pp. 128–35.

16 See Cipolla, *Fighting the Plague*, ch. 2; Christine Werkstetter, "Die Pest in der Stadt des Reichstags: Die Regensburger 'Contagion' von 1713/14 in kommuni-kationsgeschichtlicher Perspektive," in Johannes Burkhardt and Christine Werkstetter (eds), *Kommunikation und Medien in der Frühen Neuzeit*, Histor-ische Zeitschrift Beihefte, n.s., 41 (Munich, 2005): 267–92.

17 Mario Infelise, "From Merchants' Letters to Handwritten Political Avvisi: Notes on the Origins of Public Information," in Francisco Bethencourt and Florike Egmond (eds), *Cultural Exchange in Early Modern Europe, III: Corres-pondence and Cultural Exchange in Europe 1400–1700* (Cambridge, 2007): 33–52; Brendan Dooley (ed.), *The Dissemination of News and the Emergence of Contemporaneity in Early Modern Europe* (Aldershot, 2010); "News Net-works in Early Modern Europe," Queen Mary, University of London, http://newscom.english.qmul.ac.uk/about/index.html; on flexibility of the manuscript medium and circulation of printed reports, see Filippo de Vivo, *Information and Communication in Venice: Rethinking Early Modern Politics* (Oxford, 2007), pp. 57–63; and see Bettina Bosold-DasGupta, *Traiano Boccalini und der Anti-Parnass: Frühjournalistische Kommunikation als Metadiskurs* (Amster-dam and New York, 2005), esp. ch. 2.

18 For numerous *political* avvisi written to a humanist naturalist, Gian Vincenzo Pinelli, see Biblioteca Ambrosiana (Milan), Manoscritti, D 491 inf.

19 Tadino, *Raguaglio della gran peste*, p. 43.

20 Tadino, *Raguaglio della gran peste*, pp. 81–82. ASM, Sanità, P.A., Carton 278 Peste/Certificati di sanità/Processi di untori, 1576–1720, Envelope 5.

21 ASCM, Gride, Carton 6, Fasc. 106, instruction dated 12 July 1628.

22 ASM, Sanità, P.A, Carton 67 Protomedicati, e.g., Conservatori di sanità instruction to anciani, 1588.

23 Anita Hipfinger et al. (eds), *Ordnung durch Tinte und Feder? Genese und Wir-kung von Instruktionen im zeitlichen Längsschnitt vom Mittelalter bis zum 20. Jahrhundert* (Vienna, 2012).

24 ASM, P.A., Carton 278 Peste/Certificati di sanità/Processi di untori, 1576–1720, 4 July 1630. Supplies lay in the purview of the Tribunale di Provvisione rather than the Tribunale di Sanità.

25 For examples of interdependence among public offices in Milan, see ASM, Sanità P.A., Carton 282 Peste, stranieri, svizzeri, e.g., letter dated 22 June 1630, written by the health board secretary to the Tribunale di Provvisione regarding suspect corn shipments from the infected area of Graubünden; see also Tadino, *Ragua-glio della gran peste*, pp. 45, 79–83.

26 Tadino, *Raguaglio della gran peste*, pp. 77–78. ASM, Sanità, P.A., Carton 279 bis Previdenza generale 1576–1629, *avvertimento* dated 25 November 1629.

27 ASM, Sanità P. A, Carton 278 Peste/Certificati di sanità/Processi di untori, 1576–1720, certificate dated 19 August 1600; Tadino, *Raguaglio della gran peste*, pp. 30–54.

28 On the authority of *conservatori di sanità* to make *grida*, see Tadino, *Ragua-glio della gran peste*, p. 89; ASM, Sanità, P.A., Carton 278 Peste/Certificati di sanità/Processi di untori, 1576–1720.

29 See discussion and references in Mendelsohn, "Public Practice," Chapter 1 of this volume.

30 Ferdinand de Saussure, *Course in General Linguistics*, ed. Charles Bally, Albert Sechehaye, and Albert Reidlinger, trans. Wade Baskin (New York, 1959), chs. 3–4.

31 On recruitment from outside, see Schlegelmilch, "Promoting a Good Physician," Chapter 3 of this volume; for *medici condotti*, see Pugliano, "Accountability, Autobiography, and Belonging," Chapter 7 of this volume.

32 See Selvatico, *Collegii mediolanensium*; Tadino, *Venerabilis Collegii Physicorum*.

33 For reflections and recent research on inns and taverns as places of public communication, see Gerd Schwerhoff, "Stadt und Öffentlichkeit in der Frühen Neuzeit: Perspektiven der Forschung," in Schwerhoff (ed.), *Stadt und Öffentlichkeit in der Frühen Neuzeit* (Cologne, 2011): 1–28, pp. 13–17.

34 Filippo de Vivo, "Pharmacies as Centres of Communication in Early Modern Venice," *Renaissance Studies*, 21 (2007): 505–21; Sandra Cavallo, *Artisans of the Body in Early Modern Italy: Identities, Families and Masculinities* (Manchester, 2007).

35 On "public sphere" before the eighteenth century, see Mendelsohn, "Public Practice," Chapter 1 of this volume, n. 37; Brendan Dooley and Sabrina A. Baron (eds), *The Politics of Information in Early Modern Europe* (London, 2001); Peter Lake and Steven Pincus, *The Politics of the Public Sphere in Early Modern England* (Manchester and New York, 2007); leaky Venetian secrecy: de Vivo, *Information and Communication in Venice*, esp. ch. 2.

36 Exemplary as a study of both together: de Vivo, *Information and Communication in Venice*; see also Joop W. Koopmans (ed.), *News and Politics in Early Modern Europe, 1500–1800* (Leuven and Paris, 2005); on manuscript communication in the early age of print: Asa Briggs and Peter Burke, *A Social History of the Media: From Gutenberg to the Internet*, 3rd edn (Cambridge, 2009), ch. 2; Harold Love, *Scribal Publication in Seventeenth-Century England* (Oxford, 1993).

37 Examples like these can be found in the sources referenced in note 8 and note 24 above.

38 See Mendelsohn, "Public Practice," Chapter 1 of this volume, n. 54.

39 See Silvia Rota Ghibaudi, *Ricerche su Ludovico Settala: biografia, bibliografia, iconografia e documenti* (Florence, 1959). ASM, Sanità, P.A, Carton 67 Protomedicati, on Settala's election.

40 ASCM, Codex 1709, *consilia* by Tadino and Settala.

41 ASM, Sanità, P.A, Carton 291 Ordinazioni di Sanità.

42 Tadino, *Venerabilis Collegii Physicorum*, p. 40; Paolo Pissavino, "Per un'immagine sistemica del Milanese Spagnolo: Lo Stato di Milano come arena di potere," in Pissavino and Gianvittorio Signorotto (eds), *Lombardia Borromaica, Lombardia Spagnola 1554–1659* (Rome, 1995): 163–231.

43 ASCM, Codex 1709, *responsi* by Tadino and his collegues to the Senate, which was also a penal court.

44 See ASM, Sanità, P.A, Carton 278 Peste/Certificati di sanità/Processi di untori, 1576–1720; Tadino, *Raguaglio della gran peste*, 30–54.

45 Sandra Cavallo and Tessa Storey, *Healthy Living in Late Renaissance Italy* (Oxford, 2013), p. 79.

46 See Gianna Pomata, "Sharing Cases: The *Observationes* in Early Modern Medicine," *Early Science and Medicine*, 15 (2010): 193–236; J. Andrew Mendelsohn, "The World on a Page: Making a General Observation in the Eighteenth Century," in Lorraine Daston and Elizabeth Lunbeck (eds), *Histories of Scientific Observation* (Chicago, 2011): 396–420.

47 Silvia De Renzi, "Witnesses of the Body: Medico-Legal Cases in Seventeenth-Century Rome," *Studies in the History and Philosophy of Science*, 33 (2002): 219–42; Jacalyn Duffin, "Questioning Medicine in Seventeenth-Century Rome: The Consultations of Paolo Zacchia," *Canadian Bulletin of Medical History*, 28 (2011): 149–70.

48 On bureaucratic and academic practices: Becker and Clark (eds), *Little Tools of Knowledge*; see generally the research agenda outlined in Volker Hess and J. Andrew Mendelsohn, "Paper Technology und Wissensgeschichte," *NTM – Zeitschrift für Geschichte der Wissenschaften, Technik und Medizin*, 21 (2013): 1–10.

49 Pomata, "Sharing Cases"; Siraisi, *Communities of Learned Experience*.

50 See note 47 above and, for the earlier period, Mario Ascheri, "'Consilium sapientis' perizia medica e 'res iudicata': diritto dei 'dottori' e istituzioni comunali," in Stephan Kuttner and Kenneth Pennington (eds), *Proceedings of the Fifth International Congress of Medieval Canon Law, Salamanca 21–25 September 1970* (Vatican City, 1980): 533–79.

51 Thereafter *conservatori di sanità* were appointed only as advisors, and the posts went to the medical professors at the University of Pavia rather than the *nobili physici collegiati*; ASM, Sanità, P.A., Carton 186 Medica/Piani/Sistemi; ASCM, Dicasteri, Carton 340 Sanità.

52 Lodovico Settala, *Avertenze et osservationi appartenenti alla compositione de i medicamenti. Tradotte dal nono libro delle Osservationi del sig. Lodovico Settala medico collegiato, [...] da Alessandro Tadino medico collegiato milanese* (Milan, 1630).

53 Lodovico Settala, *Animadversionum, & cautionum medicarum, libri duo. Septem alijs iam editis additi, Animadversiones, quae ad vulnera curanda, & quae ad componenda medicamenta pertinent, continentes* (Milan, 1629).

54 Tadino, preface to Settala, *Avvertenze*: "carico di Protofisico del Sig. Settala."

55 Tadino, preface to Settala, *Avvertenze*, fols. 1–4.

56 Harold J. Cook, *The Decline of the Old Medical Regime in Stuart London* (Ithaca, 1986); Laurence Brockliss and Colin Jones, *The Medical World of Early Modern France* (Oxford and New York, 1997), chs. 3 and 8.

57 Lodovico Settala, *De peste et pestiferis affectibus libri quinque* (Milan, 1622).

58 Lodovico Settala, *Preservatione dalla peste scritta dal sig. protomedico Lodovico Settala* (Brescia, 1630), p. 4.

59 Tadino, *Raguaglio della gran peste*; on early modern *historia epidemica*, see Pomata, "A Sense of Place," Chapter 8 of this volume.

60 As enduring symbol of decline: D'Amico, *Spanish Milan*, p. 2; for Tadino's views on the plague-spreader theory and investigation: Sabine Kalff, *Politische Medizin der Frühen Neuzeit: Die Figur des Arztes in Italien und England im frühen 17. Jahrhundert* (Berlin, 2014), ch. 5; see also Ann G. Carmichael, "The Last Past Plague: The Uses of Memory in Renaissance Epidemics," *Journal of the History of Medicine and Allied Sciences*, 53 (1998): 132–60.

61 Michael Bernhard Valentini, *Pandectae medico-legales, sive Responsa medico-forensia ex archivis academiarum celebriorum [...] latinitate donata* (Frankfurt am Main, 1701).

62 Tadino, *Raguaglio della gran peste*, f. A2r: "Perché l'immortalità dell'anima nostra non sà trovare frà le mortali felicità il proprio, et adequato contento; perciò quante piú dispositioni nobili in se richiude, tanto meno delle ordinarie grandezze si satolla. [...] Armato di tal zelo questo mio parto, nato dal commando, nodrito dalla curiosità, & aggrandito frà i stupori; desidera immortalare la sua gloria, non già perchè sia ornato da un dire romanzo, che á ciò non mira l'Auttore, mà ben sì, perchè seco apporta d'un meravigliossisimo racconto

la schietta, pura et netta verità necessaria per il conquisto di questa immortalità."

63 These and other charges run throughout the *Raguaglio della gran peste*, for example, in chs. 5, 19, 56; for a comprehensive analysis of Tadino's and other accounts of the epidemic of 1629–1630, see Kalff, *Politische Medizin*, ch. 5, noting charges of greed and corruption on p. 303, 328, 387.

64 ASCM, Codex 1709, manuscript by Tadino, "Raguaglio di Parnaso," dated 1644.

65 Bosold-DasGupta, *Traiano Boccalini*.

66 Tadino, "Raguaglio di Parnaso."

6 Negotiating on Paper

Councilors, Medical Officers, and Patients in an Early Modern City

Annemarie Kinzelbach

One day in mid-1594, a note was entered into the session of the town council of Nördlingen under the guise of a medical certificate, headed *Schauzettel* ("inspection note"), as such certificates normally were. Yet the heading was misleading. Most of the text was not the usual brief report by medical officers on a sick person. Instead, it reported a conflict among medical officers. It described one medical officer tearing apart a *Schauzettel* written by another—a scandalous act. We learn about this act from the town-appointed barber-surgeon, Thomas Greiffenstein (or Greiffensteiner), whose note had been expedited into council by its heading. In so far as he had copied a certificate into his note, the heading *Schauzettel* was properly applied, but two-thirds of the note was devoted to defending himself and denouncing the town-appointed physician, Hieronymus Reusner, by evoking the following scene. Greiffenstein had sent word to Reusner suggesting that the physician join him in fulfilling the burgomaster's request for a third medical examination of a sick woman, Els Mößlerin. The physician declined to join in the examination and asked the surgeon to issue the certificate on his own, to which the physician would simply add his signature. The following day, when Greiffenstein went to pick up the signed certificate, he learned that Dr. Reusner had torn it apart and had decided that two certificates would have to be submitted to the town council: one by the physician and one by the surgeon. Greiffenstein continued his account of this conflict by recommending to the councilors that they check the text of his own allegedly offending certificate, which he had copied into his note, disguised under the *Schauzettel* heading. He thus proposed a way for the council to exonerate him immediately of any charge regarding his certificate for the sick woman. Moreover, he cited the patient as a witness to threats made against him by Dr. Reusner, implying that the doctor planned to appeal to the council for dismissal of Greiffenstein from his office as official town barber-surgeon.

The opponents in this conflict—two medical officers, one a university-educated physician, the other an artisan-trained barber-surgeon—and the various other actors (burgomaster, councilors, the person responsible for the records office in the town hall, and the examined woman) belonged to

DOI: 10.4324/9781315554693-9

different layers of Nördlingen society.[1] The physician and the surgeon had been appointed to their offices by the council of this Imperial town. Both were involved in officially examining sick inhabitants. Both provided medical services in the town and beyond. The burgomasters and members of the council considered themselves as the sovereign government of a medium-sized "republic," including territory beyond the town.[2] Nördlingen preserved an autonomous status until the early nineteenth century, despite its small size of less than 10,000 inhabitants, continuous competition with neighboring territorial sovereigns, and direct relationship (as an Imperial town) with the Holy Roman Emperor.[3] This status makes the community of Nördlingen an excellent object of study for linking general history to the history of science and medicine, because most administrative and many private papers were kept in the town's archive, mostly under surveillance of the council clerk ("Rath-Schreiber"), who was in charge of written and documented oral communication in and around the town hall.[4]

Historical studies on the symbolic modes of acting on paper and acting by paper have offered insights into social and political processes by looking closely at the forms of such acting, especially in conflicts in their community contexts.[5] Analysis of such papers and of the ways they were manipulated can assist in grasping processes of (oral and written) communication.[6] Communication among persons in disparate layers of society has been characterized as "negotiating."[7] In addition, exploring how the writing was performed and what it implied provides evidence of the significance such papers embodied and the meanings they had for members of the society in and beyond the city.[8]

This chapter focuses on paper power and its limits. Several thousand *Schauzettel* (certificates) were written in Nördlingen between the late fifteenth and early nineteenth centuries. Samples from different decades help characterize such official papers and paper power, the writing and reading process, the actors, and the communication involved. This is followed by an in-depth analysis of papers produced during a conflict in the year 1594, which shows ongoing negotiations and their dynamics in this early modern society and the limits of paper power. Finally, I discuss a paper link between the dynamic of communication in the small world of Nördlingen and writing for and in the wider European world of scholars.

Various samples of these certificates have been analyzed in the context of gendered healthcare, poor relief, and social policy in connection with epidemic disease.[9] The intense context analysis in this chapter focuses on a crucial period when practices of medical examination were not only established, but also well documented, showing a number of characteristics such as formal structure and writing in the vernacular, which did not change until the early nineteenth century.[10] The "Republic of Letters" was well established in Europe, and new genres of learned discourse and knowledge creation were developing; many town physicians were involved in these.[11] The paperwork around the conflict documents the practices used before the impact of the Thirty Years' War, which changed aspects of such practices by, for example, destroying buildings in which examinations had been carried out and certificates written.[12]

Acting with Paper in Administrative Processes

The *Schauzettel* were official documents and important enough for councilors and inhabitants of Nördlingen to archive them separately in numbered folders with the heading *Medicinisch-Chirurgische Berichte und Schauzettul* (Medical-Surgical Reports and Certificates).[13] Each numbered folder contained the paper slips from a period of two to nine years. With mediatization and the passing of sovereignty from the town to the Bavarian duke, this heading was changed to *Acta. Schauzettel vnd medizinische Berichte über arme Kranke* ("Files. Certificates and Medical Reports on Poor Sick Persons"), thus explicitly turning these files into an archive of social policy.[14] Thus the transition from autonomous town to part of a territory corresponded to an explicit alteration of the political focus from reports for a community to reports on poor subjects.[15]

The earlier heading displays no specific purpose for the preservation of these documents; they definitely were not kept because of their forensic relevance. Files containing evidence for the courtroom were only temporarily part of this collection; traces—such as single papers with consecutive numbering—and later archiving practice suggest that forensic paperwork was filed elsewhere. From the seventeenth century juridical cases concerning, for example, accidents and suspicion of suicide were preserved separately, despite including *Berichte* (reports) and *Schauzettel* (certificates) as part of the documentation of evidence.[16]

The certificate shown in Figure 6.1 is representative of most *Schauzettel* from the sixteenth through the nineteenth centuries in several respects. To the skilled eye, the paper reveals details of its significance and clues to the administrative processes involved. The prevailing format of these sixteenth-century certificates indicates routine problems important enough to be documented in the form of a letter.[17] Half-page slips of paper were sufficient for the rather short statements, suggesting that all persons involved knew how to communicate everything necessary for the administrative context in a condensed manner.[18] In undisputed cases, the examiners did no more than refer to the request by the burgomasters or councilors, name the examined person, and characterize the disease. During the second half of the sixteenth and the earlier seventeenth century, most examiners also suggested treatment or support, though this characteristic changed over time. The size of these documents also changed, increasing to a full page by the end of the seventeenth century, though without necessarily more detailed notes; whereas, generally, the size varied with the complexity of the content and could, in some cases, cover more than two pages.[19] Despite such conformity of form, suggestions for how to write these

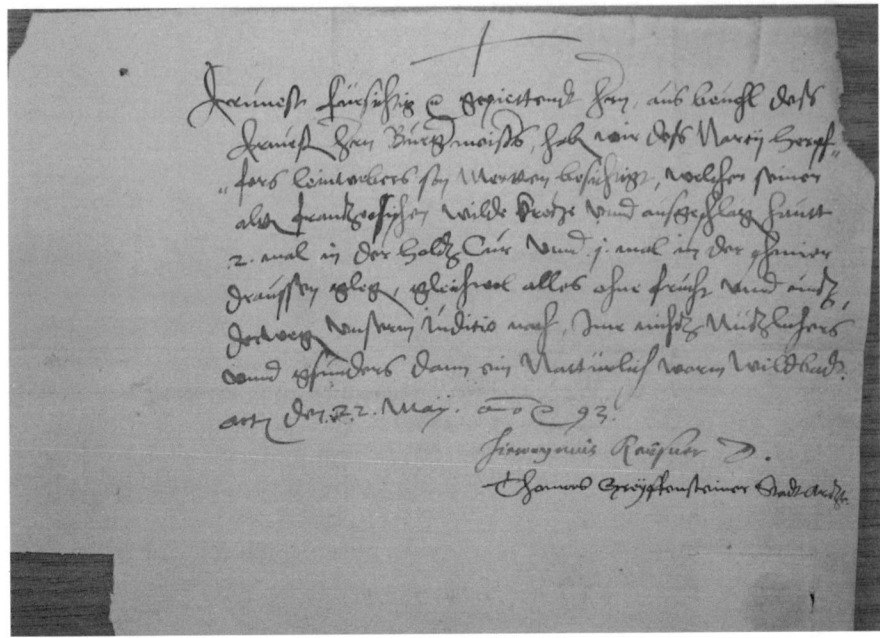

Figure 6.1 Typical sixteenth-century medical certificate (*Schauzettel*). Courtesy of
Stadtarchiv Nördlingen: R39 F2 No. 28, 22 May 1593.

certificates cannot be found in earlier sample books, but only in the early
seventeenth century. Moreover, no explicit administrative instructions for
the writing of these documents have survived from the sixteenth century.[20]

In their address, the certificates seem to convey who had the formal
power to initiate the examination and reporting process. Burgomasters and/
or the councilors are usually referred to as ordering the examination of the
sick or ailing person and demanding a report of the results to the council.
A closer look, however, makes clear that the process was often initiated by
patients, because the writing tends to obfuscate the initiative of oral or written communication between the inhabitants and the councilors of the city.[21]
In a sample of 1593, one in seven patients are indirectly named as initiators
of the examination because the usual reference to the order from the authorities is missing or because the text reveals that the respective person had first
consulted the burgomaster or councilors and demanded to be examined. By
analyzing detailed reports in conflicts and by considering reappearing
patients, it becomes apparent that many inhabitants were initiating the
examination. Obviously, either this fact was not important enough to be
recorded or this initiative was against the intentions of the town's government and, therefore, not mentioned in the certificates.[22]

Although many characteristics of the form were only slightly altered over the centuries, the content did change. Analysis of the content suggests a shift from "scandalized" sickness, such as leprosy or the "French disease," to "scandalized" poverty, which began in the later sixteenth century and was fully developed during the eighteenth century.[23] And in this shift, the texts suggest that most examinations were based on requests of sick and ailing inhabitants of Nördlingen who made the signing persons their spokesmen.

The signatures in Figure 6.1 provide evidence regarding the offices of the medical practitioners who examined the sick persons. The official designations of the offices of medical doctors and artisanal surgeons were still developing during the early modern period: a Christian name, a surname, and the abbreviation "D." for "doctor" came first and signaled one of the two *physici* (town physicians).[24] Each physician was responsible for examining the sick persons for only parts of the respective years, and they took turns after six months. During the sixteenth century, their self-labeling changed with the individual doctor in office, whereas starting in the eighteenth century they generally differentiated between *physicus ordinarius* (second physician) and *physicus senior* (first physician). Differing from such alternation, the *Stadtarzt* testified during the whole year. The title *Stadtarzt* ("town physician") referred here to an artisan: the *Wundarzt* (barber, barber-surgeon, surgeon).[25] He was usually the one writing the text of the certificate. However, we should keep in mind that terms were not yet fixed during the sixteenth century and that this has caused distortions. Sometimes the term *Stadtarzt* was also used for medical doctors. Whereas some medical doctors applied the title *physicus* rather early for themselves, scribes writing contracts and legislative texts did not differentiate consistently between the office of *Stadtarzt* for (barber-)surgeons and the office of *physicus* for medical doctors. It took all of the seventeenth century for the term *physicat* to become established.[26] Such fluidity of terms has caused confusion, and many authors (from the late eighteenth century to historians in the twentieth century) have applied the title of *Stadtarzt* erroneously to physicians only, omitting artisans in office.[27]

Some texts reveal the location of the *Schau*-office in a complex outside of Nördlingen and connect the writing of these certificates to the tradition of leper testimonies.[28] So complex motives of traditional charity, as well as issues of segregation, loomed in the background.[29] Yet the composition of the leper house with a mineral bath, the plague hospital, and the French pox house underscores its association with medical care.[30] These houses had the task of re-establishing an organic function of the city by healing the inhabitants.[31] In the complex's *Blatterstube* (pox room) and behind a curtain, the patient was typically examined within listening proximity of the inmates in this room. From the context of a supplication, we learn that during the sixteenth century, following the routine procedure meant that the patient came into the office of the barber-surgeon for examination and that the medical doctor joined there.[32] A minority of patients were examined in doctors' houses. Sick persons who were unable to walk to the office received a home visit from the doctor and surgeon. Further studies are necessary to determine whether the changes of location—first enforced by the destruction of the complex at the end of the Thirty Years' War and then continued after the reconstruction—relate to changes in local politics.

The wax seal remained a feature of certificates through the end of the town's Imperial status and underscored the official character of these paper slips. Moreover, sealing was supposed to ensure that the content remained confidential and could not be faked.[33] Most certificates were closed with a surgeon's personalized seal, displaying either surgical tools, initials of name and surname, or allusions to the name (for example, a swan for a surgeon by that name).[34] In addition to the fact that examinations were held in the surgeon's office and that he himself handwrote the certificate, the use of surgeons' own seals underscores their significance for these processes of certification. The seal also secured the certificate on its way to the council. The route from the office of the surgeon went from the boundaries of the town, outside its walls, to the center of communication: the town hall.[35] Symbolically as well as bodily, the small problem of one sick inhabitant was thus transferred from the margins to the center of power and authority by means of paper and writing. In the above-mentioned case of conflict, the patient was carrying the paper to the doctor, whence the surgeon wanted to deliver it to the town hall the next day. Such a delivery of official paper provided the surgeon—residing in his office outside the city walls—with an opportunity to enter the political communication center under the cover of office. In conflicts, the surgeon had to try to increase the frequency of his verbal or written exchange with the person in charge of the record office, the *Rath-Schreiber*, or with members of the council, so as to have a chance for such exchange in a society dominated by merchant families.[36]

The extent and limits of power and influence are also preserved on these slips by marks hinting at the following administrative procedures in which the paper was used. In Figure 6.1, the left side shows an excision; the clipping is still covering a seal. Moreover, at the top of the paper, we see a cross. Together with the back of the slip, as displayed in Figure 6.2, this signals the hand of another person in office, the *Rath-Schreiber*. This town official directly linked the burgomaster, the councilors, and the inhabitants of Nördlingen. It was the *Rath-Schreiber*, not the physician or the surgeon or the sick person, who communicated such cases to council in session. Thus the writing of surgeons and physicians was filtered by another person in office who was in everyday exchange with the councilors. Moreover, in preparing these meetings, the *Rath-Schreiber* broke the seal and, in the earlier period, wrote headings on the back of the slip.[37] The surgeon as *Stadtarzt* adopted this administrative writing technique, as illustrated in Figure 6.2, when he wrote the heading "SchauZettul," the name "Mertten Herpffner," the occupation "leinweber" (linen-weaver), and the examination date.

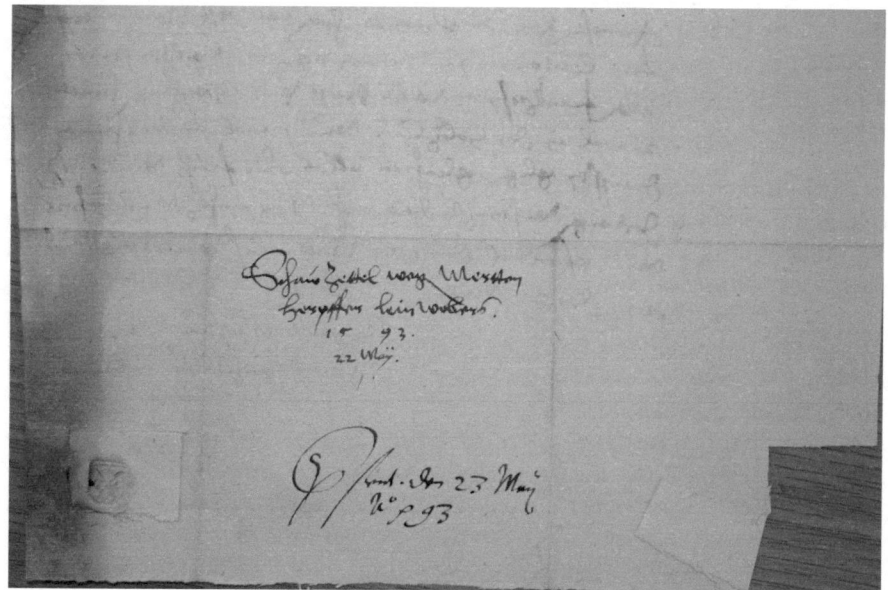

Figure 6.2 Reverse side of certificate in Figure 6.1. Courtesy of Stadtarchiv Nördlingen: R39 F2 No. 28, 22 May 1593.

Figure 6.2 also shows the short interim between writing a certificate and processing it in administration: the *Rath-Schreiber* presented the case to the council one day after examination (May 22–23, 1593). He documented this on the back of the certificate with a corresponding remark ("presented at"), giving the date of the session. The short interval signals priority given to bodily complaints and their certification, and it hints at knowledge the councilors needed either for controlling their subjects or for enacting their bonds with the community.[38] The result of such communication in council is rarely noted down on the certificate. Until the nineteenth century, the *Rath-Schreiber* signaled with a cross on the inside that the content and decisions were documented in separate, daily minutes of the proceedings in the town hall. The details of this administrative writing were supposed to remain secret. Yet entries recorded evidence, and their symbolic value is conveyed by the ornate binding of the bulky registers passed down through the ages in most Imperial towns.[39]

In these ways, the paper slips belonged to a mixture of oral and written administrative processes. Whereas doctor and surgeon had to write down their results, the writing and reporting official in the town hall communicated the case orally to the council. The decisions seem also to have been communicated orally to practitioners and patients. Separate paper slips providing this information were introduced in specific (mostly forensic) cases as extracts from the minutes and filed with the certificate and the proceedings.

The political dimension is underscored by the fact that the content of the *SchauZettul* was discussed by the councilors and then transferred into the minutes of the council to be kept forever. Furthermore, the medical practitioner as writer in office became simultaneously a stakeholder in the outcome of interaction between the authorities and sick inhabitants.[40] This procedure of oral and written communication lasted for centuries and was not fundamentally altered until the nineteenth century, when the Bavarian administration—after mediatization—introduced the practice of writing bodily examination results and council decisions together on a single sheet. A large centralized state needed more concise documentation.[41]

All in all, this long story of certification underscores the importance of ongoing oral communication—mediated by medical officeholders—between persons in power and other citizens in Nördlingen. This mid-sized Imperial town displays continuity rather than the discontinuity in politics characteristic of bigger cities.[42] The councilors and burgomasters seem to have remained in need of the symbolic capital they earned by dealing with inhabitants' everyday concerns.[43]

Acting with Paper in Conflicts

The foregoing discussion of the forms of writing and administrative processing showed how the writing of these certificates was an integral part of local politics. The political dimension and social dynamics become more obvious when analyzing the acts and writings occurring in the specific circumstances of a conflict. The implications for the medical doctors, surgeons, examined persons, councilors, and early modern society more generally can be seen by zooming in on the year 1594, especially on the aforementioned conflict appearing in certificates, on the content of other *SchauZettul* that diverged from the usual short form, and on additional reports of conflicts.

The first conflict to be analyzed is the scandalized behavior of the medical doctor (*physicus* Reusner) who ripped apart the certificate written by the surgeon (*StadtArzt* Greiffenstein), as mentioned at the beginning of this chapter. The text of the ripped certificate, as reproduced by Greiffenstein, provides clues to Reusner's motivation in tearing the paper:

> [...] we have now for the third time inspected Els Mößlerin, who according to our inspection and advice has been using the May Bath, but could not attend for the full term because she developed a new and evil rash on body and thigh. Because of this, the Wood Cure would have been not inappropriate, but considering her very old age,

that (according to the Doctor) would have been too hard and intolerable, therefore the Hand Cure in the Upper Room is considered to be advisable, actum 23 May [15]94.[44]

The surgeon suggested the "Wood Cure," a complex treatment during which "Holy" or guaiac wood was to be cooked and consumed.[45] Acting with discretion, he was applying the double-negative "nicht vndienstlich" ("not un-appropriate") to his suggestion. Moreover, Greiffenstein hinted in parenthesis at diverging opinions concerning the proper treatment of the patient. No matter how cautious, Greiffenstein thus disclosed disagreement over the appropriate cure, and Reusner reacted by tearing the surgeon's certificate apart, probably in the presence of the patient.

The fury of the doctor concerning the surgeon's insubordinate attitude can be attributed only partly to questions of the medical doctor's status, whose peers were striving to be accepted as part of the social elite.[46] Ripping the document was a symbolic act. It aimed at making the rupture between the doctor and the surgeon visible and the disagreement more public, and thereby at forcing the authorities to act and come to a decision. The surgeon's account in the context of another conflict underscores the doctor's success. The disagreement described above was just an interlude in a much more complex smoldering conflict concerning contested medical expertise, which was archived in a different context.[47]

The quarrel had started about two months earlier on April 4, 1594, and continued through July. According to their reports, which were also processed in the council, Reusner and Greiffenstein exchanged mutual accusations, which included severe allegations of malpractice. Reusner accused the surgeon of deceptively hiding an imperfect therapy of a boy's injured leg during an examination, thereby severely endangering the health of the boy. Reusner made use of the instrument of the certificate, enriched with testimonies of other surgeons, to justify his allegations.[48] The controversy intensified after a hearing in front of Senior Councilors. This hearing occurred in the aftermath of Reusner's symbolic tearing apart of the certificate. According to the surgeon, he was taken by surprise, whereas the doctor was well prepared. To these circumstances Greiffenstein attributed his official reproof six weeks later on July 1. At the end of July, Greiffenstein sent in his final and "repeated supplication" to the council, which launched a sweeping attack on the medical doctor.[49] In six tightly and diligently written pages, he accused Reusner of being reluctant in fulfilling his tasks in the examination and inspection office. Moreover, Greiffenstein charged Reusner with intrusion into the art of surgery without proper knowledge. The surgeon contrasted the doctor's incomplete knowledge gained from reading books with his own supreme surgical and anatomical knowledge gained from observing and practicing. The accusations culminated in allegations of malpractice, implying that Reusner had caused the death of several prominent persons with his aggressive cures. Among the victims, the surgeon named citizens and inhabitants of neighboring territories, including burgomasters and a prelate. Finally, he accused the doctor of acting against "order" by alienating patients from the surgeon with hollow promises because he envied the surgeon's success in and beyond the city.

With such allegations, Greiffenstein endangered the trust of inhabitants and neighbors in the competence of the council, whose members had chosen Reusner as town physician. Charging malpractice by a town physician in foreign territory endangered the always fragile balance between this Lutheran Imperial town and its neighboring Catholic territories.[50] Therefore, such severe accusations must have arisen from sheer desperation, explained partly by Greiffenstein's allusion to his fears concerning his reputation at the council. Such fears were based on the more general knowledge that the councilors would disapprove of his communicating a disagreement between persons who were intertwined closely with evidence-finding by the authorities. Councilors preferred to be heard as one voice.[51]

Additionally, severe conflicts had become a potential danger for the whole community. Shortly before the quarrel between physician and surgeon, tensions and clashes between other inhabitants of Nördlingen had culminated in a considerable surge in witch-hunting. In 1593, the hunt had spread through all layers of society; those executed included members of the medical trade and wives and widows of socially well-established families, even relatives of councilors.[52] Therefore, it was hardly a coincidence that after Greiffenstein's severe allegations, in which he also included a critique of the barber-surgeon in the pestilence house, he lost favor with the councilors and was punished as a troublemaker: two years later his contract as *Stadtarzt* was not renewed, and he was offered the less prestigious office of pestilence surgeon.[53] The medical doctor's punishment was even more indirect. Into the first decade of the seventeenth century there are only a few certificates he signed alone; instead, he often had to sign with a team, either the second physician and a surgeon or two (barber-) surgeons. Moreover, Reusner was not promoted to the office of senior physician.[54]

The consensus of medical practitioners in office was also crucial because their role as *experts* was by no means established. Neither the councilors nor the other inhabitants accepted the certificates as final expertise; the results were, rather, to be negotiated. The third examination of the diseased women (Els Mößler), occasioning the disagreement discussed in this chapter, is just one example of many repeated medical examinations ordered by the council. The burgomaster or councilors frequently demanded another examination in order to gain more detailed information concerning, for example, why a suggested cure had not had the expected success; what alternative might restore health; what prognosis justified further expenses; or why the authorities were to support a person.[55] Repeated processes of certification were also initiated by sick persons wanting to get a specific treatment or a different medical label for their sickness.[56]

Publicly known disagreement between medical doctor and surgeon in office was also unacceptable for the governors of Nördlingen because it invited attempts of fraud by patients. Hardly by coincidence, Greiffenstein reported such an attempt a couple of months after his conflicts with Reusner, and he used this occasion to display an ideal harmony between himself and another doctor, the second physician in office. According to Greiffenstein's account, Maria Adam appeared in his office in October 1594 with skin problems (*geflecht*) and assured him (in the presence of his wife and daughters) that her body showed no other signs of disease. Greiffenstein's account stresses that he assured her these complaints could be cured in a couple of weeks in the *Oberstube*, a room in the leprosy complex. Maria Adam then went to the newly appointed second town physician, Dr. Johann Graff, supposedly complaining of differing ailments. Graff and Greiffenstein, however, were in touch and discovered the differing complaints. Together they wrote a certificate recommending a "sweat bath" (*Schweißbad*). Greiffenstein reported that this caused Maria Adam to go to the surgeon in charge of the pestilence house and, finally, to Reusner.[57]

As mentioned above, patients challenging medical expertise were by no means unusual, and many patients would consult several medical doctors or surgeons if they disagreed with the suggested treatment.[58] But concealing or feigning signs of sickness was considered to be attempted fraud. Unfortunately for Maria Adam, the four medical practitioners in office agreed to report her to the council, underscoring that their *Schauzettel* recommended a couple of weeks cure in the "upper room" (*Oberstube*), at much less expense than the winter months spent in the pox house. They suggested that the latter was what Maria Adam had in mind.

By writing this report, the doctors and surgeons in office wanted to display not just a re-established harmony but, additionally, their consideration of the common welfare—a quality that jurists tried to claim exclusively for themselves.[59] For the authorities, such a prospect of keeping costs down was rather important because the 1590s culminated in the "crisis" of the late sixteenth century, with high food prices and, in 1593–94, epidemic diseases looming in neighboring Imperial towns, threatening to diminish communal finances.[60]

Assessing in Town, on Paper, and in the World of Scholars

The conflict between Reusner and Greiffenstein also points to a tension caused by a hierarchical superiority of the medical doctor, understood in terms of status, yet a de facto equality in practice, including the writing of certificates. Moreover, *equality* here also refers to social practice, bonding and networking in such mid-sized towns as Nördlingen.

Physicians' and surgeons' traces in Nördlingen go back to the Middle Ages. Until the last third of the sixteenth century, the office of physicians was rather limited compared with that of (barber-)surgeons. Physicians were asked to provide advice on how to prevent epidemic disease, whereas the medical treatment of the diseased was in the hands of surgeons in the office of *Pestbarbier* (pestilence surgeon).[61] Series of certificates in Nördlingen reveal that, through the late 1580s, a minority of testimonies (mostly concerning suspected leprosy) were written by physicians or by teams of physicians and (barber-)surgeons. In contrast, most certificates were signed by the man in office at the leprosy complex.[62] This surgeon was also in charge of cures in the *Blatterhaus* (pox house), where those suspected of suffering from the French disease were cured.[63] Moreover, before the end of the Thirty Years' War, the *Blatterstube* (pox room), where most examinations were performed, recalls a tradition in which the surgeon, not the doctor, was the person in charge. Such appreciation for specific services of surgeons was not a distinctive trait of the Nördlingen councilors. During the sixteenth century, the neighboring large Imperial City of Nuremberg regularly paid surgeons high compensation for their assurance to provide surgical services to Nuremberg's burghers for short, limited periods. Among those practitioners in Nuremberg who came from nearby Imperial towns was the surgeon family Greiffenstein from Nördlingen. The Nuremberg council paid Thoman Greiffenstein 20 florins per year for practicing as *Augenarzt* (eye specialist) for just a couple of days around Easter and Michaelmas.[64]

Physician and surgeon were similar in their association with communities that transcended the local, but they differed regarding their social bonding and networks in the town.[65] The family of the surgeon Greiffenstein had been established in local society for generations. Prior to Thomas, Caspar and Thoman also served as *Stadtarzt* in Nördlingen and had been sought after by neighboring bigger towns, which added to their prestige.[66] Although a deep embedding in local society was typical for barbers, barber-surgeons, and surgeons, their journeymen tours helped them avoid limiting their medical and social experience, as did their visiting contracts with other towns.[67] In communicating with the Nördlingen council, Thomas Greiffenstein even suggested his superior experience by emphasizing that he knew the anatomy of the human body from familiarity with teaching at German and French universities, from observing and assisting famous surgeons, and from experience at European courts.[68] The physician Reusner, coming from Löwenberg (Lwówek) in Silesia, had to rely on social relations developed mostly outside Nördlingen, albeit ever more densely in southern areas of the German-speaking lands. After studies in Leipzig, he began his doctorate in Basel and solidified bonds through publishing and through kinship and matrimony. His well-established relative, the jurist and Imperial Poet Nicolaus Reusner (1545–1602) in Lauingen (Danube), supported him during a first residence there.[69] Nicolaus's reputation helped in arranging his marriage to Waldburg Medelin, daughter of a councillor in Lauingen.[70] In this way, a twofold network to neighboring Augsburg was established: Nicolaus Reusner had lived in Augsburg for a couple of years as a participant in the Reichstag and as a teacher at the St. Anna secondary school, and Waldburg Medelin's sister was married into the influential apothecary and merchant family Welsch in Augsburg. The Welsch family provided links into the elite of Nördlingen.[71]

Reusner's professional activities illustrate how writing and publishing could become a means to establish and secure networks. Such activities could compensate for a missing, deeper integration into a town's society, thereby also laying foundations for prestige and authority. During Reusner's first year in Lauingen, the medical doctor established a friendship with the Paracelsian author Martin Ruland the Elder, who was town physician in Lauingen and personal physician to the Palatine duke, Philipp Ludwig.[72] Ruland's connections to the Palatine court most probably provided Reusner with the opportunity to study the collection of Paracelsus's manuscripts in nearby Neuburg (Danube).[73] In Reusner's dedication to the first edition of *Pandora*, an elaborately illustrated alchemical book he published in 1582, he emphasized Ruland's contributions.[74] A contemporary reader noted that *Pandora* quickly became extremely rare on the market and could only be bought for a fortune. Also in 1582, Reusner published a urinary manuscript by the Bohemian scholar Jodocus Willich.[75] In so doing, he signaled eastern scholarly ties on which he may have counted when corresponding with the Silesian Melchior Sebisch (1539–1625), who was professor of medicine in Strasbourg, another big Imperial city. In 1583, again in Lauingen, while establishing contact between Sebisch and his relative Nicolaus Reusner, he expressed his hopes of finding a post in Strasbourg.[76]

Certificates and Knowledge

Reusner's decades of practice as town physician in Nördlingen showed very limited impact on his printed publications. Explicitly for his employers in Nördlingen, he produced only one small booklet concerning directives ("Ordnung") in times of pestilence.[77] Moreover, Reusner's style was far removed from the new genre of observation literature.[78] He often disguised his own observations in an abundance of citations from traditional and recent medical literature. Furthermore, he tended not to give detailed information, for example, regarding his remedies for scurvy.[79] He also included case studies from other authors and did not name his patients apart from family members or prominent personalities.[80] In his book on scurvy, which also proliferated in bigger Imperial towns, he did not mention even one of the certified sick persons.[81] Rather differently from his successors, Reusner also hardly ever diagnosed scurvy in his certificates.[82] This indicates that medical terms had to be well established in public in order to be included in the writing of certificates. Despite the fact that writing certificates might be considered medical practice, experience from such practice was not transferred into books; rather, books had to make experience well known before it could make its way into certificates.

In Reusner's books and shared manuscripts of observations produced during his more than 30 years as a physician in office in Nördlingen, only one case from his hundreds of written certificates was found worthy of appearing in print. Significantly, this was the conflict from the year 1594. In the printed version, the case of the boy suffering from an injured leg was not about contested medical expertise; instead, it was turned into a medical observation. In the manuscript that he shared with others and that was post-humously published, Reusner simply pointed to mistakes ("male curato") of unnamed practitioners and the immediate success of his own prescriptions.[83] This manuscript case also indicates that sharing observations was not Reusner's primary aim. He wanted to document his superiority in surgery and in practice, exactly the field in which he had been challenged by the surgeon.

However, rather differently from colleagues publishing at universities and many decades later, neither Reusner nor his posthumous publisher directly named or criticized the surgeon.[84] Despite the conflict, the sources indicate that a joint examination and writing practice prevailed in mid-size communities until the beginning of the nineteenth century. In writing certificates, surgeons and physicians in office participated in the day-to-day communication between members of the council and other members of the community. The official form of these certificates and their prompt processing testify to the importance given to these papers. Changes in form suggest a knowledge transfer over time from administration to medical officers. This seems to have affected the surgeons most, as most certificates displayed their handwriting.

In analyzing the language and medical content of Reusner's and other *Schauzettel* of Nördlingen, we find continuities beyond what has been described above and elsewhere. Medical terms, even in Latin, were used, yet not those of the scholarly discussions of the day but, rather, those of "scandalized" diseases. Descriptions of symptoms and vivid metaphors (for example, that frost and heat had attacked) prevail.[85] In phrases such as "he complains of," the patient is increasingly named as the source of such descriptions.[86] Moreover, phrases such as "she begs the high magistrate to provide her with the lazaretto aid" suggest that medical officers increasingly became the voice of ailing, sick and needy persons.[87] However, a thorough and comparative analysis of language and medical content of *Schauzettel* for the centuries of their existence remains a *desideratum*.

Notes

Acknowledgments: This chapter was developed during my participation in the ERC-funded project "Ways of Writing: How Physicians Know, 1550–1950," and I thank my colleagues for the discussions. The article also benefited from comments and discussions of participants in the three workshops leading up to this volume. I am indebted to Mary Terrall (University of California, Los Angeles) and Alfred Weiß (University of Salzburg) for their supportive and critical comments during the final workshop.

1 For a detailed analysis of this society, see Christopher R. Friedrichs, *Urban Society in an Age of War: Nördlingen, 1580–1720* (Princeton, 1979).

2 For the complex meaning of "republic," see Ruth Schilling, *Stadtrepublik und Selbstbehauptung: Venedig, Bremen, Hamburg und Lübeck im 16.–17. Jahrhundert* (Cologne, 2012), pp. 1–6.

3 Alexander C.H. Bagus, *Schwäbische Reichsstädte am Ende des Alten Reiches: Zeiten des Umbruchs in Nördlingen, Aalen und Schwäbisch Gmünd* (Aachen, 2011), pp. 122–23.

4 These men in office were often notaries and sometimes also councillors; see *Notariatbuch: Wes einem Schreiber oder Notarien [...] zu wissen sey [...]* (Frankfurt, 1535). On archives, see Markus Friedrich, *Die Geburt des Archivs: Eine Wissensgeschichte* (Munich, 2013).

5 Christoph Dartmann, "Furor: Konfliktpraktiken und Ordnungsvorstellungen im kommunalen Siena," in Christoph Dartmann, Marian Füssel and Stefanie Rüther (eds), *Raum und Konflikt: Zur symbolischen Konstituierung gesellschaftlicher Ordnung in Mittelalter und Früher Neuzeit* (Münster, 2004): 129–53, pp. 144–47.

6 Jeannette Rauschert, "Gelöchert und befleckt: Inszenierung und Gebrauch städtischer Rechtstexte und spätmittelalterlicher Öffentlichkeit," in Karl Brunner (ed.), *Text als Realie* (Vienna, 2003): 163–81.

7 The concept of "negotiating" was developed in the 1990s and is useful for analyses of early modern societies; more recently see Stefan Brakensiek, "Herrschaftsvermittlung im alten Europa: Praktiken lokaler Justiz, Politik und Verwaltung im internationalen Vergleich," in Stefan Brakensiek (ed.), *Ergebene Diener ihrer Herren? Herrschaftsvermittlung im alten Europa* (Cologne, 2005): 1–21, pp. 4–5; James Lee, "Political Intermediaries, Political Engagement and the Politics of Everyday Life in Urban Tudor England," in Rudolf Schlögl (ed.), *Urban Elections and Decision-Making in Early Modern Europe, 1500–1800* (Newcastle upon Tyne, 2009): 179–95.

8 Hagen Keller, "Vorschrift, Mitschrift, Nachschrift: Instrumente des Willens zu vernunftgemäßem Handeln und guter Regierung in den italienischen Kommunen des Duecento," in Hagen Keller, Christel Meier and Thomas Scharff (eds), *Schriftlichkeit und Lebenspraxis im Mittelalter: Erfassen, Bewahren, Verändern* (Munich, 1999): 25–41, pp. 27–35.

9 Annemarie Kinzelbach, "Konstruktion und konkretes Handeln: Heilkundige Frauen im oberdeutschen Raum, 1450–1700," *Historische Anthropologie* 7 (1999): 165–90; Mitchell L. Hammond, "Medical Examination and Poor Relief in Early Modern Germany," *Social History of Medicine*, 24 (2011): 244–59; Annemarie Kinzelbach, "Armut und Kranksein in der frühneuzeitlichen Stadt: Oberdeutsche Reichsstädte im Vergleich," in Konrad Krimm, Dorothee Mussgnug and Theodor Strohm (eds), *Armut und Fürsorge in der frühen Neuzeit* (Ostfildern, 2011): 141–76; Annemarie Kinzelbach, "*an jetzt grasierender kranckheit sehr schwer darnieder:* 'Schau' und Kontext in süddeutschen Reichsstädten der frühen Neuzeit," in Carl C. Wahrmann, Martin Buchsteiner and Antje Strahl (eds), *Seuche und Mensch* (Berlin, 2012): 269–82.

10 Kinzelbach, "Schau," pp. 271–73.

11 Reusner's network, for example, stretched into Eastern Europe, beyond the usual boundaries; Gábor Almási, *The Uses of Humanism: Johannes Sambucus (1531–1584), Andreas Dudith (1533–1589), and the Republic of Letters in East Central Europe* (Leiden and Boston, 2009), p. 75. For genres and town physicians, see Gianna Pomata, "Observation Rising: Birth of an Epistemic Genre, 1500–1650," in Lorraine Daston and Elizabeth Lunbeck (eds), *Histories of Scientific Observation* (Chicago, 2011): 45–80, p. 59; Michael Stolberg,

"Medizinische *Loci communes:* Formen und Funktionen einer ärztlichen Aufzeichnungspraxis im 16. und 17. Jahrhundert," *NTM Zeitschrift für Geschichte
der Naturwissenschaften, Technik und Medizin,* 21 (2013): 37–60.

12 See Annemarie Kinzelbach, *Gesundbleiben, Krankwerden, Armsein in der
frühneuzeitlichen Gesellschaft* (Stuttgart, 1995), pp. 43–46, 125–31, 194–98;
Annemarie Kinzelbach and Patrick Sturm, "Der Siechenhauskomplex vor
den Toren Nördlingens: Entwicklung, Funktion und bauliche Gestalt vom
13. bis zum 18. Jahrhundert," *Jahrbuch Nördlingen,* 33 (2011): 25–54, pp.
36–46.

13 For the political, social, and cultural implications of archiving, see Friedrich,
Geburt.

14 For this change, see Kinzelbach, "Schau," pp. 278–82.

15 Examples of file titles and numbering: StadtANoe R39 F2 No. 28–33; example
of changed file title: R39 F3 No. 63. On political aspects of poor relief in the
context of early modern Imperial Towns, see Kinzelbach, *Gesundbleiben,* with
references consultable from the index entries on pp. 478 and 483; Claudia
Stein, *Die Behandlung der Franzosenkrankheit in der Frühen Neuzeit am Beispiel Augsburgs* (Stuttgart, 2003), pp. 172–83; Hammond, "Examination"; Kinzelbach, "Armut."

16 StadtANoe R39 F2 No. 7–9; see now also J. Andrew Mendelsohn and Annemarie Kinzelbach, "Common Knowledge: Bodies, Evidence and Expertise in
Early Modern Germany," *Isis* 108/2 (2017): 259–79.

17 StadtANoe R39 F2 No. 12–33.

18 For condensed communication, see Hagen, *Vorschrift.*

19 StadtANoe R39 F2 No. 42–46; No. 12, 1549; No. 29, 20 November 1594,
28 May 1596; No. 46, 11 February 1712, 4 October 1713.

20 For templates for official letters and contracts, see *Cantzleybüchlein. Zeiget an
Wie man Schreiben sol [...]* (Straßburg, 1522) and later editions by Moritz
Breunle; Alexander Machholth, *Formular oder Schreiber Buch* (Eisleben,
1559); templates for examination results: Johann R. Sattler, *Thesaurus Notar-
iorum* (Basel, 1614), 816–17.

21 Patrick Oelze, "Decision-Making and Civic Participation in the Imperial City
(Fifteenth and Sixteenth Century): Guild Conventions and Open Councils in
Constance," in Schlögl, *Urban Elections,* 147–78, p. 177.

22 StadtANoe R39 F 2 No. 28; No. 28, 1593.05.22./23, 1593.07.22, 1593.12.17,
1593.12.24; No. 29, 1594.11.20. For problems identifying the initiator, see
Fritz Dross and Annemarie Kinzelbach, *"nit mehr alls sein burger, sonder alls
ein frembder*: Fremdheit und Aussatz in frühneuzeitlichen Reichsstädten," *Medizinhistorisches Journal,* 46 (2011): 1–23, pp. 7–12.

23 Alfons Labisch suggested the term "scandalized" (*skandalisiert*) for diseases
like syphilis, in which high public attention must be seen alongside rather low
demographic relevance; see Kinzelbach, "Schau," pp. 278–82. Further comparative analyses are necessary.

24 See Dross, "'De Officiis'," Chapter 4 of this volume; and Schlegelmilch, "Promoting a Good Physician," Chapter 3 of this volume.

25 For the complicated professional differentiation of these artisans, see Annemarie Kinzelbach, "Erudite and Honoured Artisans? Performers of Body Care
and Surgery in Early Modern German Towns," *Social History of Medicine,* 27
(2014): 668–88.

26 StadtANoe R39 F1 No. 10–13; F2 No. 12 – F3 No. 63. During the sixteenth
and seventeenth centuries in neighboring Imperial towns, contracts for medical
doctors appointed them to the office of *Statt Leibarzt* (1511, 1530), or *Arzat*
for the inhabitants (1573), or *Statt Arzet* (1595), as well as to the combination

of *physico und/ald Stattarzet* (1583–1687), Überlingen StadtA Rp 21.09.1511; 2,20,1022; 2,21,1031; Ulm StadtA A[4403]; Philipp Ludwig Wittwer, *Entwurf einer Geschichte des Kollegiums der Aerzte in der Reichsstadt Nürnberg* (Nuremberg, 1792).

27 In 1780, Adelung's encyclopedia does not provide an article under the keyword *Stadtarzt*; instead, Adelung refers the reader to the keyword *Physikat*. There, however, he applies the neutral term *Arzt*, under which he also included the artisans. In contrast, in 1837, the detailed encyclopedia of Krünitz referred to medical doctors exclusively; see Johann Christoph Adelung, *Versuch eines vollständigen grammatisch–kritischen Wörterbuches der hochdeutschen Mundart* (Leipzig, 1774 and 1780), vols. 1 and 4; Johann Georg Krünitz, *Oeconomische Encyklopädie, [...]* (1773–1858; online, Trier: Universitätsbibliothek, 2001), vol. 167 (http://opacplus. bsb–muenchen.de/search?oclcno=643049918), accessed September 17, 2013; historians have generally followed suit, though some have differentiated, such as Gerhard Naber, "Der Arzt als städtischer Amtsträger im alten Amberg" (Diss. Univ. Erlangen–Nürnberg, 1967), p. 3.

28 Kinzelbach, "Schau."

29 Carole Rawcliffe, *Leprosy in Medieval England* (Woodbridge, 2006).

30 Kinzelbach and Sturm, "Siechenhauskomplex."

31 Carole Rawcliffe, "The Concept of Health in Late Medieval Society," in Simonetta Cavaciocchi (ed.), *Le interazioni fra economia e ambiente biologico nell'Europa preindustriale, secc. XIII–XVIII* (Florence, 2010): 317–34, p. 317.

32 StadtANoe R39 F1 No. 11, 1594.07.31.

33 Gabriela Signori, "Einleitung," in Signori (ed.), *Das Siegel: Gebrauch und Bedeutung* (Darmstadt, 2007): 9–20.

34 StadtANoe R39 F2 No. 12 (Hans Hörzog), No. 27, 28 (Stephan Schwan), No. 33 (Veit Gentzler).

35 See Christopher R. Friedrichs, "Das städtische Rathaus als kommunikativer Raum in europäischer Perspektive," in Johannes Burkhardt and Christine Werkstetter (eds), *Kommunikation und Medien in der Frühen Neuzeit* (Munich, 2005): 159–74, pp. 164–66.

36 StadtANoe R39 F1 No. 11, 1594.07.31, Greiffenstein insinuated that Reusner preferred to frequent the drinking hall of the merchants on Sundays, instead of joining in on the examinations in the leprosy complex outside town.

37 For duties in this office, see Manfred J. Schmied, *Die Ratsschreiber der Reichsstadt Nürnberg* (Nuremberg, 1979), pp. 84–55, 137–38.

38 Michael Aumüller, "Informationsverdichtung als Herrschaftsintensivierung?" in Anja Horstmann and Vanina Kopp (eds), *Archiv – Macht – Wissen: Organisation und Konstruktion von Wissen und Wirklichkeiten in Archiven* (Frankfurt a.M., 2010): 39–54, pp. 42–88; Schilling, *Stadtrepublik*, pp. 222–37.

39 For secrecy, see Friedrichs, "Rathaus," p. 167; for symbolic context, see Schilling, *Stadtrepublik*, pp. 61–105.

40 For politics as "empowering interaction," see Randolph C. Head, "Modes of Reading, Community Practice and the Constitution of Textual Authority in the Thurgau und Graubünden, 1520–1660," in Wim Blockmans, André Holenstein and Jon Mathieu (eds), *Empowering Interactions: Political Cultures and the Emergence of the State in Europe, 1300–1900* (Farnham, 2009): 115–29, p. 128.

41 See, for Prussia, Cornelia Vismann, *Akten: Medientechnik und Recht* (Frankfurt a.M., 2000), pp. 204–16.

42 The focus is also on corporations in Philip R. Hoffmann-Rehnitz, "Discontinuities: Political Transformation, Media Change, and the City in the Holy Roman Empire from the Fifteenth to Seventeenth Centuries," in Jason P. Coy,

Benjamin Marschke and David W. Sabean (eds), *The Holy Roman Empire, Reconsidered* (New York, 2010): 11–34, pp. 16–21.

43 Alexander Schlaak, "Overloaded Interaction: Effects of the Growing Use of Writing in German Imperial Cities, 1500–1800," in *Holy Roman Empire*, 35–47, p. 44.

44 In translating, I have kept as close as possible to the German text and original punctuation; StadtANoe R39 F2 No. 29, 23/24 May 1594.

45 The Wood Cure was first used for the treatment of the French disease; see Annemarie Kinzelbach, "*Böse Blattern* oder *Franzosenkrankheit*: Syphilis–konzept, Kranke und die Genese des Krankenhauses in oberdeutschen Reichsstädten der frühen Neuzeit," in Martin Dinges and Thomas Schlich (eds), *Neue Wege in der Seuchengeschichte* (Stuttgart, 1995): 43–69, pp. 58–59. Then the Wood Cure was expanded to various diseases; see Jon Arrizabalaga, John Henderson, and Roger French, *The Great Pox: The French Disease in Renaissance Europe* (New Haven, 1997), pp. 187–90. All in all, it was one of the more popular New World remedies; Harold J. Cook and Timothy D. Walker, "Circulation of Medicine in the Early Modern Atlantic World," *Social History of Medicine*, 26 (2013): 337–51, pp. 340–41.

46 Marian Füssel, *Gelehrtenkultur als symbolische Praxis: Rang, Ritual und Konflikt an der Universität der Frühen Neuzeit* (Darmstadt, 2006).

47 StadtANoe R39 F1 No. 11, reports by Greifenstein and Reusner, from May 2 to July 31, 1594.

48 StadtANoe R39 F1 No. 11, 30 April 1594.

49 StadtANoe R39 F1 No. 11, 31 July 1594.

50 This balance remained a challenge to the end of the town's Imperial status; Bagus, *Reichsstädte*, pp. 122–23.

51 Friedrichs, "Rathaus," p. 167.

52 Kinzelbach, "Konstruktion," pp. 168–74; Sonja Kinzler, "Hexenprozesse in Nördlingen," in *historicum.net* (www.historicum.net/themen/hexenforschung/lexikon/alphabetisch/h-o/art/Noerdlingen_He/html/artikel/1641/ca/516b55ca5f/), accessed December 18, 2013.

53 StadtANoe R39 F2 No. 03, 15 December 1596; No. 6, 3 November 1597; No. 12, 19 December 1580; F1 No. 20, 14 November 1576, 28 March 1600; F1 No. 11, 31 July 1594.

54 StadtANoe R39 F2 No. 31–33; F1 No. 10, quarterly receipts of Reusner, 1590–1623.

55 StadtANoe R39 F2 No. 28, 16 January 1592, 18 January 1592, 9 May 1592, 30 June 1592, 16 October 1592, 21 October 1592, 5 December 1592.

56 Cf. Hammond, "Examination," p. 250; Kinzelbach, "Schau," p. 274.

57 StadtANoe R39 F2 No. 29, 20 November 1594.

58 Decades of research into patients' histories have made this clear; see Gianna Pomata, *La promessa di Guarigione* (Rome, 1994); Robert Jütte, *Ärzte, Heiler und Patienten* (Munich, 1991).

59 See Sabine Holtz, *Bildung und Herrschaft: Zur Verwissenschaftlichung politischer Führungsschichten im 17. Jahrhundert* (Leinfelden–Echterdingen, 2002), p. 93.

60 For the crises, see Wolfgang Behringer, "*Kleine Eiszeit* und Frühe Neuzeit," in Wolfgang Behringer, Hartmut Lehmann and Christian Pfister (eds), *Kulturelle Konsequenzen der "Kleinen Eiszeit"* (Göttingen, 2005): 415–508; for epidemic diseases, see Patrick Sturm, *Leben mit dem Tod in den Reichsstädten Esslingen, Nördlingen und Schwäbisch Hall. Epidemien und deren Auswirkungen vom frühen 15. bis zum frühen 17. Jahrhundert* (Ostfildern, 2014), pp. 33–71.

61 Sturm, *Leben*, pp. 275–90.

62 StadtANoe R39 F2 No. 12.
63 Kinzelbach and Sturm, "Siechenhauskomplex."
64 Stadtarchiv Nuremberg (hereafter: StadtAN), A1 1573.09.29 (three-year contract); special thanks to Fritz Dross, who shared this and other contracts.
65 Georg Simmel, *Soziologie: Untersuchungen über die Formen der Vergesellschaftung* (Leipzig, 1908), pp. 410–12; I am grateful to Alexander Kästner whose comments reminded me of this study.
66 StadtAN A1 1573.09.29; StadtANoe R39 F1, No. 03; F1, No. 19, 1571–1580; F2 No. 12, 1547–1550.
67 Kinzelbach, "Artisans."
68 StadtANoe R39 F1 No. 11, 31 July 1594.
69 Hieronymus Reusner, *Decisiones praecipuorum aliquot aporhematon iatrophilosophikon* (Basilea, 1582); dedication to D. Nicolao Revsnero; Hermann Wiegand, "Reusner, Nikolaus von," in Walther Killy (ed.), *Literaturlexikon* (Gütersloh, 1988–1991): vol. 9, 400–01.
70 Gustav Wulz, "Verzeichnis der Leichenpredigten der Stadtbibliothek Nördlingen," *Blätter des Bayerischen Landesvereins für Familienkunde* 12 (1934): 21–27, 37–42, 54–66.
71 Melchior and Hieronymus Welsch were councillors; see Friedrichs, *Society*, pp. 171, 330–31. Hieronymus Reusner and Georg H. Welsch, *Curationes et observationes medicae* (Augsburg, 1668), p. 3; Lucas Schroeck, *Memoria Welschiana, sive Historia vitae viri celeberrimi, Du. Georgii Hieronymi Welschii, Augustani [...]* (Augsburg, 1678); Wolfgang Reinhard and Mark Häberlein, *Augsburger Eliten des 16. Jahrhunderts: Prosopographie wirtschaftlicher und politischer Führungsgruppen, 1500–1620* (Berlin, 1996), pp. 778–79. For the mechanisms of application, see Schlegelmilch, "Promoting a Good Physician," Chapter 3 of this volume.
72 For Martin Ruland the Elder, see Gianna Pomata, "Sharing Cases: The *Observationes* in Early Modern Medicine," *Early Science and Medicine*, 15 (2010): 193–236, p. 214.
73 Hugh Trevor-Roper, "The Court Physician and Paracelsianism," in Vivian Nutton (ed.), *Medicine at the Courts of Europe, 1500–1837* (London, 1990): 79–94.
74 Hieronymus Reusner, *Pandora, das ist die edelste Gab Gottes [...]* (Basel, 1582), BSB Res/Alch. 88, exlibris annotation.
75 Hieronymus Reusner and Jodocus Willich, *Urinarum Probationes, D. Iodoci Wilichii Reselliani* (Basileae, 1582).
76 Many thanks to Sabine Schlegelmilch who provided the relevant files from the database of "Ärztebriefe."
77 Hieronymus Reusner, *Nvtzliche Artzneyordnung wie man sich zur zeit regierender Pestilentz verhalten solle. [...]* (Lauingen, 1597).
78 Pomata, "Observation."
79 His nephew, however, published the secretive prescription in his annotations; see Welsch, Reusner, *Curationes*, p. 63.
80 Welsch, Reusner, *Curationes*, pp. 30–31, 40, 42, 53, 56, 70, 82, 100–05, 108.
81 Hieronymus Reusner, *Diexodicarum Exercitationum Liber de Scorbuto [...]* (Frankfurt, 1600); Gregor Horst, physician in Ulm, cited frequently from Reusner; see Gregor Horst, *Büchlein von dem Schorbock [...]* (Giessen, 1615), pp. 5–7, 15–18, 45, 47, 49–50, 54, to cite some examples.
82 StadtANoe R39 F2 No. 38, 1664, April 22; No. 45, 1701.
83 Welsch, Reusner, *Curationes*, p. 17.

84 Johann J. Baier and Ferdinand J. Baier, *Introductio in Medicinam Forensis* (Frankfurt and Leipzig, 1748), pp. 36–69.

85 "[...] vergangenen donnerstag überfallen, mit frost und Hitz, nebst diesem [...] Starcke Entzündung und Hartte Geschwulst [...]," StadtANoe R39 F1 No. 11, 1766.05.06.

86 "er klagt": StadtANoe R39 F3 No. 56, 1771.06.27, 1766.04.20, 1766.02.11.

87 "sie bittet einen Hoch Edlen [...] Magistrat man möchte ihre die Lazareth Hülffe angedeihen lassen": StadtANoe R39 F3 No. 55, 1765.01.14.

Part III
Documenting, Locating

7 Accountability, Autobiography, and Belonging

The Working Journal of a Sixteenth-Century Diplomatic Physician between Venice and Damascus

Valentina Pugliano

Diario di condotta

Damascus, 29 August 1542. Cornelio Bianchi, physician to the Venetian Consul, returns to his lodgings in his nation's *fondaco* after attending a local court hearing. Once there, he fetches his journal and summarizes the morning's unpleasant events. The presiding Ottoman judge (*kadı*) had just settled an accusation of misconduct presented against him by a resident "Turk," by ordering the foreign doctor to pay 8 *maidini* in "forced alms" or, as Bianchi computed, *Lire* 1 *soldi* 12. The claim concerned the payment for a standard purgative treatment Bianchi had ordered for his patient at the consular apothecary, a laxative drink made with dates and two syrups. Whereas the Turk claimed the doctor had pocketed the money meant for the apothecary and demanded reimbursement, Bianchi believed the real reason for the quarrel to be his own unwillingness to enter into a contract of cure (*patto di guarir*) with the man. As a "French disease" sufferer, the latter probably promised an undesirably long and uncertain case. Bianchi followed this entry with a "Resolution": never again to treat "Turks or Moors or similar scoundrels." This vow was destined to be short-lived, however, and Damascene Muslims continued to form part of his clientele alongside Christians and Jews. Similarly, his commitment to contracts remained low.[1]

This scene will look familiar to most historians of European medicine: a learned physician; a dissatisfied patient; a contract for cure; a claim for redress before the civic authority; and, throughout, the use of writing to negotiate and stabilize a medical encounter. Its setting and actors, however, may not. Bianchi's case provides the opportunity to explore from a vantage point this volume's central preoccupation—namely the interaction between physicians, state administration, and the civic sphere, documented in the writing of medical officeholders. Practicing as part of a religious-ethnic minority outside the sovereignty of the state to which its members belonged, where the ties to one's polis of provenance and the

DOI: 10.4324/9781315554693-11

relationship between officeholding and political power were felt more acutely, the diplomatic physician will illuminate the extent to which locality was not only a Hippocratic determinant of medical perception but influenced the act of writing itself.

Bianchi's journal illustrates how displacement made strange the familiar. Historians of science, and more recently medicine, have mostly focused on paper technologies as tools to gather, organize, and generate knowledge within a rather homogeneous European literate environment.[2] Providing a counterpoint, this chapter contends that we should examine how the transplanted officeholder made medical paperwork an agent of socio-cultural mediation and used the lessons from a flourishing Italian documentary culture to negotiate the practical challenges and expectations surrounding a polity across the sea.

Bianchi's experience will also be instrumental in introducing a context of analysis and a category of practitioners little-known to historians of medicine and science. Far from exceptional in fact, Bianchi was a *medico condotto* and part of an infrastructure of medical provision gradually developed by Venice in its Mediterranean possessions (the *stato da mar*) and those Near Eastern emporia where it had diplomatic bases and a strong mercantile presence—notably Constantinople and the Arab regions of Syria and Egypt. From the early 1400s to the early 1700s, we find physicians, surgeons, barbers, and apothecaries serving, with some continuity, the embassy (*casa bailaggia*) in Constantinople; the consulates and Venetian nations of merchants in Alexandria and Damascus; and the surrounding vice-consular detachments in Cairo, Aleppo, Tripoli, and Beirut. Many arrived from the Venetian mainland and contiguous Italian regions; some from the Venetian Greek colonies of Cyprus and Crete; others were Ottoman subjects from the communities of Levantine and Sephardim Jews already resident in the region.[3] Retained as personal physicians to the consuls, Levantine *condotti* were paid with the taxes levied on the resident merchant colony, who also benefited from their presence.[4] Their clientele was far more varied, however. For a fee, they regularly extended their care to any transiting Christian and non-Christian resident. Like the Consul, the *condotti* were engaged initially for two years, though the policy governing their appointment varied across the region in response to the republic's agenda. While the Damascene Consul had been entitled to choose his doctor since 1507, usually from among Padua's graduates,[5] for political expediency the ambassadors (*baili*) in Constantinople were advised to employ Jewish physicians already settled in the capital and with access to the Ottoman court and—the Senators hoped—the prime information and contacts within it.[6] The office indeed carried with it an expectation of allegiance, consolidated by the *condotto*'s privileged position in the diplomatic household. He belonged to the *famiglia alta*, the Consul's circle of closest collaborators, alongside the chaplain, secretary, treasurer, apothecary, and the interpreters or dragomans.[7] The *famiglia* resided with

Venetian merchants and pilgrims in the *fondaco* (*fundūq/han*), a warehouse built around a square courtyard, with storage vaults for merchandise at the bottom and lodgings at the top. Locked at night and guarded by janissaries during the day, this had been the basic unit of foreign presence in the Levant since the twelfth century.[8]

Bianchi was appointed to accompany the newly elected Consul of Syria Niccolò Bon in 1542 for a good salary of 160 ducats.[9] His position was renewed in 1544 for another two years and the additional responsibility of the *condotta* in Tripoli by Bon's successor, the patrician merchant Domenico da Molin. Excepting this Levantine stay, Bianchi led the unremarkable life of an average practicing physician. Originally from a small town in the Veneto, Marostica, he studied at Padua with Vettore Trincavella. He married after his return from Syria, sired several children, and took up practice in Venice. He died there in 1576, struck down by one of the century's worst plague outbreaks, while assisting the sick poor on orders of the health board.[10]

He is exceptional, however, in that one of the two notebooks he used to record expenses and *notabilia* during his appointment abroad has survived. This is a slim, physically unassuming manuscript of 64 quarto leaves in the vernacular. Bianchi started it a month before departure, on 1 March 1542, and ended it on 7 February 1543. He wrote on the galley that over three months carried him from the lagoon along the Balkan and Greek coast to Crete, Cyprus and thence to Tripoli, where he remained some weeks; while riding with an armed caravan across the Lebanese mountains into Syria; and finally from the comfort of his bedroom in Damascus. This is so far the only full-length manuscript we know of that charts the daily life of a *condotta medica* in the early modern Levant.

Culturally, Bianchi's journey eastward sits between two important cultural trends that defined the Italian medical Renaissance and its view of intellectual travel to the Near East: on the one hand, fifteenth-century humanism and its philological endeavors; on the other, the vogue for natural history from the later sixteenth century frequently accompanied by an antiquarian interest in Graeco-Roman and Egyptian art and architecture.[11] Both trends counted representatives among the *condotti*. Two of Bianchi's predecessors in Damascus, Girolamo Ramusio (*condotto* 1483–86) and Andrea Alpago (*condotto* 1487–1517), used the experience to learn Arabic and to attempt a translation of Avicenna's oeuvre.[12] Prospero Alpino published his bestselling *De Medicina Aegyptiorum* (1591) after three years in Cairo (1580–84) and several excursions along the Nile.[13] Overall unaffected by these developments, I believe Bianchi represents a type of sixteenth-century *condotto* for whom the backdrop of Levantine travel still mostly concerned trade, pilgrimage, and politics.

Accordingly, we should not expect to find in his notebook that programmatic impetus for recording observations for later use, for detailed measurement and attention to the changing landscape, that historians have documented for the journals of grand tourists and eighteenth- and nineteenth-century travelers.[14] Bianchi produced a basic tool of rationalization of one's

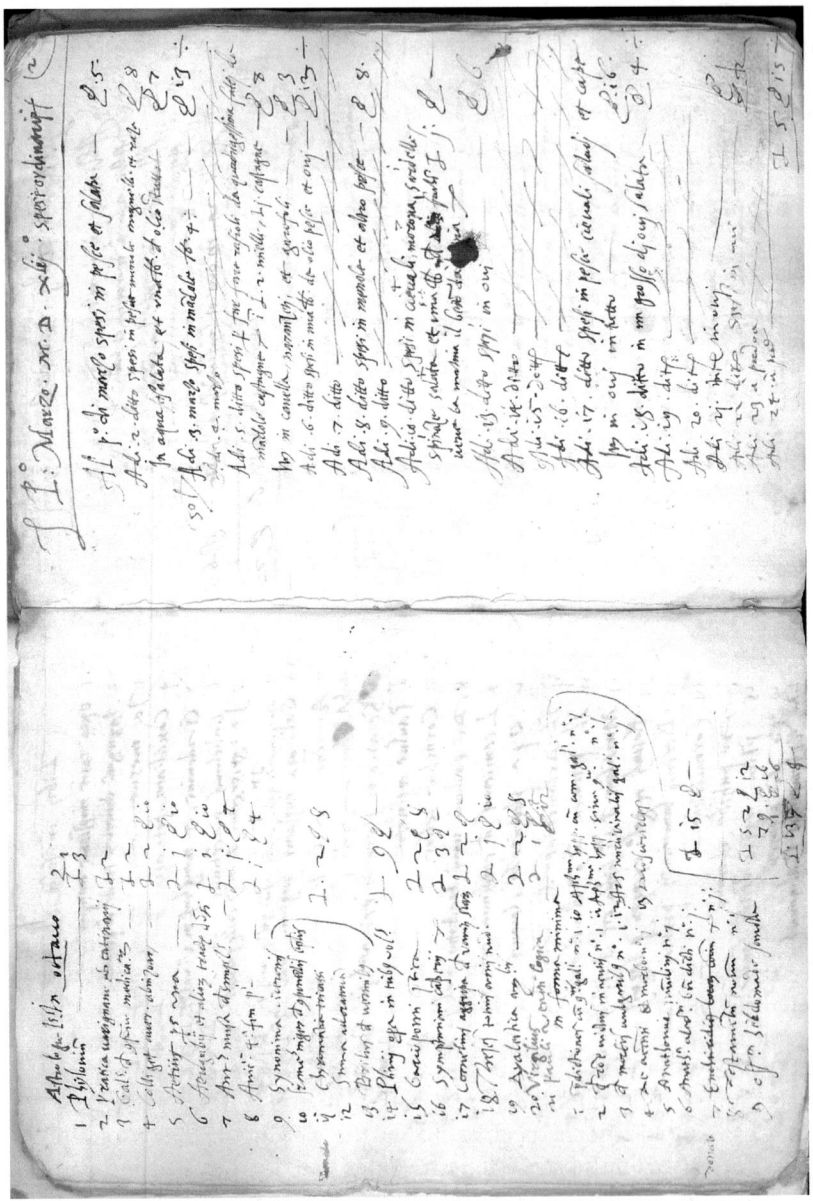

Figure 7.1 Opening pages of diary of sixteenth-century Venetian diplomatic physician Cornelio Bianchi. On the left: inventory of books in octavo, listed with their value. On the right: Bianchi begins his accounting of "ordinary expenses" (BMC, Cicogna 1117, cc. 1v–2r). Courtesy of the Biblioteca del Museo Civico Correr, Venice.

medical practice and economic life, rather than textual knowledge or the world of particulars. The notebook is primarily an account book, notwithstanding several narrative entries that seemingly stretch the genre. It opens with inventories of the items that accompanied the doctor to Syria: drugs, linens, and books.[15] (See Figure 7.1.) Like many contemporaries heading eastward, Bianchi spent a preparatory month in Venice to procure essentials: a mattress for his ship cot, garments, dry food, reference texts for his practice and a medicine chest to use on board and get him started in Damascus. To keep in contact with family and trading partners, he also bought 12 unbound booklets of 20 pages each (*quinterni*), possibly aware of the shortage of paper in Syria following the industry's decline the previous century.[16] The remaining manuscript consists of credits and debts entered according to date in no thematic order, like a merchant's wastebook or a household daybook.

The format is hardly surprising. Bookkeeping was one of the main uses of literacy among early modern professionals and artisans, and one of the first places scholars looked to find an instrument of intellectual ordering.[17] The entries record the money Bianchi spent for his daily upkeep during travel and the few tourist excursions undertaken en route to Damascus, from groceries to translator fees; the cost of self-medication and hygiene routines; income from his medical practice; dues with the apothecary; and shopping notes, from the "white beret" bought in Tripoli as a gift for his sister-in-law,[18] to items that helped him reconstruct his study abroad: a desk covered by a carpet, a document box, an inkpot and fresh lemons to erase the blots, perfume, and a bolt for the door to ensure privacy.[19] Yet this study evokes an image of *medicus ac philosophus* that fails to capture the diversity of activities undertaken by this type of officeholder. Indeed, numerous entries concern petty trading, one of the main incentives of the appointment abroad. Acting as intermediary, Bianchi utilized the renowned metalworking expertise available in Damascus, hiring Jewish and Muslim craftsmen like "Bubach" and "Hameth the Lame" to decorate "in the Turkish manner" items imported from Venice and Cyprus. Once transformed into fashionable commodities, fabrics, candelabra, daggers, and basins were shipped back to the metropolis to be resold at a profit.[20]

The daybook's heterogeneous focus resulted not only from its material nature as portable aid during travel and practice, but also from the habit of medical authors and scholars of recycling existing and often mundane writing models, slowly adapting them to serve new purposes.[21] Bianchi had at his disposal several scribal traditions developed between the late medieval and early modern period in both learned and trade milieux, which combined note-taking and day-by-day chronicling with a new emphasis on self-narrative: from merchant handbooks to domestic chronicles or "libri di famiglia" to spiritual and New World travelogues.[22] Much could be said of the influence on Bianchi and his contemporaries of late medieval accounts of pilgrimages to the Holy Land and their tourism of the sacred. Directing the attention to religious customs and architecture, these remained the main source of knowledge on the Turks until the mid-sixteenth century, when a new generation of secular accounts appeared, notably Girolamo Ramusio's *Navigationi et Viaggi* (1550–1606), Pierre Belon's *Les Observations des plusieurs singularitez* (1553), and the *Turcicae epistolae* (1581) of the Habsburg ambassador to Constantinople, Augier Ghislain de Busbecq.[23] Two pilgrim narratives (*itinerarii*) indeed accompanied Bianchi on his voyage alongside a few good reads, including Petrarch's *Canzoniere*, Boccaccio's *Decameron*, Plutarch's *Lives*, and an instructive *History of the Turks*, possibly Paolo Giovio's popular *Commentario delle cose de' Turchi* (1531).[24]

This chapter will focus on the journal's medical entries, interrogating the doctor's compulsion to write them through the double lens of the challenges of displacement, and of the relationship governing medical writing and state administration. Speaking to the growing reappraisal of medicine's scribal cultures, Bianchi's eclectic, non-narrative daybook provides an example of how practitioners wrote for their profession in daily life.[25] This activity seldom occurred programmatically or strictly by genre but was frequently conditioned by material constraints and the pressures of wider contexts. For the diplomatic physician, one such context was the need to manage one's health during a perilous transit and to acclimatize to a new environment. The chapter considers this aspect first, connecting it to the rising importance of first-person experience in sixteenth-century medical writing. A second context is provided by the insitutional framework of the *condotta medica* abroad. The displacement of one's medical practice produces specific silences and moments of unevenness in the diary. The chapter examines how the physician's identification with the Venetian community abroad rendered writing on the latter almost superfluous, while it compelled close accounting of the reality beyond the *fondaco's* walls. In doing so, Bianchi not only embraced the writing imperative of an administrative culture that regularly ran checks on its urban medical practitioners. He also satisfied the documentary needs of a republican government that famously viewed the acquisition of information as a mainstay of politics, and, as the century progressed, betrayed increasing anxiety about the might of the Ottoman Empire.

Writing's Reassurances

Back from his *condotta* of seven years in Aleppo (1578–1586), Tommaso Minadoi thanked God for his safe return to "Christian lands" and proffered the manuscript he had just completed on the latest Turco-Persian war to the Pope as an ex-voto: "as sailors and pilgrims hang a candle or a rope, a lamp, a statue, an image and similar things, to the sacred altars as a sign of dangers and misfortunes past, so I bring these papers of mine [to you]."[26] Bianchi, too, often took up the quill to keep under control a voyage undertaken to guard his countrymen's health, but which was fraught with risks to his own safety and logistical problems. His diary is not only a rich source for a learned healer's approach to self-medication, but also highlights his uses of medical knowledge to place into a recognizable framework the anxieties of uprooting.

The Mediterranean crossing prompted Bianchi, who suffered acutely from sea sickness ("vomito et turbatio"), to monitor closely the pulse of his health (and the cost of maintaining it). This form of medical autobiography is not yet one of preemptive or serial recordings. Records appear only when there is a crisis, a moment of bodily imbalance. On April 28, for example, finding himself blocked in the harbor of Pola because of adverse winds, Bianchi paid to be ferried to land for a walk "so that my body [bowels] may loosen." As he noted the following day, the exercise had been helpful: his body "moved" and he "benefited" six times. On April 30, he managed to accompany the other gentlemen traveling on the galley on an impromptu hare hunt organized by the *podestà* of Parenzo. He passed some fecal blood, painlessly, and "took no further remedy."[27] Once in Syria, he continued logging any indisposition and the steps taken to counteract it. In October he spent two worrying days in bed, with little sleep, a painful headache and "sweat on the forehead." After passing urine tinged with red on the second day, he resolved to write to a colleague in Cyprus for advice.[28] Never straying from Galenic humoralism, Bianchi's therapy of choice was frequent purging complemented by small changes in diet, including fasting. A painful hangover after an evening of libations in Tripoli prompted him to purge himself with some cassia and vow complete abstinence from wine.[29]

Bowel movements and a sensitive stomach ("crudità") remained a source of constant concern for the doctor, who feared the moment that "nature gave in, defeated by the superfluous evacuation" as he described the demise from dysentery of the consulate's chaplain, Niccolò Pettinello.[30] The stomach, as Rebecca Earle reminds us in her study of the Spanish conquistadors in the New World, was a central preoccupation for Europeans traveling across distances and cultures. Any change in environment represented a threat, as Hippocrates taught, because it brought a change not only in climate, but also in the foodstuffs available to nourish one's body and its humoral make up—to the point where diet became a source of identity and ingestion of indigenous foods the path to creolization.[31] The Venetians' long familiarity with the Near East and its edible imports complicates the picture, I would suggest, and indeed Bianchi's intense supervision of food and weather effectively evaporates once the sea voyage is over. The local fare fails to hold his interest except for citrus fruits and raisins confectioned with lye (*cebibi damasceni*), a delicacy for which he received a recipe from an Ottoman envoy.[32] Though centered around the gaster—indigestion, constipation, colic, vomiting, bilious discharge or "colera," diarrhea or "fluxo," in addition to chills, fevers, phlegm, and heaviness of head—Bianchi's catalog of discomforts betrays rather his alertness to those diseases routinely associated with the Levant: plague, dysentery, and malarial fevers.[33]

We can speculate about the extent to which this *condotto* subscribed to and reinscribed an existing negative discourse on the Levantine healthscape that circulated in the Venetian administration and found support in a number of personal stories. Leaving aside the recurrent state of war, many died during the journey eastward or soon after arrival, defeated by spoiled food and water, the intense heat, and the blades of robbers. Shocked "ob multa itineris pericula," including the stormy weather and corsairs, Girolamo Ramusio wrote a will the moment he touched the shore of Alexandria in 1483. Somewhat ironically, he died three years later after overindulging in apricots, which he had previously labeled *mazafranchi*, "Christian murderers," precisely for their treacherousness to the Europeans' stomach.[34] With this cautionary tale probably in mind, before departure Bianchi spent almost 4 lire to purchase the best-known preservers of health: theriac and mithridate.[35] He also remained alert to rumors of epidemic outbreaks, for instance, recording during the stopover in Cyprus that in Aleppo the plague was allegedly killing 300 people a day.[36] The Venetian Health Board had taken increasingly strict measures from the mid-fifteenth century to curb the risks of contagion from incoming Levantine goods and individuals.[37] Over the following century the association between Ottoman lands and plague became established, with the latter often described as endemic to Constantinople and seasonal, appearing there every spring.[38] As Eric Dursteler notes, while often inserted in a wider rhetoric of sacrifice for the *patria*, these preoccupations were foremost in the minds of the patricians chosen to serve in the eastern consulates, and often reason sufficient for declining the position.[39] The records of the "Cottimo of Alessandria e Damasco" similarly testify to the routine difficulty of filling the position of *condotto* because of the prospect of recurrent outbreaks and a salary considered by many practitioners to be too low for the risk.[40]

Writing helped exorcise this uneasiness. Weaving together accounting and confession like many of his contemporaries, Bianchi took his fate into his hands one entry at a time. The diary shows that he kept returning to his notes, including the occasional episode of illness. He highlighted entries of interest with a few words in the margin, added to pre-existing paragraphs, underlined the names of localities visited, and balanced accounts in spare corners in a manner of textual appropriation and re-elaboration common among early modern readers.[41] (See Figure 7.2.) Rather than a prelude to publication, the resulting system of annotation was a convenient retrieval framework that, *inter alia*, would have helped the physician consult this empirical repository of medical precedents, including his own personal chronology of illness and health.

As a paper technology, the daybook is symptomatic of a wider phenomenon of consolidation of the biographical and autobiographical voice in early modern medical writings.[42] An interest in one's life, Vivian Nutton observed, was already pronounced in the father of Renaissance medicine, Galen, whose entire works Bianchi dutifully dragged across the Mediterranean.[43] But this turn to the individualization of experience and its retelling finds its clearest example in the sixteenth century in the new prosopographical genres of *curationes* and *observationes*. Significantly, Pomata ties their emergence to the notes-on-the-go that medical students were now encouraged to take during visits, and to which Bianchi's daybook probably bore more than a passing resemblance.[44] The extent to which said daybook circulated among the physician's family and acquaintances in Marostica, Padua and Venice remains difficult to assess. For

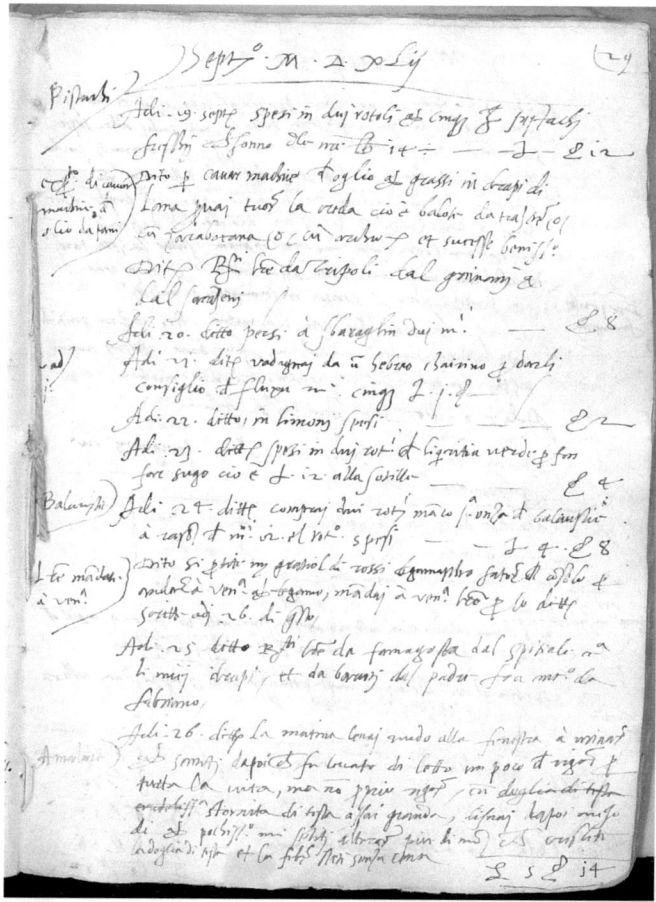

Figure 7.2 Diary of Cornelio Bianchi. Bottom of page: the entry of September 26, 1542 is summed up with "Amalare" (BMC, Cicogna 1117, c. 29r). Courtesy of the Biblioteca del Museo Civico Correr, Venice.

his part, Bianchi tied it firmly to the idea of posterity by drawing (poorly) the family coat of arms on its title page. (See Figure 7.3.) The gesture transforms a transient set of notes into a finished product that might be passed on for didactic purposes, aligning it to the many *libri di famiglia* produced in the period.[45]

Conversely, the journal's legacy for the wider medical and scholarly audience, familiar with copying and sharing knowledge in handwritten form, would have been its potential use as a rhetorical tool, providing material for anecdotes and *exempla* in medical and natural historical treatises.[46] Explicative storytelling was experiencing a resurgence in precisely the kind of literature that Bianchi had taken with him to Damascus: *practicae*, pharmacopoeias, and treatises on

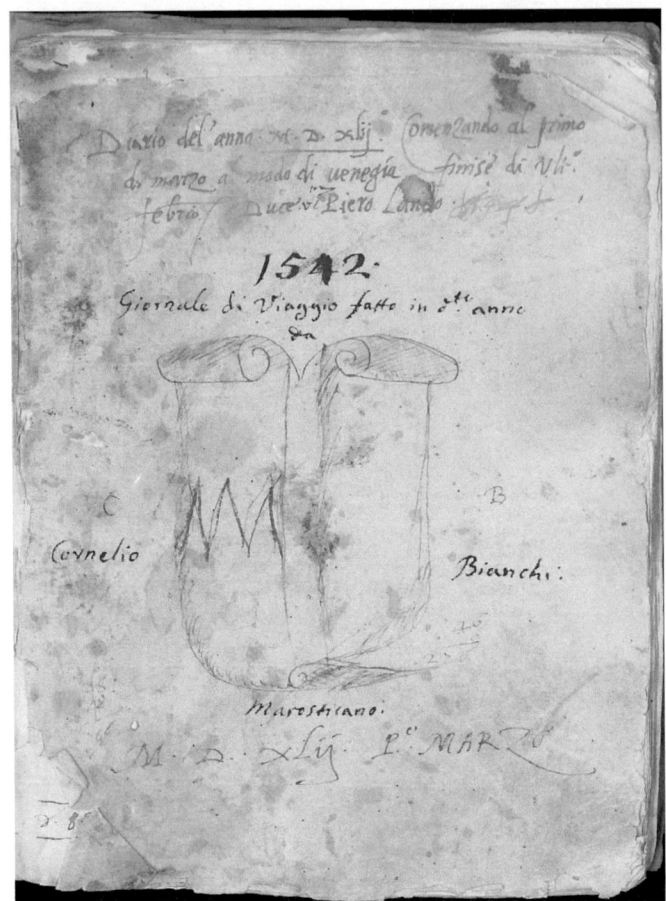

Figure 7.3 Cornelio Bianchi packages his "Diary" or "Travel Journal" (BMC, Cicogna 1117, frontispiece). Courtesy of the Biblioteca del Museo Civico Correr, Venice.

epidemiology.[47] If not actively constructing the imagery of an unhealthy Levant, Bianchi's medical repository would certainly reinforce the widespread concern among professionals and laymen that the region held dangers to health. These manifested themselves most often as a weakness in the stomach and the head that could lead to violent and fatal humoral imbalances, from which, as the notes on his practice testified, not even the locals were safe. At times intimate, at times folkloric, the *condotto*'s records could thus foster knowledge exchange not only between Europe and the Levant, but also between genres and spheres of writing, between the academic and the domestic, the intellectual and the prosaic, unveiling that dialog which scholarship is increasingly employing to problematize our traditional view of the medical "professions."[48]

Paper Republic, I: Writing Acts

Writing not only reassured but insured. Reflecting a different kind of anxiety, the *condotto*'s records of his medical practice strongly responded not only to the written culture of European medicine, but also, I argue, to the perceived challenges posed by the adoptive locality. We read, for example, that on 23 October 1542 Bianchi visited Jacob the Jew, giving him one dram of rhubarb for an unspecified ailment and leaving with his wife a medicine to administer the following morning. For this he received 5 *maidini*. On October 30, he earned 1 gold ducat medicating for colic Messer Renaldo, one of two French gentlemen who were visiting the Venetian Consul after completing the pilgrimage to Jerusalem.[49] As was the case in Italy, the doctor charged different rates according to the patient's status. Christian merchants and Ottoman military officers paid the most, while local artisans the least, and often only for the drugs prescribed. Rarely exceeding three lines, these entries barely resemble the formal case histories of medieval medicine or the narrative *curationes* that would soon be popularized in print by another Italian-educated physician mobile across the Mediterranean, Amatus Lusitanus (1511–1568).[50] There is little circumstantial data about the patient and no general doctrinal excursus on the illness at stake. In contrast with the detailed entries Bianchi devotes to himself, key pieces of information, whether symptoms, diagnosis or therapy, are routinely missing. Only occasionally are we informed of the outcome.

One of the longer entries drives this point home. In July 1542, after riding a second time 14 miles out of the city to visit a "spahi Turco" (*sipahi*, cavalryman) suffering from pneumonia, Bianchi recorded:

> He gave me maidini 26 that are Lire 8 soldi 4. *Item* he gave me towards the account of the apothecary for the mixture and ointment 10 maidini. On my return I spent for the dragoman Lire 1 soldi 4. *Item* I gave to prepare the syrups and date-based purge soldi 16. I remain debtor to the apothecary of Lire 2.[51]

A month later, as we saw in the opening of this chapter, the *sipahi* sued him.

While this "shopbook" with some work might have become a "casebook,"[52] its primary function, I suggest, was accountability. The physician was creating a folder with data to fall back on in case of contention. The records track specific kinds of information: earnings, treatment administered and drug dosage, and dues with the apothecary and other collaborators. A parallel, unsurprisingly, can be drawn with Bianchi's accounting for his commercial transactions which—funded by third-party capital, involving orders yet to fulfill, and spanning months and the width of the Mediterranean—were premised on uncertainty. As the amateur merchant safeguarded himself against risk by registering sums anticipated and debts, together with the flow of related paperwork such as invoices for goods (*polize*) and memoranda of orders (*ricordi*), so his medical note-taking would help consolidate his position and insure against wrongdoing.[53]

Bianchi's receipts of payment and records of operational choices resemble what anthropologists of writing call "writing acts"—a use of paper and ink that relies on the performativity of language and the capacity of words to take control of things and actions, both in process and in potentia as "act models."[54] Thus, rather than monologic or static, we should see his accounts as written with an eye to the future and in virtual dialog with customers and collaborators. This dialog was triggered whenever further advice was requested, a claim was filed, or a patient relapsed. The diary tells of this process graphically, through marginalia and crossed-out lines as in the entry of 2 November 1542, begun as "I lent to the apothecary 6 maidini," subsequently flagged with "credit with the apothecary," and finally struck out when the debt was extinguished.[55]

At a basic level, this bookkeeping reflects a European medical environment where practitioners were increasingly taken to task by patients, colleagues, competitors, and the overseeing civic authorities.[56] And, increasingly, they were expected to respond with paperwork. Thus, apothecaries were required to file away the prescriptions that physicians sent to their shops, and account for the drugs sold and their quantities. Physicians could try to ensure payment and avoid litigation by contracting a cure, although the practice was losing ground among Italy's collegiate physicians, who eventually left it to empirics and non-corporative healers.[57] The extant records of litigation cases in north-Italian towns involving dissatisfied and non-paying clients reveal that these journals and bills were indeed consulted by the protomedicato and the civil courts called upon to judge on the matter.[58]

Yet, the emerging culture among fifteenth- and sixteenth-century physicians of documenting one's practice, often framed by scholarship as a product of the writing imperative of a humanist education, should be situated in a larger institutional context that saw the rise of administrative paperwork and the archive. Medieval Venice was at the vanguard of this bureaucratization on the Italian peninsula. Filippo De Vivo ties this triumph of paperwork to the nature of Venetian government, an oligarchy ruling through a multitude of deliberative bodies. Each decision was voted upon based on proposals and counter-proposals; then copied with all its supporting documentation and sent to other committees for ratification and implementation; and continuously updated through emendations, comments, and erasures until the accumulation of glosses forced the clerks to transcribe everything anew. From the fifteenth century, the chancery staff proliferated alongside documents in duplicate and triplicate.[59] In fact this process was nurtured by a crucial new appreciation of written evidence, which Laurie Nussdorfer connects to developments in the law faculties of medieval Italy and the rise of the notaries' *scriptura publica*. This shook up the process of decision-making among the ruling elites, making it document-dependent and creating a culture of intertextuality in the use of records.[60] It would have a palpable impact on the early modern medical world too.

This recording imperative reverberated across the lower corporative levels and is well-attested for the three Venetian Colleges of Physicians, Surgeons, and Apothecaries. Representing the largest groups of medical practitioners in the city, these bodies hired professional clerks and kept books of expenditures and minutes of meetings, rolls of apprentices and elected officers, and copies of the legislation relevant to their group taken from the registers of overseeing bodies like the *Giustizia Vecchia* and *Provveditori alla Sanità*.[61] The city fostered a medical culture accustomed to reporting to the authorities and administering itself through autograph documents also at the individual level. Charlatans submitted supplications for licenses to practice. Apothecaries filed signed declarations of their holdings for fiscal purposes and testified about the income of neighboring shops. Physicians and surgeons petitioned to have their "secrets" rewarded.[62] Officeholders, as this volume illustrates, were expected to contribute a variety of documents that required the mastering of several audiences and rhetorical conventions.[63] Their writing output, however, strongly depended on the nature of their appointment and adoptive polity. Unlike their peninsular counterparts, Levantine *condotti* had no predetermined responsibility for the collective problems of the *civitas*—be it the allocation of poor relief, the licensing of practitioners, or the management of group responses during epidemics. It was only after his return from Syria that Bianchi experimented with formal administrative writing at the health board's request, producing with two colleagues a "peritia" on a new method for disinfecting clothes during the 1576 plague that took his life.[64] Contrariwise, his colleagues in Constantinople would have advised on a genre of official paperwork strictly related to the difficulty of controlling the recurrent outbreaks in the region: the bills of health issued by the *bailo* to Venetian travelers and valid across the Levant.[65]

Bianchi operated with this urban, professional framework in mind. It is, therefore, ironic that on the occasion when his accounts should have served him, when sued by the *sipahi*, they failed him. This occurred not because they went unacknowledged—Bianchi insisted the *kadı* knew he was in the right—but probably in order to avoid clashes, a reminder of the highly politicized setting outside the notebook's pages.[66] Venetian merchants operating across the Syrian emporia were regularly imprisoned for unpaid debts and other alleged fiscal misdeeds toward their Mamluk and Ottoman counterparts (frequently a contrived method for the local governor to raise revenue).[67] We may wonder whether Bianchi was reminded of the moral utility of accurate bookkeeping when he visited three such compatriots in jail in October 1542: Daniel Bragadino, Zuanfrancesco dalla Riva, and Anzolo Nicolai.[68] Generally, Shaw and Welch's assessment on the bookkeeping of Italian apothecaries offers a helpful perspective: "The carefully maintained account books survived, not as a testimony to the success of this system, but to the constant fear of its failure."[69]

While in keeping with a European accounting tradition, Bianchi's note-taking patterns conceal a dynamic that has all to do with locality and the Levantine officeholder's exceptional position. At a closer look, we find that most of his medical notes concern visits outside the diplomatic household and its satellite Venetian colony. They document the *condotto*'s practice among traveling European Christians, among the Ottoman Empire's communities of Jews, Armenians and Orthodox Greeks, and among several sets of its Muslim majority interchangeably labeled as "Turks" or "Moors," including its peripatetic military, resident notables and, to a smaller degree, craftsmen. All are carefully identified in the journal by their confession (often at the expense of personal names), not surprisingly the most significant marker of identity for someone writing with the Mediterranean specter of renegades as well as the Reformation in mind.[70] The diplomatic physician's adoptive polity, in other words, was mixed for social status, political allegiance, provenance, and confession in even greater proportions than those displayed by cosmopolitan yet mostly Catholic Venice and its restrictive definition of "foreigner" (anyone from outside the city).[71] These differences were marked outwardly by clothing, customs, and especially language. We should not forget that to navigate the city Bianchi, like most temporary consular servants, hired one of the consulate's interpreters, usually the Syriac Jew Nesin, who became the linchpin of medical practice at one remove.

The nature of this mediated "bedside" practice still needs to be examined, together with the amalgam of expectations regarding the management of the body, illness and cure, to which such a mixed polity exposed the *condotto*. Yet Bianchi's appeal as a healer to the Damascene population was probably familiarity rather than novelty. His popularity certainly confirms the impression of historians of Ottoman medicine that Hippocratic-Galenic humoralism filtered by Arabic authors—what most *condotti* peddled in the fifteenth and sixteenth centuries—was the primary choice of Ottoman elites and urban communities.[72] In Bianchi's case this approach was vividly epitomized by the crate of 62 medical books he embarked with him, filled with theoretical texts from his student days at Padua and tomes with practical knowledge for his stay in the Levant. The works of Galen, Avicenna, Rhazis and Averroes were packed together with *practicae* by fifteenth-century Italian surgeons; treatises on epidemiology, fevers, and uroscopy; the pharmacopoeias of Serapion and Mesue; and the newly rediscovered classics of Dioscorides and Pliny.[73]

One of the clearest effects of this heterogeneous polity, I would argue, was a radical departure from the customary credit economy of European corporative medicine. The accounts testify how Bianchi demanded and usually succeeded in being paid for his services upfront. Credit was probably a risk he could not afford in a context where professional networks and personal connections formed through kinship and neighborhood ties were not there to help him assess the reputation of potential patients, especially in the first months of residence that the diary documents.[74] Deprived of small-town ways of accrediting trust, however, the small-town doctor seems to have tempered this uncertainty by curing those with whom he had at least a passing acquaintance. Most of his clientele came either from his consular contacts among local notables, or from the social network he was building daily through his forays in the bazaar. The above-mentioned Jacob, for example, decorated for him basins for barbering.[75] Only slowly could the *condotta* abroad become the kind of community-based medicine that a physician on retainer encountered in the average Italian town, however, and it is unfortunate that Bianchi's second notebook has not survived to support or disclaim this development.[76]

Accounting, therefore, was a means to harness risk when faced with an unwieldy clientele and in a context of isolation from usual forms of professional authority and solidarity, embodied by a health board, a college, a set of colleagues and former teachers, which, however restricting they may have felt at home, also provided a supporting infrastructure. It should not surprise that the *condotto* fell back on other tried and tested paper tools and their established epistemologies. The diary mentions two *consilia* (though there were likely more), a genre particularly apt to serve remotely the Venetian detachments in Syria and Egypt. The first was requested in November 1542 by a merchant evidently used to this form of therapeutic writing back home. Bedridden with quartan fever in Aleppo, Niccolò Mozanico desired written advice about his deteriorating condition, especially instructions to alleviate "the cruelest shaking and chill" caused by the malarial fever. Two months earlier Bianchi had produced another *consilium* for a Jew of Cairo suffering from dysentery.[77] It is not clear whether the latter belonged to the Venetians' extended network, and this raises interesting questions about the stability that these technologies were seen to possess across space and societies. The *condotto* certainly seems to have viewed their conservative nature as a promise of their reliability as legal and epistemic instruments across borders. A history of the transregional use of medical paper technologies would probably revise our notion of, *inter alia*, the *consilium* as a quintessentially European medical tool, and reveal paper trails that followed human diasporas across the Mediterranean.[78]

It was indeed a shared documentary practice, combined with the lesson of using paperwork to one's advantage imparted by the flourishing bureaucratic culture of Venetian medicine, that turned Bianchi to contracts. He demanded that a Greek-born janissary, whom he believed beyond saving, obtain from the *kadı* a certified statement that would exonerate the physician from the responsibility of his death.[79] Taken together with our opening anecdote of the failed contract with the Turk, this entry confirms an intriguing involvement in the European doctor's practice of the Ottoman religious-judicial administration, both as a legal system that could be called upon as guarantor by the foreign practitioner and an authority that could regulate his activity. Like international commerce, medical practice brought the foreigner in close, operative contact with the Empire's residents. It thus took him outside the scope of Venetian civil law dispensed by the Consul and within that of the *kadı* court which regularly judged *zimmis* (non-Muslim subjects) and *müste'min* (visiting foreigners) of the Empire following sharia law.[80] This juridical liability or "sociolegal ambiguity," to borrow from Natalie Rothman's definition of Veneto-Ottoman trans-imperial subjects (in-betweens like interpreters, commercial brokers, converts), would have given the physician an additional reason for preventative note-taking and writing acts.[81] But the Ottoman administration's involvement was possible also because it was premised on a shared medical practice. Not only were "contracts of consent" drawn up before the *kadı* widely used by Ottoman healers to prevent litigation when risky surgical operations were at stake. Ottoman patients and their families were equally accustomed to suing their practitioners if treatment failed.[82] This conveys a further insight. Rather than a route of exclusion, litigation before the *kadı* sanctioned the view that both local authorities and population saw the *condotto* not as an exception but as a natural addition to the sizable pool of non-Muslim practitioners that had been populating the medical marketplace of Syria and Egypt for centuries.[83] As they document the *condotto*'s readiness to turn to the local administration as he would have done to the magistracies back home, these contracts (and legal-medical writing at large) also normalized his position in the eyes of the adoptive polity.

Still, the question of whether locality engendered a fear of the foreign in the *condotto* remains a plausible one. Given that both of Bianchi's contracts were concerned with Muslim militia men (a group little-loved by foreign nations),[84] one could argue that they were used to inscribe difference. Bianchi after all came from an Italian administrative environment increasingly anxious about dissimulation and public unrest, and invested in recording the identity of those who inhabited and crossed its lands through the help of documentation: passports, portraits, safe conducts.[85] In fact, written contracts seem to have been the exception rather than the rule for this *condotto*, again probably because they worked on credit (payment was settled upon delivery of the promised cure) and forced on him a set of obligations from the outset.[86]

Yet, undoubtedly, both formal and informal writing are used by Bianchi to construct a position of safety and authority in the new civic sphere. This process, I would argue, is part of a larger history of medical paperwork as an agent of mediation. So far this mediation has been considered mostly in relation to court trials and narratives of malpractice, of impingement on guild monopolies and fiscal misconduct, all linking individual practitioners and patients to the authority within fairly homogeneous socio-cultural formations.[87] Bianchi is clearly operating with these cases as a referent. Once in the Levant, however, the traditional instances of paperwork to which he is led by both his learned habitus[88] and urban documentary culture—*consilia, regimina, responsa*, contracts, and especially accounts—become objects of mediation between communities across markedly different religious, cultural, social and political borders. The story of this border-crossing mediation still needs to be told.

In similar transplanted contexts in fact, "European" paperwork has been examined, notably by cultural geographer Miles Ogborn, for the role of written trading instruments within larger imperial and colonial developments, which apply uneasily to the Venetians' "provisional" presence in the Levant.[89] Conversely, historians of science and medicine have preferred to study how European scholars dealt with knowledge transfers between different medical and cultural systems through the medium of print and publication projects.[90] The *condotto*'s conservative paper technologies, however, are not primarily designed to master unfamiliar data but social relations and social authority over medical transactions. They negotiate power relationships and translate from one medical system and its patient–practitioner relationship to another similar but not identical one. They often do so materially—think of the contract for the janissary which, archived by the *kadı* court presumably in Arabic or Turkish, was no longer intelligible to the doctor—suggesting parallels with epistemological practices of gift-giving within both diplomatic and pre-colonial contexts that are worth exploring further.[91] To do so it might be useful to adopt Ogborn's suggestion of retracing the writing's avenues of material production and distribution, as well as to understand these writing acts as a problem of communication.[92] Most of Bianchi's notes after all were vestiges of cross-cultural encounters, concealing underneath the doctor's inked words the local patient's speech and demands.

Paper Republic, II: Polis in Motion

How to read then the note-taker's comparative silence about his practice *within* the *fondaco*? This too lay outside his contractual salary's remit, yet the records are few, often no more than a quick line with a name and a sum of money: "I visited the merchant Messer Agustin de Anzelieri and the Magnifico Domenico da Molin. I earned a ducat"; "I earned 2 cecchini [...] for medicating Messer Jacopo Priuli."[93] In a Levantine world where both doctors and merchants relied on written safeguards, the graphic void should be taken as a signifier of tight-knit relations. *Nostran*, "from our land," is the term by which Bianchi distinguishes subjects from the Veneto.[94] The officeholder draws a line between what he views as his immediate "civic community," the transplanted nation of (male) merchants and consular servants gravitating around the *fondaco*, and the larger city into which he is also led by his practice. Note-taking (or its absence), in other words, becomes a means to enact "the actual location of socio-cultural boundaries," an activity synonymous with those who, like Rothman's trans-imperial subjects, straddled two geopolitical realities.[95]

As has been noted for the minorities of early modern Europe, including the mobile trading nations of Germans, Dutch and Florentines, credit-worthiness and trust were bred through confessional uniformity as well as insularity and clear-cut distinctions between "friends" and "strangers."[96] Unlike the strangers outside the *fondaco* whose patient profile needed to be sketched with care, the *nostrani* were not only familiar faces but indi-viduals whose patronymics and offices embedded them in an easily identifi-able web of relations across both mainland and colonial republic. Full records were superfluous. (Rather, probably concerned about the weight of his own credentials in this enclave, or aware that official documents were becoming a source of identity, it was Bianchi who made sure to carry to Syria a copy of his doctoral certificate.[97]) This social network would offer support in case of problems with one of its own. Bianchi reciprocated with generosity: when Anzolo del Piero, secretary to Alvise Grimani, died of fever and "colera" after spending a night outside in the cold following an altercation with a bricklayer, the physician noted he had attended to him for 11 days but "I did not ask for anything." He could also devote an empathetic note to the progress of a colleague's illness: "Our chaplain left the bed after suffering from intermittent [malarial] fever for 8 days."[98] Within the *fondaco's* walls, it seems, the doctor could establish that moral economy of obligation (and credit) that had been elusive outside.[99]

This narrative of belonging, which Bianchi articulates in terms of prov-enance (Veneto) and confession (Christian), becomes explicit in the few entries dedicated to the religious "customs of the Moors," which are com-pared to those of home. To commemorate their dead, for example, every October the Turks bake *focaccie* with butter and give them to the children "for the love of God." They also give alms and fast "as we Christians in Italy do on November 2, and they lay myrtle and other fragrant herbs on the graves, and the neighborhoods resonate with celebrations."[100] Ponder-ing through similitudes on the commensurability of Islamic and Catholic customs, Bianchi engages in an exercise of cultural translation that also sharpens his sense of belonging.[101] If not necessarily a homogeneous Ven-etian identity, what the doctor finds in the *fondaco* is a solidarity built through collective forms of living; mutual dealings; acts of sociability like a meal "al fresco with all the company (*compagnia*)"; and a shared lan-guage in an early modern world increasingly conscious of linguistic identity.[102] The civic sphere in which the diplomatic physician operates is thus layered. Surrounded by the demands of the physical city of Damascus, his polis, the political and cultural referent dictating his allegiances remains Venice, whose contours are no longer near nor taken for granted, but need to be reaffirmed.

Along these lines, the *diario di condotta* betrays another important connection to the Venetian polis. Its writing was sustained and elicited by a specific conception of statecraft. Historians have long recognized the Venetian administration's inquisitorial alertness and systematic investment in the acquisition of information about threats to its stability from within and without.[103] The specter of Ottoman advance in eastern Europe underscored by the fall of Constantinople (1453) and the tense political situation in the peninsula put on hold with the Peace of Lodi (1454) triggered both an explosion of diplomatic writing across the Italian states and a need for sustained intelligence-gathering. As state chanceries began to devise new ways of archiving the resulting data, news about commerce, political decisions, court intrigues, and military campaigns became a vital commodity.[104] The Doge and Great Council of Venice regularly paid travelers to hear reports of their experiences. In 1508 the Bolognese pilgrim Lodovico Varthema earned 25 ducats in this manner, recounting his travels to India and, through them, the Portuguese eastward expansion.[105] Not only were the Levantine communities considered perfectly positioned for such reporting, but the Venetian political class expected its citizens to be familiar with, and contribute to, the government's overall aims even though they were excluded from participation in it.[106]

Bianchi left for Syria at a delicate moment in the political and economic life of Venice, which found itself sliding from the dominant position held throughout the fifteenth century to one of marginalization. Only five years earlier, an infamous defeat by the Turks off the Aegean coast at Preveza (1538) had marked the beginning of Venice's territorial decline in the Mediterranean, and a turning point for the government's approach to the Ottoman problem. Direct confrontation was abandoned for a careful politics of diplomacy, achieved through resident embassies, the cultivation of personal relationships with Ottoman officials, lavish gift giving, and the building of an ever-larger information network of which medical practitioners would become an integral part.[107]

Bianchi did not set out to broker intelligence. Yet, perhaps to instruct himself in the manner of correctly reporting to officials or anticipating the possibility of secretarial work for the Consul, he took with him Cicero's *Synonyma* and a style manual teaching letter composition to chancery staff by the Paduan professor of rhetoric Francesco Negri (*De componendis epistulis*, 1488).[108] Behind his attention to certain incidents, moreover, we can discern the republic's informational imperative and its heightened anxiety toward the Ottomans. To understand the potential relevance of his notes we must recall his position within the diplomatic household. In Constantinople, the *famiglia* regularly participated in the opportunities for sociability fostered by the open-door policy of the *bailo*, who for the sake of networking wined and dined Christian diplomats as much as Ottoman officials and individual Muslim neighbors almost daily.[109] References to the Consul's expenses and material possessions in late fifteenth-century

Damascus, from payments for singing darvishes to inventories of elaborate furnishings, paint a similar picture.[110] Bianchi was certainly a regular participant in convivial occasions inside and outside the *fondaco*, attesting to the officeholder's socialization, if not necessarily integration, into the adoptive community that other contributions in this volume describe.[111] In July 1542, shortly after his arrival, he accompanied the Consul to the "Signor bassà" (*paşa*, provincial governor) for a banquet and was allowed to visit his court, "very beautiful and with a great number of slaves and janissaries." Such encounters often fostered personal relationships between foreign doctors and Damascene residents and provided opportunities to scout for future patients. A few months later we find him curing the *paşa*'s son Habilei.[112] But they also made the *condotto* a privileged observer of potentially sensitive occurrences. Of interest to Venice, for example, would have been the gruesome case of stabbing involving a group of the *paşa*'s Mamluk slaves and the Sultan's janissaries that Bianchi recorded on 7 January 1543. The incident followed an Ottoman victory against the Habsburgs, for which Sultan Süleyman I had ordered universal celebrations for seven days and nights. Shops were kept open and people allowed to drink. The foreigners, we are told, worried about "garbugli," clashes. Equally, the pageant of some of Damascus's most influential notables, which Bianchi witnessed when a caravan heading for Mecca passed through the city, would have interested an oligarchy that made ample use of ceremonial displays of power and specifically sought to remain updated on the chain of command in the Ottoman provinces.[113]

Analyzing artisan autobiography, Amelang has argued that in the act of recording public events and social conflict, there was often an expression of dissent, as the author claimed participation in a political discourse traditionally beyond her/his reach. I read the *condotto*'s diary writing as a more literal performance of citizenship.[114] Though Bianchi's service to the state is still undeveloped and informal, his journal previews a much tighter relationship between *condotti* and political power that unfolded from the second half of the sixteenth century, particularly in the centers of power in Constantinople, when the practitioners were handpicked to serve as informers to the republic.[115]

The information thus gathered must often have been exchanged orally between *condotto* and Consul, and there is evidence that anecdotes and news gathered by the former regularly trickled into the diplomat's weekly confidential dispatches and final *relazione* to the senate (the latter unfortunately lost for the consuls to Syria and Egypt prior to 1575).[116] *Relazioni* were themselves a hybrid genre: a textual record of a speech that every *bailo* and consul was expected to deliver upon return. In order to put together the speech, which lasted up to five hours, while abroad these diplomats took notes in portable journals very much like Bianchi's.[117] But the physician may have found another model for this type of reporting in a distinctive genre of diary writing that emerged in Venice during the upheavals of the second half of the fifteenth century. Patricians and minor nobles took to chronicling events and news relevant to one's *patria* and the public good, Marin Sanudo's *Diarii* being probably the best-known result.[118] These diaries relied on precisely the kind of information gathered by the *condotto*. Indeed, the only reason we possess the Damascene letters of Andrea Alpago is because Sanudo transcribed them as evidence of the disruption caused by the Portuguese in the Indian spice trade, and of the Safavid Kingdom's expansionist aims in the 1510s.[119]

The private and static nature of the *condotto*'s journal should not be overestimated also given the republic's political culture. Recent studies have demonstrated both the oligarchy's preference for the manuscript form as a medium for political discussion,[120] and the widespread use of diplomatic and chancery records as sources for historical narratives on Venice alongside private letters, journals and merchant handbooks.[121] While some records were obtained illicitly by bribing well-placed scribes, the archives of medieval and early modern towns, Ketelaar stresses, were seen as embodying the community's identity and thus meant to be accessible to citizens.[122] And if not verbatim, Bianchi's journal may have entered the vast machinery of Venice's urban historiography through oral excerpts. The city was renowned for its lively oral political culture, which saw all manner of men and women congregating to opine and gossip in piazzas, churches, and (not least) pharmacies and barber shops.[123] As Robert Schwoebel has remarked of pilgrims, most did not write down their experiences upon return, but nonetheless would have recounted them to neighbors and family, becoming for many the main link to a Levantine world still far from the life of the average European.[124]

Conclusion

Bianchi did not set out to write an exclusively medical notebook, nor did he fashion a paper technology that would serve as a storehouse of *notabilia*. His *diario di condotta* is interesting not because it embodies a novel genre of medical writing, but because it illuminates the professional uses to which the category of diplomatic physicians could put ink and paper. All *condotti* who were new to the Levant faced the perils of a new healthscape and the need to adjust their understanding of what city and polis were. All had to unpack the issues of professional isolation and accountability to an expanded clientele and recalibrate their view of the duties and prerogatives of officeholding. Bianchi's answer was to turn to traditional paperwork and traditional ways of organizing medical practice on the page, which, however, acquire new meaning once transposed from the European town. Writing becomes an act designed to help the doctor negotiate his role at a crossroads of religious identities, cultural laws, and political loyalties; and cope with a civic sphere endowed with different degrees of trust and risk. In doing so, the *condotto* carries the republican polis with him in terms not only of political allegiance, but also of the writing models of a new bureaucratic culture. Yet while Bianchi's referent scribal community remains the Venetian administration and his colleagues, in practice his interlocutors were increasingly Ottoman officials. The diary offers a glimpse of an alignment in the use of writing technologies in matters of health between European and Ottoman healers and administrations that remains to be explored. Generally, the journal reminds us that even the most banal medical script was a "situated" practice, and that for diplomatic physicians writing itself was an operation deeply entangled with the notions and emotions of self-preservation and belonging.

Notes

Acknowledgments: This chapter stems from and was written during my project, "Venetian Medicine and Science in the Mamluk and Ottoman Levant, ca. 1400–1750," undertaken in 2012–2015 at the University of Cambridge, Department of History and Philosophy of Science, and funded by Wellcome Trust Grant WT100278MA. I wish to thank for their helpful comments Lars Behrisch, Laura Di Giammatteo, Lauren Kassell, Harun Kuçuk, Margaret Pelling, Natalie Rothman, Gabriella Zuccolin, participants in the "3P" workshops, and the editors of this volume.

1 Biblioteca Museo Civico Correr, Venice (BMC), MS Cicogna 1117, "Giornale o Diario di Cornelio Bianchi del viaggio suo in Tripoli nella Siria M.D.X.L.I. I. Essendo Doge Pietro Lando," c. 26v. For an excellent overview of Bianchi's biography and manuscript, I am indebted to Francesca Lucchetta and Giuliano Lucchetta, "Un medico veneto in Siria nel Cinquecento: Cornelio Bianchi," *Quaderni Studi Arabi*, 4 (1986): 1–56.
2 See Ann Blair, *Too Much to Know: Managing Scholarly Information Before the Modern Age* (Chicago, 2009) and bibliography; also, this volume's Introduction.
3 Although the records are patchy, contractual provisions for some of these Levantine *condotti* can be found in the registers of the "Cottimo di Alessandria e Damasco," the body overseeing the expenses and income of Venice's consulates in the Levant. For the fifteenth and sixteenth centuries, see Archivio di Stato, Venezia (hereafter: ASVe), *Cinque Savi alla Mercanzia*, bb. 27, 27bis.
4 An established system across the Italian peninsula, the *condotta medica* enabled smaller communities to retain a practitioner's services and ensure accessible care to its *civitas* by offering him a salaried residential appointment; Donatella Bartolini, *Medici e comunità: Esempi dalla terraferma veneta dei secoli XVI e XVII* (Venice, 2006), pp. 9–35; Richard Palmer, "Physicians and the State in Post-Medieval Italy," in Andrew W. Russell (ed.), *The Town and State Physician in Europe from the Middle Ages to the Enlightenment* (Wölfenbuttel, 1981): 47–61.
5 Guglielmo Berchet, *Relazioni dei consoli veneti nella Siria* (Turin, 1866), p. 40.
6 Francesca Lucchetta, "Il medico del bailaggio di Costantinopoli: Fra terapie e politica (secc. XV–XVI)," *Quaderni Studi Arabi*, 15 (1997): 5–50.
7 See the contractual provisions in note 3 above. Eric R. Dursteler, *Venetians in Constantinople: Nation, Identity, and Coexistence in the Early Modern Mediterranean* (Baltimore, 2006), p. 32.

8 Olivia R. Constable, *Housing the Stranger in the Mediterranean World: Lodging, Trade, and Travel in Late Antiquity and the Middle Ages* (Cambridge, 2003), pp. 270–75.

9 Early sixteenth-century *condotte* in Italy commanded a salary of 70–110 ducats (Bartolini, *Medici*, p. 29; Lucchetta, "Medico," p. 6).

10 Lucchetta and Lucchetta, "Cornelio."

11 Nancy G. Siraisi, *History, Medicine, and the Traditions of Renaissance Learning* (Ann Arbor, 2007), pp. 225–60; Sonja Brentjes, "The Interests of the Republic of Letters in the Middle East," *Science in Context*, 12/3 (1999): 435–68; Amanda Wunder, "Western Travelers, Eastern Antiquities, and the Image of the Turk in Early Modern Europe," *Journal of Early Modern History*, 7/1–2 (2003): 89–119.

12 Francesca Lucchetta, *Il Medico e filosofo bellunese Andrea Alpago (d. 1522) traduttore di Avicenna* (Padua, 1964); eadem, "Girolamo Ramusio profilo biografico," *Quaderni Storia Università Padova*, 15 (1982): 1–60.

13 Siraisi, *History*, p. 233ff.

14 Marie-Noelle Bourguet, "A Portable World: The Notebooks of European Travellers (Eighteenth to Nineteenth Centuries)," *Intellectual History Review*, 20/3 (2010): 377–400.

15 BMC, Cicogna 1117, cc. a–r, c–v, 1r–v.

16 Ibid., c. 8r. Eliyahu Ashtor, *Studies on the Levantine Trade in the Middle Ages* (London, 1978), VI, pp. 25–26.

17 Peter F. Grendler, *Schooling in Renaissance Italy: Literacy and Learning, 1300–1600* (Baltimore, 1991), pp. 306–31; Anke te Heesen, "Accounting for the Natural World: Double-Entry Bookkeeping in the Field," in Londa Schiebinger and Claudia Swan (eds), *Colonial Botany: Science, Commerce, and Politics in the Early Modern World* (Philadelphia, 2005): 237–51.

18 BMC, Cicogna 1117, c. 15v.

19 Ibid., cc. bv–cr, 26r, 28v.

20 Lucchetta and Lucchetta, "Cornelio," pp. 23–26.

21 Valentina Pugliano, "Specimen Lists: Artisanal Writing or Natural Historical Paperwork?" *Isis*, 103/4 (2012): 716–26; Fabian Krämer, "Ein papiernes Archiv für alles jemals Geschriebene: Ulisse Aldrovandis *Pandechion epistemonicon* und die Naturgeschichte der Renaissance," *NTM: Zeitschrift für Geschichte der Wissenschaften, Technik und Medizin*, 21/1 (2013): 11–36.

22 For an overview, Jacob Soll, "From Note-taking to Data Banks: Personal and Institutional Information Management in Early Modern Europe," *Intellectual History Review*, 20/3 (2010): 355–75; on autobiography, James Amelang, *The Flight of Icarus: Artisan Autobiography in Early Modern Europe* (Stanford, 1998), pp. 133–35; Raul Mordenti, *I libri di famiglia in Italia*, Vol. 2 (Rome, 2001).

23 Giuliano Lucchetta, "Viaggiatori e racconti di viaggi nel Cinquecento," in Girolamo Arnaldi and Manlio Pastore Stocchi (eds), *Storia della cultura veneta* (Vicenza, 1980), 3/II: 433–89; François Tinguely, *L'écriture du Levant à la Renaissance: Enquete sur les voyageurs français dans l'empire de Soliman Le Magnifique* (Geneva, 2000).

24 BMC, Cicogna 1117, c. 8r.

25 See Stolberg, "The Many Uses of Writing," Chapter 2 of this volume.

26 Tommaso Minadoi, *Historia della guerra fra Turchi et Persiani dall'anno 1577 al 1585* (Rome, 1587), sig. α2r-v; Lucia Samaden, "Giovanni Tommaso Minadoi (1548–1615): Da medico della 'Nazione' Veneziana in Siria a professore universitario a Padova," *Quaderni Storia Università Padova*, 31 (1998): 91–164.

27 BMC, Cicogna 1117, c. 14v.
28 Ibid., c. 29v.
29 Ibid., c. 20r.
30 Ibid., c. 38v.
31 Rebecca Earle, *The Body of the Conquistador: Food, Race and the Colonial Experience in Spanish America, 1492–1700* (Cambridge, 2012).
32 BMC, Cicogna 1117, c. 28v.
33 Lucchetta and Lucchetta, "Cornelio," p. 26; Nükhet Varlik, "From 'Bête Noire' to 'le Mal de Constantinople': Plagues, Medicine, and the Early Modern Ottoman State," *Journal of World History*, 24/4 (2013): 741–70.
34 Lucchetta, "Girolamo," pp. 40–41.
35 BMC, Cicogna 1117, c. 8r.
36 Ibid., c. 17r.
37 Jane Stevens-Crashaw, *Plague Hospitals: Public Health for the City in Early Modern Venice* (Aldershot, 2012), Ch. 6.
38 See the anonymous sixteenth-century letter in BMC, *Provenienze Diverse*, MS C.98, fasc. 5, cc. 168r–169v; and the comments made on the outbreak of 1600 by the bailo Agostino Nani (ASVe, *Senato, Dispacci, Costantinopoli*, filza 52, cc. 189r, 236r, 258v).
39 Eric R. Dursteler, "The Bailo in Constantinople: Crisis and Career in Venice's Early Modern Diplomatic Corps," *Mediterranean Historical Review*, 16/2 (2001): 1–30, pp. 16–17.
40 See for example BMC, *Provenienze Diverse*, MS C.2329, fasc. X, c. 44r (27 Sep 1524).
41 See generally Blair, *Too Much to Know*.
42 Siraisi, *History*, pp. 107–19.
43 Vivian Nutton, "Galen and Medical Autobiography," in Vivian Nutton (ed.), *From Democedes to Harvey: Studies in the History of Medicine* (London, 1988): 50–62.
44 Gianna Pomata, "Sharing Cases: The *Observationes* in Early Modern Medicine," *Early Science and Medicine*, 15 (2010): 193–236, pp. 205–06.
45 Amelang, *Flight*, p. 182; Mordenti, *Libri*, p. 23.
46 For extensive use of the anecdotes gathered by a *condotto* in Crete in the 1580s, Onorio Belli, and circulated via his correspondence, see the local flora of the Veronese apothecary Giovanni Pona, *Monte Baldo descritto* (Venice, 1617).
47 Chiara Crisciani, "Histories, Stories, Exempla, and Anecdotes: Michele Savonarola from Latin to Vernacular," in Gianna Pomata and Nancy G. Siraisi (eds), *Historia: Empiricism and Erudition in Early Modern Europe* (Boston, 2005): 297–324.
48 See Mendelsohn, "Public Practice," Chapter 1 of this volume.
49 BMC, Cicogna 1117, cc. 32r–v.
50 Pomata, "Sharing"; for a casebook, Michael Stolberg, "Empiricism in Sixteenth-Century Medical Practice: The Notebooks of Georg Handsch," *Early Science and Medicine*, 18/6 (2013): 487–516.
51 BMC, Cicogna 1117, c. 21r.
52 I thank Margaret Pelling for the turn of phrase.
53 Alfred W. Crosby, *The Measure of Reality: Quantification in Western Europe, 1250–1600* (Cambridge, 1997): 199–224.
54 On the model of J.L. Austin's speech acts, Béatrice Fraenkel, "Actes écrits, actes oraux: la performativité à l'épreuve de l'écriture," *Études de communication*, 29 (2006): 69–93.
55 BMC, Cicogna 1117, c. 33r.

56 See Margaret Pelling, *Medical Conflicts in Early Modern London: Patronage, Physicians and Irregular Practitioners, 1550–1640* (Oxford, 2003).

57 Gianna Pomata, *Contracting a Cure: Patients, Healers, and the Law in Early Modern Bologna* (Baltimore, 1998): 25–55.

58 Ibid., p. 95, for physicians and barber-surgeons. For apothecaries: James Shaw and Evelyn Welch, *Making and Marketing Medicines in Renaissance Florence* (Amsterdam, 2011), p. 137.

59 Filippo De Vivo, "Ordering the Archive in Early Modern Venice (1400–1650)," *Archival Science*, 10 (2010): 231–48, pp. 234–36.

60 Laurie Nussdorfer, *Brokers of Public Trust: Notaries in Early Modern Rome* (Baltimore, 2009), pp. 1–31.

61 See the guild-books of Apothecaries and Surgeons: BMC, MS Cl. IV, 209/1, "Mariegola dei Spicieri"; Biblioteca Nazionale Marciana, Venice, Cod.Marc. Ita. Classe VII, 2329 (=9723), "Collegio Medico-Chirurgico. Libro dei Priori D (1549–1628)."

62 ASVe, *Dieci Savi sopra le Decime in Rialto*, bb. 157bis, 158, 166 (1581 tax census); David Gentilcore, *Medical Charlatanism in Early Modern Italy* (Oxford, 2006).

63 See Di Giammatteo and Mendelsohn, "Reporting for Action," Chapter 5 of this volume.

64 Lucchetta and Lucchetta, "Cornelio," p. 41.

65 Durlster, "Bailo," p. 7.

66 On the tensions between the Venetians and Mamluk and Ottoman governors, Eric Vallet, *Marchands Vénitiens en Syrie à la fin du XVe siècle* (Paris, 1999).

67 Georg Christ, *Trading Conflicts: Venetian Merchants and Mamluk Officials in Late Medieval Alexandria* (Leiden, 2012).

68 BMC, Cicogna 1117, c. 30r.

69 Shaw and Welch, *Making*, p. 123. Upon his return to Venice, the Consul of Damascus was required to submit the account book and journal drawn up during his consulate to the Cottimo of Alexandria and Damascus (BMC, *Provenienze Diverse*, MS C.2329, Fasc. X, c. 43r).

70 Religious faultlines held equal importance for Ottoman subjects: Suraya Faroqhi, *Subjects of the Sultans: Culture and Everyday Life in the Ottoman Empire from the Middle Ages until the Beginning of the Twentieth Century* (London, 2000), pp. 80–100.

71 For the few Mamluks and Turks walking Venice's streets (amid large colonies of Armenians and Greeks), Paolo Preto, *Venezia e i Turchi* (Florence, 1975), pp. 118–31.

72 Miri Shefer-Mossensohn, *Ottoman Medicine: Healing and Medical Institutions, 1500–1700* (Albany, 2009), pp. 24–37.

73 BMC, Cicogna 1117, c. 1r-v. Lucchetta and Lucchetta, "Cornelio," pp. 48–56, provide a catalogue raisonné.

74 This parallels the reluctance to extend credit to foreigners and those without relations found in their study of Renaissance pharmacy by Shaw and Welch, *Making*, pp. 81–85. For the similarities with long-distance trade, Peter Mathias, "Risk, Credit and Kinship in Early Modern Enterprise," in John J. McCusker and Kenneth Morgan (eds), *The Early Modern Atlantic Economy* (Cambridge, 2001): 15–35.

75 BMC, Cicogna 1117, c. 24v.

76 Lucchetta and Lucchetta, "Cornelio," p. 3 n. 2.

77 Ibid., c. 29r.

78 Advice literature in the form of *responsa*, for example, was widespread among the Jewish communities: Silvia Nagel, "Il *consilium* nella letteratura

ebraica medievale: la tradizione dei *responsa* rabbinici," in Carla Casagrande et al. (eds), *Consilium: Teorie e pratiche del consigliare nella cultura medievale* (Florence, 2004): 299–324.

79   BMC, Cicogna 1117, c. 44v.

80   Dursteler, *Venetians*, pp. 135–36; Najwa Al-Qattan, "Inside the Ottoman Courthouse: Territorial Law at the Intersection of State and Religion," in Virginia H. Aksan and Daniel Goffman (eds), *The Early Modern Ottomans: Remapping the Empire* (Cambridge, 2007): 201–12.

81   Natalie Rothman, *Brokering Empire: Trans-Imperial Subjects Between Venice and Istanbul* (Ithaca, 2012), p. 11.

82   Ali H. Bayat, "Şer'ye sicilleri ve Tıp Tarihimiz I: Riza Senetleri," *Türk Dünyasi Araştimalari*, 79 (1992): 9–19. I thank Nükhet Varlik for the reference. On the *kadı*'s role in health matters, Nükhet Varlik, *Plague and Empire in the Early Modern Mediterranean World: The Ottoman Experience, 1347–1600* (Cambridge, 2015). The sixteenth-century Ottoman administration was also displaying a new concern for archiving and preserving paperwork (Al-Qattan, "Inside").

83   Peter E. Pormann and Emilie Savage-Smith, *Medieval Islamic Medicine* (Edinburgh, 2007).

84   Ashtor, *Studies*.

85   Valentin Groebner, *Who Are You? Identification, Deception, and Surveillance in Early Modern Europe* (New York, 2007), esp. pp. 65–94.

86   Patient–practitioner agreements, both written and oral, were still widely used in late seventeenth-century Veneto (Bartolini, *Medici*, pp. 139–40).

87   On the uses of manuscript writing to mediate between different social settings and aspirations of social mobility, see Silvia De Renzi, "A Career in Manuscripts: Genres and Purposes of a Physician's Writing in Rome, 1600–1630," *Italian Studies*, 66/2 (2011): 234–48.

88   See Stolberg, "The Many Uses of Writing," Chapter 2 of this volume.

89   Miles Ogborn, *Indian Ink: Script and Print in the Making of the English East India Company* (Chicago, 2007).

90   Harold Cook, *Matters of Exchange: Commerce, Medicine, and Science in the Dutch Golden Age* (New Haven, 2007), pp. 339–77.

91   See Carina L. Johnson, *Cultural Hierarchy in Sixteenth-Century Europe: The Ottomans and Aztecs* (New York, 2011).

92   Ogborn, *Indian*, p. 21; James A. Secord, "Knowledge in Transit," *Isis*, 95/4 (2004): 654–72, pp. 666–68.

93   BMC, Cicogna 1117, c. 21r.

94   On the "sense of community" uniting the Venetian merchant network across Syria, Vallet, *Marchands*, pp. 191–211.

95   Rothman, *Brokering*, p. 13.

96   Mathias, "Risk," pp. 24–33.

97   BMC, Cicogna 1117, c. 8r.

98   Ibid., c. 27v.

99   Craig Muldrew, *The Economy of Obligation: The Culture of Credit and Social Relations in Early Modern England* (Basingstoke, 1998).

100 BMC, Cicogna 1117, c. 31r.

101 For further examples, Lucchetta and Lucchetta, "Cornelio," pp. 33–34. On contemporary discourses of commensurability and fascination for Islam, Nancy Bisaha, *Creating East and West: Renaissance Humanism and the Ottoman Turks* (Philadelphia, 2004).

102 See Peter Burke, *Languages and Communities in Early Modern Europe* (Cambridge, 2004), pp. 15–42; Eric R. Dursteler, "Language and Identity in the

Early Modern Mediterranean," in John Watkins and Kathryn L. Reyerson (eds), *Mediterranean Identitites in the Premodern Era: Entrepôts, Islands, Empires* (Aldershot, 2014): 35–52.

103 Filippo De Vivo, *Information and Communication in Venice: Rethinking Early Modern Politics* (Oxford, 2007).

104 Paul M. Dover, "Deciphering the Diplomatic Archives of Fifteenth-Century Italy," *Archival Science*, 7 (2007): 297–316, pp. 299–300.

105 Joan-Pau Rubiés, *Travel and Ethnology in the Renaissance: South India through European Eyes* (Cambridge, 2002), p. 125.

106 Lester J. Libby, "Venetian Views of the Ottoman Empire from the Peace of 1503 to the War of Cyprus," *The Sixteenth Century Journal*, 9/4 (1978): 103–26; Eric R. Dursteler, "Describing or Distorting the 'Turk': The *Relazioni* of the Venetian Ambassadors in Constantinople as Historical Source," *Acta Histriae*, 19/1–2 (2011): 231–48.

107 Libby, "Venetian."

108 BMC, MS Cicogna 1117, c. 1v. On Negri, Lucchetta and Lucchetta, "Cornelio," p. 53.

109 Dursteler, *Venetians*, pp. 173–85.

110 Deborah Howard, "Death in Damascus: Venetians in Syria in the Mid-Fifteenth Century," *Muqarnas*, 20 (2003): 143–57, p. 147; Constable, *Housing*, p. 76 (Alexandria).

111 See Pomata, "A Sense of Place," Chapter 8 of this volume.

112 BMC, Cicogna 1117, cc. 22v, 40v.

113 Ibid., cc. 39v, 40r; Libby, "Venetian," pp. 109–10.

114 Amelang, *Flight*, pp. 196–98.

115 See Lucchetta, "Medico."

116 Berchet, *Relazioni*, pp. 23–24.

117 Dursteler, "Describing," pp. 233, 237; Dover, "Deciphering," p. 311.

118 Christiane Neerfeld, *"Historia per forma di diaria": La cronachistica veneziana contemporanea a cavallo tra il Quattro e il Cinquecento*, Memorie Istituto Veneto Scienze Lettere Arti 114 (Venice, 2006).

119 Lucchetta, *Medico*, pp. 17–20.

120 Caroline Callard, "Diplomacy and Scribal Culture: Venice and Florence, Two Cultures of Writing," *Italian Studies*, 66/2 (2011): 249–62.

121 Neerfeld, *Historia*, pp. 8, 215.

122 Eric Ketelaar, "Records Out and Archives In: Early Modern Cities as Creators of Records and as Communities of Archives," *Archival Science*, 10 (2010): 201–10, pp. 206–07.

123 See De Vivo, *Information*, and bibliography therein.

124 Robert Schwoebel, *The Shadow of the Crescent: The Renaissance Image of the Turk (1453–1517)* (Neuwkoop, 1967), p. 177.

8   A Sense of Place

Town Physicians and the Resources of Locality in Early Modern Medicine

Gianna Pomata

A manuscript in the University Library of Bologna seemed quite a disappointment when I examined it for the first time. Described in the library inventory as the *diario* compiled between 1585 and 1611 by Petronio Fabrazzi, physician of the small town of Minerbio in the territory of Bologna,[1] I opened it with the eager expectation of finding a record of his practice—case reports, notes about local disease, weather observations, and so on. Nothing of the kind. To my surprise, the manuscript contained what looked like the field notes of a modern anthropologist intent on tracing the kinship pattern of a tribe. Together with local events (births, deaths and local crime, such as brawls, thefts, and murders), the physician meticulously noted, year after year, all the marriages that were contracted among the village families, and the ties of affinity thus created. Since weddings were routinely recorded by the parish priest, one wonders what the purpose was of creating such a document. The answer is that the physician, a native of Minerbio, was interested in the shifting dynamics of local politics and economic power, as reflected through the lens of marital alliances.[2]

Though definitely idiosyncratic, this document speaks of an aspect of early modern medical practice that was far from rare—the strong ties that bound physicians to a specific place because of their contractual agreement to serve a community as civic doctors. We know that early modern medical practitioners worked typically on retainer, under hiring terms set down by contract with a city, town or village, and they were obliged by contract to reside permanently in that place. A residency requirement was a regular feature of such contracts, or *patti di condotta*, as they were called in Italy. The physician was not supposed to be absent from the community that hired him for any significant amount of time—not even for a night, in fact—without his patients' express leave (*licencia egrotantium, licencia ipsius infirmi*) or the assent of the local authorities.[3] A deep need for stability seems to be a *desideratum* of the patient–doctor relationship as reflected in these contracts. Early modern patients often mentioned being "abandoned" by their physician as a serious breach of trust.[4] For town physicians, it was worse than that: it was literally a breach of contract, with legal consequences. So the civic doctor was contractually sedentary, so to speak, at least for

DOI: 10.4324/9781315554693-12

a certain period of time, since he could, of course, move from *condotta* to *condotta*, seeking better payment and life conditions.

In this chapter, I will investigate the significance of place in the paper record left by early modern physicians who authored and published case collections (*observationes* and *curationes*), a new medical genre that developed in the late sixteenth and early seventeenth century.[5] Was place a significant element in these practitioners' case records and in their understanding of disease? Early modern case collections presented a strong emphasis on individual patients and individual variation in health and illness. Did attention to place imply a shift toward a new understanding of disease as affecting not just individuals but entire communities? I will examine the attention to local conditions in the case literature of this period, suggesting that we see the emergence of a more population-oriented notion of disease. This new orientation, I argue, was related to the fact that the authors of *observationes* often worked as town physicians, with strong ties to a specific locality. Indeed, these doctors' tie to place is also indicated by the fact that we often find them in the role of local historians (or local "ethnographers," as in the case of Dr. Fabrazzi described above).[6] I will focus in particular on the significance of place in the medical work of Epifanio Ferdinando the Elder, a town physician from seventeenth-century Mesagne, a small town in Southern Italy. In Ferdinando's writings, as we shall see, we find a significant example of the early modern trend that associated a specific disease with a specific place.

The Town Physician as Case Collector

Town physicians feature prominently among the authors of *observationes*. For the most important early collections (late sixteenth century), this is true for instance of Martin Ruland the Elder, town physician in Lauingen, Swabia, and the author of *Curationes empiricae et historicae* (a thousand cases, published in installments, a hundred at a time, over the course of several years, 1578–1595).[7] It is also true of Pieter van Foreest, the author of *Observationes et curationes medicinales*, published in 32 volumes from 1584 to 1609 (for a total of 1180 cases). Van Foreest was first public physician of his home town, Alkmaar in northern Holland, and later of the Delft municipality, which he faithfully served for about 40 years and to which he dedicated the first volume of his *Observationes*.[8] Working as a town physician was also part of the profile of most authors of the collections of *observationes* published in the first half of the seventeenth century. To quote just a few representative examples, it is the case of Felix Platter, who was throughout his life the main town doctor of Basel; of Philipp Hechstetter, town physician at Augsburg, whose *Observationes* (1624) were dedicated to the civic authorities; of the *practicus celeberrimus* Gregor Horst, town doctor at Ulm; of Nicolaes Tulp, the protagonist of Rembrandt's *Anatomy Lesson*, town doctor in Amsterdam;[9] and of Epifanio Ferdinando the Elder, town doctor of Mesagne, of whom more anon.

The role of the town physician was particularly well suited to the enterprise of gathering and publishing cases. Case collections offered medical practitioners the possibility to advertise their clientele, emphasize their claim to successful practice and display their understanding of disease patterns, based on years of experience in a specific local context. This case literature allows us to reconstruct various aspects of early modern medical practice, in particular the physicians' handling of individual patients. Most importantly, the *observationes* clearly indicate that early modern medical care was individualized, that is, centered on understanding the patient's specific temperament, bodily habit, and nature. The early modern *observationes* were written with a focus on the individual case and they reflect a casuistic style of thinking, with only limited interest in nosological classification and generalization.[10] This is indicated by the very format of the new genre, in which cases are presented sequentially in numerical order, within a simple list-like framework. In the early examples of the genre, no nosological organization is apparent: Ruland's cases, for instance, are arranged in *centuriae*, or groups of hundreds, following the model of Amatus Lusitanus' *Curationes*, the first printed example and the recognized model of the new genre.[11] Within each of Ruland's *centuriae*, cases are entered in a miscellaneous manner (as in Amatus) with no apparent nosological grouping, though sometimes cases of the same condition appear in a sequence. The attention seems to be on individual variation in disease and consequent adjustment of therapy (again, as in Amatus). Van Foreest, in contrast, systematically organized his *observationes* by type of disease (the first seven books are on fevers) and by body part (books 8 to 28). Books 29–32 are on specific illnesses and conditions (arthritic diseases, poisonings, venereal diseases). He did not adopt the *centuria* convention, and the number of cases in each of his books varies considerably, based on the significance he attributed to the condition. Fevers, for instance, get a lot of space, extending to 248 cases, while the section on venereal disease has only 36 cases.

But even when cases were grouped by type of disease, as in van Foreest, they were not conceived as individual items to be aggregated into general taxonomic disease classes. Reasoning did not stress classification into fixed kinds, but rather the use of analogy to locate individual precedents along a continuum of similarity and difference. In other words, cases were collected under flexible, symptom-based categories meant for bedside consultation—documenting, for instance, various configurations of a certain illness in different individuals. Nor did the nosological organization of the case collection, as adopted by van Foreest, become paradigmatic. Ferdinando's *Centum historiae* (1621), for example, went back to the *centuria* model: he offered a hundred cases listed simply in chronological order, by year and month of their occurrence, independently of the type of disease.

There is no doubt that the early modern case collections, from the late sixteenth century to the early decades of the seventeenth, were focused on individualized diagnosis and especially individualized treatment.[12] The patient's temperament, idiosyncrasies, and personal life (including factors such as gender, age, social class, life circumstances) were perceived by the physicians as fundamental to understand genesis and treatment of disease. The prescription was supposed to be uniquely suited to the patient and his or her symptoms, the stage of the disease, his or her normal conditions of health, the weather, the season, and so on. The authors of these case collections opposed a rigid adherence to any standardized form of therapy. In fact, they poured scorn on generic remedies, which they saw as the sure mark of the charlatan.[13] They believed that only a learned physician could deliver the kind of complex diagnosis and individually tailored prescription that represented the best kind of medical care, and they designed their case collections to show how a competent doctor could steer his therapeutic course to fit each new situation. Offering individualized therapy bolstered their self-image and sense of professional standing, while also matching their patients' expectations. The early modern *observationes* reflect not only the resilience of the Hippocratic-Galenic ideal of individualized treatment, but also the preference of the patients themselves (especially elite patients) for personalized care.

And yet in these very same case collections, we see the emergence of a new attention to diseases affecting not only individuals, but also entire communities. Most interestingly, though the very structure of the case collection was based on individualized attention to the single patient, we notice a new interest in *morbi populares* or *morbi publice grassantes*, that is, conditions affecting large numbers of people in the same locality. The new attention to place in the Renaissance *observationes* contrasts with what we find in the medieval genre devoted to individual cases, the epistolary *consilia*.[14] There was no role of place in the *consilia*, and there could not be, because the doctor was asked to give advice on a case that he had not personally seen and that was described to him by letter. So local knowledge was not a resource for the medical practitioner, as the sick person was located in some other place, often at considerable distance. Based as they were on first-hand experience, in contrast, the *observationes* allowed physicians to draw on their knowledge of place, and thus to make intellectual capital of locality, so to speak. This was especially a resource for town physicians, and increasingly they made use of it in their case collections.

Historia epidemica and the Localization of Disease

Morbi vulgares (also *populares*, and *epidemii*) were the various dictions with which early modern physicians translated the Hippocratic term *epidemiai*, as we can see from the titles of the Renaissance commentaries on the ancient *Epidemics*.[15] The medieval translations of *Epidemics* were uniformly named *Libri epidemiarum*. The new expression *morbi vulgares* (or *vulgo vagantes*) was used first in the translation of *Epidemics* by the humanist physician Manente Leontini (c.a 1513).[16] Originally, the term *historia epidemica* referred generically to the case narratives in the Hippocratic *Epidemics*, which do not all refer to what we would now call epidemic diseases.[17] But soon it came to indicate in Renaissance medicine only those conditions that affected a locality and a community, suggesting the emergence of a new connection between place and disease.

This trend also reflected the growing influence of another Hippocratic work, the treatise *Airs Waters Places*, whose impact, like that of *Epidemics*, was a Renaissance phenomenon, unprecedented in the Middle Ages. Historians have highlighted the significance of *Airs Waters Places* as a primary factor of the new emphasis on place we find in early modern medicine.[18] *Airs Waters Places* stressed the importance of understanding peculiarities of place in the diagnosis and treatment of patients. Particular configurations of soils and wind, season and climate were supposed to produce particular patterns of morbidity. Therefore, doctors were expected to have detailed knowledge of the local climate and weather patterns in order to understand the peculiar interaction between place and person that determined health and disease.

These ideas, very influential in Renaissance learned medicine, as Nancy Siraisi has shown, were echoed and emphasized also in the vernacular medical literature of the same period, as we learn from a recent study by Sandra Cavallo and Tessa Storey.[19] Siraisi has noted the diffusion of late Renaissance commentaries on *Airs Waters Places*, which contrasts with the scarcity of medieval commentaries on this text.[20] Some of these commentaries contained localized information: for instance, that by the Florentine Baccio Baldini (1586) included a discussion of the water of the river Arno, in relation to the projects of Baldini's patron, the Grand-duke Cosimo I of Florence, for improving the water supply in the city. Siraisi calls it an example of the "localization or domestication of Hippocratic environmental teaching" that we find in this period, when treatises on the quality of local air, local winds, and local water multiply.[21] In Rome, the physician Marsilio Cagnati wrote a treatise on the quality of the local air, in which he offered a yearly review of health conditions in the city from 1568 to 1580, based presumably on some kind of epidemiological record or diary.[22] He also described two local epidemics (as he called it, *epidemia*, or *popularis aegritudo*) that affected the Roman population in 1591 and 1593.[23] Reading the Hippocratic *Epidemics* reinforced this trend: lecturing on book two of this text led Girolamo Mercuriale to write about a recent pestilential epidemic in the Veneto area.[24]

More evidence of this new emphasis on place comes from the Renaissance transformation of a traditional medical genre, the *regimina sanitatis* (regimens of health). In the Middle Ages, these texts used to be addressed to a specific person or social group (usually from the elite).[25] In the early modern period, in contrast, they provide health advice for the people of a specific locality. This shift of the genre is evident in the first city-specific regimen to be published in Italian: the physician astrologer Tommaso Giannotti Rangoni's *Consiglio* for the Doge and the people of Venice.[26] Within vernacular health advice literature, in particular, Cavallo and Storey describe "a growing desire to relate health advice to the specific local environment in which people lived." Native place and climate, local lifestyle and custom became increasingly important considerations in order to establish what was healthy and unhealthy for entire communities. Cavallo and Storey speak of "regionalism as one of the distinctive forces of the mid sixteenth-century regimen."[27]

An important aspect of this story concerns the conceptualization of disease. The focus on place shifted medical attention from the individual aspect of illness (the patient's constitution and the specific way in which the sickness affected him or her) to the local context of disease, and therefore to the way in which it could affect a population. This issue had been debated since the late Middle Ages in the vast medical literature on the plague. Plague treatises, in fact, often referred to a particular local epidemic.[28] But what we see now is an attention to locality that goes beyond the generic notion of the plague as a universal disease, and a new focused interest in the historical description of specific epidemics. This is indicated by the many texts debating whether a certain *morbus popularis* was truly plague or not, as for instance Tommaso Somenzi's *De morbis qui per finitimos populos adhuc grassantur* (1576).[29] It is also suggested by the concomitant rise of monographs on local epidemics clearly distinguished from the plague, like Gian Battista Codronchi's study of the respiratory conditions affecting the people of Imola in 1602, which he attributed to exhalations from the maceration of hemp in the bogs around the city.[30]

The Place of "Place" in the *Observationes*

Do we find this same attention to locality in the early modern case collections? What does the *observationes* literature tell us about place and disease? In the new genre's recognized ancient model, the Hippocratic *Epidemics*, the association of illness and locality was strong, as evident from the fact that some conditions were named after a specific place, such as the famous Cough of Perinthus, minutely described in book 6.[31] But in the first case collection to be printed in the sixteenth century, Amatus Lusitanus' *Centuriae* of *Curationes*, place is not particularly important, possibly reflecting Amatus' wandering practice—from Ferrara, Florence and Rome in the 1540s to Ancona, Dubrovnik and finally Salonicco in the 1550s and 1560s.[32] Amatus does occasionally use the notion of *morbus epidemialis* or of *morbi publice grassantes*, briefly noting of a *catarrhalis affectio*, for instance, that it spread to various places with varying intensity, more serious in some communities, less so in others.[33] But overall his attention to this aspect of disease is sporadic at best. In the 1628 collected edition of Amatus' seven *centuriae* of cases, the index does not contain a category for epidemic diseases: in fact, cases are not organized by disease, but by body part, in the traditional head-to-toe model.[34] It is fascinating, however, to note that Amatus was newly struck by the significance of place at the end of his peregrinations, when he settled to live and work in Greece, in the same place where he believed that Hippocrates had lived and worked. Called to visit a woman in Larissa, he immediately recollected—and this is how he starts the case narrative—that "Hippocrates, who long practiced in this town, often mentioned that it was an unwholesome place, due to its very bad waters and to the foggy, misty, and pestilential air (*coelum*) from the various lakes surrounding it."[35] From this bad quality of the place, Amatus deduced an unfavorable prognosis for the case at hand.

The first case collection that gives sustained attention to epidemic diseases is that by the Dutch town physician Pieter van Foreest.[36] The entire book 7 of van Foreest's *Observationes* (1584–1609) is devoted to cases of "fevers raging in a community, with epidemic diseases" (*febres publice grassantes, cum morbis epidemiis*).[37] Here he described epidemics of various nature in several Dutch localities, starting with his native Alkmaar, where he set up to practice medicine in 1546. In Alkmaar, he observed and described epidemics of *variolae* (smallpox) and *morbilli* (measles) in 1551, and of "catarrhal" fevers in 1553 and 1557. In 1558, van Foreest became town physician of Delft, a community that he would continuously serve for over 37 years. In Delft, he reported an episode of the plague in 1557, several bouts of *variolae* and *morbilli* in 1561 and 1563, and an epidemic of throat and respiratory affections in 1580. In the same book of his *Observationes*, he also minutely described the plague that struck Harlem in 1573, while the town was besieged by the Spanish troops.[38] Interestingly, van Foreest's book on epidemic diseases has a different structure than the rest of his case collection. While the other sections of his *Observationes* uniformly consist of individual cases, in the book on epidemic diseases he intermixed case narratives of an epidemic's specific patients with *observationes* devoted, in contrast, to describe the general features of that same disease. The physician's point of observation shifted back and forth between the individual sick person and the common features of the disease as it affected a population.

Van Foreest also included in this book an *observatio* on the epidemic of *Sudor Anglicus*, the "English Sweate," which had memorably swept through Amsterdam in 1526. In this case, van Foreest's description of the disease was not based on his direct observation but on that of two other physicians, Iohannes Tyengius, who had practiced in Amsterdam at the time of the epidemic, and the Ghent practitioner Tertius Damianus, who had written a short treatise on it, based on first-hand experience.[39] English sweating sickness is one of several early modern diseases that took their

name from place. Another example of this association of locality and illness is the *Febris Hungarica* (also called *Languor Pannonicus*), that was
repeatedly described in the case collections written by military physicians
at the end of the sixteenth century and the beginning of the seventeenth.
The Hungarian fever appears to have been endemic in the valleys of the
Danube in the early modern period. It struck the troops in every campaign
against the Turks led by the armies of the German Emperors in the Hungarian plains. It was first described in detail by Thomas Jordan, who took
part as army physician in Maximilian II's campaign against the Turks of
1566.[40] Jordan called it *Lues Hungarica*, or *Languor Pannonicus*, noting
that it decimated the Austrian troops but that the native Hungarians
almost entirely escaped. He also noted that the disease resisted to treatment so long as the patient remained in the region, but would be cured as
soon as he escaped to a different air and diet.[41] Tobias Cober, a military
physician who collected his experiences of seven years of campaigns in his
Observationes castrenses, also described cases of the Hungarian Fever in
1597, attributing the disease to the troops' habit of sleeping on the bare
ground, or possibly to the drinking of foul beer.[42] In 1600, the disease was
also described in a specific treatise, including 30 *observationes* of individual cases, by Martin Ruland the Younger. He defined it as

> an epidemic disease (*morbus epidemius*), because it affects many
> people at one and the same time, even if they are of different tempera-
> ment, and because it derives from an epidemic, that is to say, common
> cause, be it the air or the same food for many people.[43]

Cober's *Observationes castrenses* were reissued in 1685 with a preface
by the noted physician and scholar Heinrich Meibom. Besides locating
Cober's work in the tradition of the Hippocratic *Airs Waters Places*,
Meibom stated emphatically that physicians needed to acquire "peritia
locorum," expert knowledge of places.[44] It is this knowledge of place that
we see developing in the early modern case literature. My exploration of
the *observationes* suggests that place acquired an increasingly significant
role in these texts, becoming an important factor in diagnosis and therapy,
and perhaps most remarkably in the conceptualization of those forms of
disease that affected people independently of individual temperament. The
temperies of the local air, weather and climate conditions became just as
important a conceptual tool for the physician's understanding of disease as
the patient's individual temperament had always been. It is interesting to
note that next to town physicians, we find military doctors prominently
involved in this trend, that is, doctors who not only were responsible for
taking care of a population over a certain period of time but had the additional advantage of observing this population as it was affected, individually and collectively, by the constant change of place required by military
operations. Although the *observationes* are fundamentally devoted to

individual cases and reflect an individualistic conception of treatment, they also show, like the early modern health regimens, an increasing effort to understand disease using the cognitive resources offered by the observation of locality.

The trend toward a localized concept of illness is particularly evident in the *observationes* of a town physician from the southern Italian region of Apulia, Epifanio Ferdinando's *Centum historiae* (1621).[45] In Ferdinando's case collection, we find not only systematic attention to specific local conditions (especially the local air) as the first item to be considered in each case report, but also the identification of another early modern disease associated with place—tarantism, from Taranto, the main city in the Apulia region. Ferdinando's work deserves particular attention.

Epifanio Ferdinando of Mesagne: The Town Physician as Local Historian and Eulogist

Epifanio Ferdinando the Elder (1569–1638), was the founder of a dynasty of physicians with very strong ties to their hometown, Mesagne, in the agricultural area of Apulia, the heel in Italy's "boot." His son Diego (1611–1662) and his grandson Epifanio the Younger (1640–1717) were also town doctors of Mesagne. All three wrote local history.[46]

Ferdinando the Elder graduated in medicine in Naples in 1594 and went back to his hometown to practice. He became town physician (*medico condotto*) in 1595 and held the job most of his life. His ties to Mesagne were very strong: he also held political office as town mayor. He left Mesagne only temporarily to travel to Rome as the personal physician of Giulia Farnese, the widow of Prince Giovanni Antonio Albricci, who had also been in his care.[47] There is some claim (unsubstantiated, as far as I can see) that Ferdinando was offered a teaching position at the university of Padua in 1616, and that he turned it down. In any case, he returned to Mesagne, where he resumed his duties as town physician.[48] He devoted much of his later years to writing the history of his hometown, *Antiqua Messapographia seu Historia Messapiae*, whose manuscript he completed in 1637, the year before his death.[49]

The combination of medical and antiquarian interests was fairly frequent in the early modern period.[50] In fact, Ferdinando's teacher Giovanni Maria Moricino had also written the history of his hometown Brindisi.[51] Most interestingly, Ferdinando's son and grandson, both physicians, continued to contribute to the history of Mesagne, though they did not author any medical works. Ferdinando's son Diego wrote a *Messapographia seu historia Messapiae*.[52] In turn, his grandson Epifanio the Younger left four bulky manuscript volumes of local genealogy, *Delle fameglie di Mesagne*, in which he transcribed a great number of notarial documents.[53] A present-day historian has used this source to reconstruct family strategies in the context of early modern Mesagne's social and economic history.[54] These three texts were never published but are extant in manuscript. Taken together, they testify to the deep identification with place and civic role that characterized this family of physicians.

For the purposes of this paper, I will concentrate on the role of place in Ferdinando the Elder's case collection, *Centum historiae*, which present in chronological order a hundred cases from his first 17 years of practice in Mesagne, from 1596 to 1613. Like van Foreest's text, this is an important and influential specimen of the *observationes* literature, widely read and cited over the seventeenth and eighteenth centuries. What is the role of place in Ferdinando's *Centum historiae*? Most interestingly, for each case Ferdinando made locality—in the sense of local microclimate and weather conditions—the first item in his methodic discussion of diagnosis and therapy. Ferdinando was concerned not to give simply a *historia* of each case. He wanted to be considered a "rational physician, worthy of the Hippocratic art," not just a "historian." "So that we don't appear to be mere historians,"[55] he declared at the beginning of his work that he would methodically examine each case from the viewpoint of the "non-natural, natural and preternatural" aspects of disease. Most interestingly, of the six non-naturals (that is, air, exercise and rest, food and drink, sleeping and waking, excretions and retentions, and the passions of the soul) he chose to pay special attention to one—"air, that is to say, its quality, constitution, the time of the year and the place."[56] Synthetically, he called all these factors "aeris cognitio" ("knowledge of the air"), and he argued that such knowledge was as fundamental to understanding disease as that of the patient's own temperament in health (the natural aspect of the case) and his or her pathological condition (the preternatural aspect). So for each case Ferdinando reported the specific local and meteorological conditions under which it had developed.

Ferdinando was much interested in air and water quality, as indicated by the fact that he authored a *Libellus de bonitate aquae cisternae*. He also dealt with this topic in one of his earlier publications, *Theoremata medica et philosophica* (1611), and he emphasized these issues in a health regimen he wrote for Pope Paul V, "Libellus de vita propaganda."[57] One of his unpublished works relates directly to the expert knowledge he claimed on the local air. This is a short treatise, called "De Coelo Messapiensi" (On the Air of Mesagne), which is very much in the tradition of localized *regimina* that have been described by Cavallo and Storey.[58] Though purporting to describe the quality of Mesagne's air in general terms, however, the text has an *ad personam* agenda: it is addressed to Ferdinando's patron and patient, the prince Giovanni Antonio Albricci, whom Ferdinando was hoping to persuade to move his residence to Mesagne from the town of Salice Salentino, which Ferdinando deemed unhealthy.

At the beginning of his work, Ferdinando places it in the tradition of the eulogy of a place for its salubriousness, quoting Cicero on Syracuse, Marco Antonio Sebellico on Venice, Giorgio Alessandrini on Milan, Symphorien Champier for Lyon, and so on.[59] He favorably compared Mesagne's micro-climate not only with the unhealthy Salice Salentino, where the prince resided when visiting his Apulian fiefs, but even, more daringly, with the Roman air "which gives rise to lethargic and semitertian fevers, and especially the site of the Vatican, which is extremely pestilential [*pestilentissimus*]."[60] He listed Mesagne's advantages: first of all, a semi-elevated position, on a low hill, from which the rain would naturally drain.[61] No nearby body of stagnating water. A location between the mountains and the sea, the "sparkling Adriatic," visible in the distance: an ideal position for following the Salernitan health precept, *De mane montes, de sero respice fontes*, "in the morning, look at the mountains, in the evening look at the fountains."[62] Another health advantage was the presence in town of many potteries, whose kilns, constantly operating, by day in the winter and by night in the summer, sent out a smoke, which improved the air, correcting its excessive moistness due to the prevailing southern wind. "This smoke—argued Ferdinando—brings the air [*coelum*] of Mesagne to the utmost perfection by constantly purifying and drying it."[63]

This explained, in his opinion, why epidemic diseases rarely came to Mesagne, and the fact that head wounds would heal faster there, "a most distinctive sign of air that is subtle and well-tempered, or a little leaning to be dry."[64] Further signs of the air's salubriousness were the lusciousness of the vegetation and the longevity of the local people: Ferdinando mentions his paternal uncle, as well as his maternal uncle and aunt, all centenarians.[65] Particularly healthy is the air of the fortress, where presumably the prince would reside, whose *temperies* (well-temperate condition) is ensured by "the numberless orchards surrounding it, which send out a sweet smell in various seasons."[66] In the vicinity of the fortress, the air of the Carmelitan monastery of S. Angelo is especially renowned for its bracing qualities. "The Carmelitan fathers never seem to age, never lose their appetite and I never knew them to be sick."[67] This is due to the fragrance of the great variety of aromatic plants that grow there—*myrtus, lentiscus*, the white *viola, polygonum*, anise, hyssop, savory and thyme.[68] The air of S. Angelo is especially recommended for those affected by empyema and phthisis. By ancient custom, the physicians of Lecce sent their patients to convalesce in S. Angelo, and in his case collection Ferdinando twice reports that he regularly sent patients there who were affected by tabes and dropsy.[69]

Variations in the qualities of the air, Ferdinando concludes, are more important for health than the variations of water.[70] These local differences in air quality must be investigated in all their variety. "Not only water but also earth and air vary in innumerable ways: as people say: *La terra, l'acqua e l'aria vanno a palmi*," says Ferdinando quoting a local peasant proverb. "Soil, water and air go by the palm of the hand": each bit of them may be different, and should be measured by the yardstick of the hand, the symbol of human labor and human scale.[71] For Ferdinando, it is the task of the medical practitioner to serve his community (*patria*) by investigating "the variety of the seasons, the site, the variety of particular regions, and the corresponding 'constitutions' of the air [*coeli constitutiones*]." [72] It was an appropriate creed for a town physician.

A Place, a Disease: Taranto and Tarantism

In Ferdinando's case collection, locality further emerges as a significant aspect of disease in a way that goes beyond the emphasis on air quality derived from Hippocratic environmentalism. In fact, Ferdinando's *Centum historiae* is especially famous for his description of another early modern disease named after a place—tarantism, from Taranto, the main city of Apulia. Ferdinando's account of tarantism ("on the bite of the tarantula," case no. 81 in his collection) would become famous, and would be cited by Giorgio Baglivi (also from Apulia) in his *De Anatome, Morsu & Effectibus Tarantulae* (1696) and by many other European physicians throughout the eighteenth and nineteenth centuries.[73] It became in fact a fundamental source for all interested in the phenomenon, not only among early modern and modern medical writers, but even present-day anthropologists.[74]

Ferdinando appends his discussion of the disease to a single case narrative, dated end of August 1612:

> Pietro Simeone, a Mesagne boy of hot and dry temperament, was bitten by a tarantula in the left part of his abdomen while he was in the countryside at night, as was his custom [...] Immediately, he felt a sharp pain at the spot of the bite and fell to the ground for the span of three Hail Maries—chilled all over, his body hair bristling, pain in his pubes and a penile erection. He could not stand on his legs, he cried and sighed, and felt like he was suffocating. He wanted to shout but could not. At dawn, he was taken into town, music was immediately called for, and he responded especially to the kind that is called *Catena*. Upon hearing that music, he at once started to leap and dance in a frenzied way, sweating profusely. He was sleepless for a week, during which time he would only take pure wine. He did not defecate for four days. He liked to hear funeral dirges, and tried to throw himself in water. He loved the color red, and abhorred all things blue, which he would rip to pieces and trample under his feet. [...] After a week of frenzied dancing, he was healed by the sweating and the music.[75]

Ferdinando tries to understand and explain this behavior as a form of illness caused by the tarantula's poison. He strongly disagrees with the opinion of those people who had argued that it was either a "fictive illness, a chimera," or a form of melancholy and madness. He is convinced, based on his long experience and observation, that it is "a true and real disease" ("morbus verus & realis"). Those who do not believe it, he says, "should come and see, and make the experiment [*periculum facere*] by letting themselves be bitten by the tarantula."[76]

Ferdinando localizes the disease and reconstructs its history. He argues that the tarantula is so called from the ancient city of Taranto, the main urban center in Apulia, which is infested by this kind of animal. He traces the first association of the symptoms with the bite of the tarantula in medieval sources, arguing—correctly—that the phenomenon was unknown to the ancients.[77] He reviews the previous literature on the tarantula's bite, marking as dubious all the symptoms that he has not seen himself. He always notes whether or not he has personally observed the symptoms listed in the literature. He argues, for instance, that it is not true that the symptoms stop when the *tarantatus* kills the *tarantula* that bit him, as reported by some authors:

> I know a great number of women and men, who killed the tarantula immediately after it bit them, and yet they danced for many years. Mita Lupa, who is still living, has danced for 17 years, though she killed the tarantula.[78]

His account stresses repeatedly his long, first-hand observation of the *tarantati* (those bitten by the *tarantula*) over more than 20 years of medical practice.

> I have seen *tarantati* who go and live in graves, virgins who throw themselves into a well, shouting, pulling their hair, showing their obscene parts. I have seen others sleep in coffins, hurl themselves into the sea, sing funeral songs. Some ask to be buried up to their neck, others like to be whipped on the heels, on the anus; some flagellate themselves; others bite other people. [...] They refuse to eat and subsist only on wine [...] They feel as if their bones are breaking, and they say they are *scantati & minuzati, & spezzati* (terrified, broken and ground to pieces). They often like the color red and hate blue or black things [...] They love to hear of the sea and long for those songs that speak of it. They quiet down only immersed in water, inside big clay vessels, or suspended inside wells, bound with ropes so that they don't drown.[79]

But the most striking aspect of these symptoms, Ferdinando says, is that they return cyclically once a year for long periods of time. In the summer, the time of the harvest, and also the period of most intense activity of the tarantulas, the *tarantati* feel compelled to enact their frenzied dancing, as if in commemoration of the original bite, sometimes returning to the very place where they were bitten. Again, Ferdinando offers his personal testimony:

> I know women who have danced for ten, fifteen, seventeen, twenty, even thirty years [...] always in the summer, until the effects of the poison die out. It is a poison that can last for many years, like the French disease.[80]

Each summer, he reports, it is a local custom for troupes of musicians and flute-players to wander around Apulia playing for the *tarantati*, and they make a lot of money. The disease is also a local business. Some poor people, especially women, have spent all their fortune on the music therapy, repeated year after year.[81]

Though other remedies can be used (surgical remedies as they apply to all animal bites; antidotes such as *alexipharmaca*, theriac and bezoar),[82] Ferdinando admits that the sovereign treatment for the bite is music, the local remedy. "In this region of ours, all over Apulia, no other kind of remedy is used for the *tarantati* but music."[83] Not any music, but a specific kind of local music, called *tarantella*, of which Ferdinando describes several varieties with their vernacular names (*cinque tempi, panno verde, panno rosso, moresca, catena, spallata*). The *tarantati* require a loud music with a very intense rhythm to induce the frantic dancing that releases the poison.[84] But which of the several varieties of local music will work for each person struck by the tarantula has to be ascertained on an individualized basis, with the musicians trying the various kinds until the *tarantatus* responds by starting to dance.[85] Ferdinando has no doubt that the music therapy works. "I have practiced medicine for twenty years, and I never saw a *tarantatus* die of the bite."[86] He also believes that those *tarantati* who do not participate in the orgiastic dancing for reasons of decency and shame—such as religious men and women—develop worse symptoms and fall into more serious diseases.[87]

But why does the music therapy work? And how can one understand the *mira varietas* (amazing variety) of the symptoms? Ferdinando's methodical mind arranges the things observed in a list of a hundred "why" questions, to which he tries to give an answer.[88] He draws on the natural history of the *tarantula*, in order to establish the temperament of this animal and the consequent qualities of its poison. The *tarantula* is described by natural historians as bloodless and therefore cold, dry, and full of melancholic humor.[89] It is this melancholic temperament of the *tarantula* that accounts for many of the symptoms displayed by the *tarantati*. So, for instance, why are they drawn to sepulchres and funeral dirges? Why do they long to be buried under ground? Because of the melancholic nature of the *tarantula* poison, since the atrabiliar or melancholic humor is associated with the element earth. Why do they love to hear of the sea and throw themselves into wells? Because they are eager for water, due to the dry nature of the tarantula's poison. The intensity and variety of the symptoms—such as the role of various colors and different kinds of music in the healing ritual—are explained by the varieties of the tarantulas themselves, each drawn to a certain color or music—and especially the varying ways in which the tarantula's poison affects people differently according to their individual temperament.[90] The worst symptoms develop whenever the tarantula bites somebody who has a melancholic temperament, the black bile of the animal interacting with, and reinforcing, the black bile of the patient. This also explains the variable duration of the symptoms, and why some people have to submit to the music ritual for years, until "the remnants of the poison" in their bodies are completely expelled.[91]

And yet, Ferdinando admits that there is much that cannot be explained within the humoral framework. Is the poison transmitted across the generations? Does a *tarantatus* generate another *tarantatus*? Is it a contagious (*contagiosus*) and hereditary (*haereditarius*) disease, "like dog rabies, the French disease, and leprosy?"[92] He does not know. He is especially puzzled by the topography of the disease, which exhibits a clear gender pattern. Why is it that in some places, as for instance in Brindisi, the *tarantati* are mostly women while elsewhere, as in Mesagne, they are mostly men? Here Ferdinando abandons the humoral theory for an answer that has to do with local work and life conditions. He notes that Brindisi and Mesagne have each different agricultural economies and consequently different settlement patterns. In Brindisi, there are many fruit trees and the houses are set in these orchards, where the tarantulas proliferate. Women, who live and work at home, are thus exposed to the bite of the animal. In Mesagne, in contrast, people grow wheat in fields that are far from the village, so the tarantulas are not often seen in the houses. In this case, it is the men who have a higher chance of being bitten, because they work in the fields.[93]

But the issue of the geographical locality of disease raises a more fundamental issue for Ferdinando. Why does it seem endemic in Apulia and is not found elsewhere? Ferdinando rejects the view of those who had argued that only the locals are bitten by the tarantula, and that foreigners are immune to the bite. He does not believe it, for the good reason that, as he says, "we all are made of four elements and four humors."[94] But also because his long experience in Mesagne tells him otherwise: "I knew several Spaniards who were bitten and danced; an Egyptian woman, a woman from Ethiopia and another from Albania, who were bitten here in Apulia, and they all danced."[95] But there is no denying that, while people may be bitten by tarantulas anywhere, the striking behavioral symptoms of the *tarantati* and the music healing ritual are only found in Apulia. Why? Ferdinando considers a possible humoral reason, in the framework of Hippocratic environmentalism. Can it be the sun, the climate, the quality of food? None of these answers seem persuasive to him. It is certainly not the heat of the region, because there are hotter places than Apulia, in which one does not meet with the *tarantati*. Hard pressed, Ferdinando goes back for an explanation to the idea of local variation (*varia locorum differentia*) that he also used in *De Coelo Messapiensi*. The extraordinary power of the Apulian tarantula's bite may be caused by an unknown quality of the air [*coelum*] and also, possibly, by a "mysterious [*arcana*], secret, hidden, occult quality" of the local *tarantula* itself, which does not derive from its humoral temperament, or its specific mixture of qualities, but from the "whole substance and form" (*tota substantia et forma*) of the animal.[96] Early modern physicians resorted to the concept of *tota substantia* whenever they could not explain a disease by means of the humoral theory: it was their admission that they had reached the end of the humoral tether.[97] So it was for Ferdinando, and he was aware of it. He admits that if he wanted to deal fully with the problem of local variation, he would have to be more of a historian and less of a philosopher.

> Bountiful Nature, or the Glorious God who is the maker of Nature, has chosen, with wondrous foresight, to endow different places with different and marvelous virtues, so much in their minerals and vegetables as in their living beings. Of this, I will pass over in silence innumerable examples, because if I wanted to pursue them all, I would perform the office of the historian, rather than that of the philosopher.[98]

Ferdinando did not coin the term *tarantism* but initiated a long tradition of medical writings on the phenomenon as a local disease, observed in a specific community, thus paving the way for an understanding of its cultural aspects. Ernesto De Martino, the Italian anthropologist who first led a fieldwork expedition to Apulia in the 1950s to study the *tarantati* from an ethnographic viewpoint, argued that Ferdinando was unable to understand tarantism for what it is: not a medical, but a cultural phenomenon.[99] For De Martino, tarantism could only be understood as a cultural response, individually and collectively elaborated, to the bite of the tarantula as the symbol of the hardship of peasant life—the symbol of a threat to personhood that the Apulian peasants exorcize through a music ritual.[100]

De Martino wrote a great book on tarantism, *La terra del rimorso* (*Land of Remorse*), where remorse means, as it does etymologically, remorse—the human experience of being bitten, over and over again, by the haunting memory of trauma. But if we read his masterpiece of ethnographic description after reading Ferdinando, as I have done for this essay, we can see that all the fundamental traits of the tarantati's behavior, down to the pathos of their very words—their cry of being "*spezzati, schantati, minuzzati, e rotti, e tramazzati*"[101]—were already noted in Ferdinando's work. The Apulian physician had already given a thick description of the phenomenon, and recognized, though dimly, its historical and cultural character. He had established, for instance, that both the disease and the healing rituals had developed in the Middle Ages, as confirmed by De Martino's historical research.[102] Far from encapsulating the phenomenon in the straitjacket of Hippocratic humoralism, Ferdinando admits that the humoral explanation is inadequate. At the end of his description, he is left with the rather mechanical explanation that the music ritual helps because "by inciting the *tarantati* to leap and dance, the lurking benumbed forces of the poison are stirred by the quick motion of the body and pushed out by sweating." But he knows that there is more to this process than the mere mechanics of bodily fluids. "It is a duel," Ferdinando says, "between the poison and Nature, which the latter wins thanks to music, the exercise of the soul."[103] Ultimately, it is not only the occult quality of the tarantula that explains the behavior of the *tarantati*: it is also the occult power of their soul, summoned and intensified by the power of music, that makes them raise from prostration and assert themselves in the ritual dance. Here, at the end of his *observatio* on the tarantula's bite, Ferdinando comes close to interrogating not only the mysteries of nature but the no less hard to decipher mysteries of culture.

Ferdinando's account of tarantism is first of all a localized description of disease, and it should be understood, as I suggest in this chapter, within the Hippocratic regionalism that can be widely observed in early modern medical culture.[104] But it is much more than that. It also offers a description of the disease as a cultural phenomenon, one that cannot be fully accounted for within a Hippocratic and indeed any naturalistic medical framework. The case of Ferdinando shows that, much like Dr. Fabrazzi of Minerbio, with whom this essay began, the town physician could be much more than a medical practitioner. He could also be the local historian and ethnographer—the faithful observer of the traumas and healing rites of a local culture.

Notes

1 BUB (Biblioteca Universitaria, Bologna), ms. 115: "Diario del Dott. Petronio Fabrazzi medico di Minerbio." The manuscript was so titled by a nineteenth-century compiler of the Library's inventory. Fabrazzi himself called it "vacchetta abcedaria."

2 Fabrazzi's text has been used as a source by local historians: see Camillo Zamboni, *Cronaca del castello di Minerbio* (Bologna, 1855), pp. 38–39, 53, 156.

3 Luigi Guerra-Coppioli, "Capitolati medici dei tempi andati," *Rivista di storia critica delle scienze mediche e naturali*, 1 (1910–12): 129–36, pp. 135–36; Irma Naso, *Medici e strutture sanitarie nella società tardo-medievale* (Milan, 1981), pp. 37, 40; Gianna Pomata, *Contracting a Cure: Patients, Healers and the Law in Early Modern Bologna* (Baltimore, 1998), p. 49. For the similar duties of town physicians in the German territories, see Dross, "'De Officiis'," Chapter 4 of this volume.

4 Pomata, *Contracting a Cure*, p. 49.

5 On the *observationes* see Gianna Pomata, "Sharing Cases: The *Observationes* in Early Modern Medicine," *Early Science and Medicine*, 15: 3 (2010):

193–236; "Observation Rising: Birth of an Epistemic Genre, ca. 1500–1650," in Lorraine Daston and Elizabeth Lunbeck (eds), *Histories of Scientific Observation* (Chicago, 2011): 45–80; "The Recipe and the Case: Epistemic Genres and the Dynamics of Cognitive Practices," in Kaspar von Greyerz, Silvia Flubacher and Philipp Senn (eds), *Wissenschaftsgeschichte und Geschichte des Wissens im Dialog – Connecting Science and Knowledge* (Göttingen, 2013): 131–54.

6 More in general, on early modern physician historians, see the fundamental contribution of Nancy G. Siraisi, *History, Medicine, and the Traditions of Renaissance Learning* (Ann Arbor, 2007).

7 Martin Ruland the Elder, *Curationum empiricarum et historicarum in certis locis et notis hominibus optimè, riteque probatarum & expertarum centuriae* (Basel, 1578–1595). The ten *centuriae* were first published together in Basel in 1628. Ruland the Elder (1532–1602) was later court physician to Rudolph II in Vienna.

8 Pieter van Foreest (Forestus), *Observationum et curationum medicinalium de febribus ephemeris et continuis libri duo* (Antwerp, 1584). This was the first instalment of van Foreest's *Observationes*, which was dedicated to the municipality of Delft. The various instalments were published in Antwerp 1584–1609 (books 26–32 posthumously). Van Foreest also published nine books of *Observationes chirurgicae*, with a total of 158 cases. On van Foreest (1521–1597), see Ingo Wilhelm Müller, *Iatromechanische Theorie und ärztliche Praxis im Vergleich zur galenistischen Medizin* (Stuttgart, 1991), pp. 49–52; Henriette A. Bosman-Jelgersma (ed.), *Petrus Forestus Medicus* (Amsterdam, 1996).

9 Felix Platter, *Observationum in hominis affectibus plerisque libri tres ... , in quibus eo ordine diversorum affectuum progressus, eventus, curationes ... historice describuntur* (Basel, 1614); see Katharina Huber, *Felix Platters "Observationes": Studien zum frühneuzeitlichen Gesundheitswesen in Basel* (Basel, 2003), pp. 11–15. Philipp Hechstetter, *Rararum observationum medicinalium decades tres* (Augsburg, 1624–1627). Gregor Horst, *Observationum medicinalium singularium libri quatuor priores* (Ulm, 1625); Id., *Observationum medicinalium singularium libri quatuor posteriores: his accedunt Epistolarum et consultationum medicinalium a Germaniae medicis potissimum et aliis communicatarum libri duo* (Ulm, 1628–1631). On Horst, see Claudia Ragheb, *Die Pathologie des Gregor Horstius im Vergleich zu den Galenisten seiner Zeit, erläutert am Beispiel Jean Fernels*, Dissertation (Giessen, 1996); Isabel Wilhelm, *Krankheiten von Gehirn und Sinnesorganen in Kasuistiken des Gießener Arztes Gregor Horstius (1578–1636)*, Dissertation (Giessen, 1994). Nicolaes Tulp, *Observationum medicarum libri tres* (Amsterdam, 1641); see I.C.E. Wesdorp, "The Physician Dr. Nicolaes Tulp," in Sebastien A.C. Dudok van Heel et al. (eds), *Nicolaes Tulp. The Life and Work of an Amsterdam Physician and Magistrate in the Seventeenth Century* (Amsterdam, 1998): 117–48.

10 On case-knowledge as a "style of thinking," see John Forrester, "If *p*, then What? Thinking in Cases," *History of the Human Sciences*, 9/3 (1996): 1–25.

11 On Amatus' *Centuriae curationum* as the model of the new genre, see Pomata, "Sharing cases," pp. 206–15.

12 On this aspect of the *observationes*, see my paper "The Individual in the Case: The Focus on Individuality in Early Modern European Case Collections," presented at the conference *Individualized Medicine in Historical Perspective: From Antiquity to the Genome Age*, Institute of the History of Medicine, Johns Hopkins University (15–16 May 2014). The principle of individualized treatment has survived in Arabo-Galenic medicine to the

present day: see Agnes G. Loeffler, "Individual Constitution versus Universal Physiology: Iranian Responses to Allopathic Medicine," *Body and Science*, 13/3 (2007): 103–23.

13 For an authoritative example of this view, see Paolo Zacchia, *Quaestiones medico-legales* (Rome, 1621–1651), tomus I, lib. VI, quaestio VII, "De erroris empiricorum," where it is said of charlatans that they use remedies "promiscue et indifferenter in omnibus morbis" (I have used the Lyon, 1701 edition, where the citation is at p. 474).

14 See Jole Agrimi and Chiara Crisciani, *Les "consilia" médicaux* (Turnout, 1994).

15 See, for instance, Anuce Foës, *Liber Secundus Hippocratis de morbis vulgaribus, … pene in integrum restitutus, commentariis sex & Latinitate donatus* (Basel, 1560); Herman Cruserius, *Commentarius in Hippocratis I et III de morbis vulgaribus* (Basel, 1570); Francisco Valles, *In libros Hippocratis de morbis popularibus commentaria* (Madrid, 1577).

16 Pearl Kibre, *Hippocrates Latinus: Repertorium of Hippocratic Writings in the Latin Middle Ages* (New York, 1985), no. XIX, 138–142: *Epidemics* was known to medieval Western Europe only in partial Latin translation. On Manente Leontini's humanist translation, see Innocenzo Mazzini, "Manente Leontini, Übersetzer der hippokratischen Epidemien (cod. Laurent. 73, 12): Bemerkungen zu seiner Übersetzung von Epidemien Buch 6" in Gerhard Baader and Rolf Winau (eds), *Die hippokratischen Epidemien: Theorie – Praxis – Tradition* (Stuttgart, 1989): 312–20.

17 As, for instance, in Girolamo Mercuriale, *Praelectiones Pisanae … in Epidemicas Hippocratis Historias* (Venice, 1597); see Siraisi, *History, Medicine*, p. 287, n. 47.

18 Siraisi, *History, Medicine*, pp. 72–79. On the long-term influence of *Airs Waters Places*, see Charles E. Rosenberg, "Epilogue: *Airs, Waters, Places*: A Status Report," in Special Issue on *Modern Airs Waters Places* (eds) Alison Bashford and Sarah W. Tracy, *Bulletin of the History of Medicine*, 86/4 (2012): 661–70.

19 Sandra Cavallo and Tessa Storey, *Healthy Living in Late Renaissance Italy* (Oxford, 2013), pp. 70–112.

20 Siraisi, *History, Medicine*, pp. 93–102. She mentions four major commentaries by L'Alemant, Cardano, Baldini and Settala. During the Middle Ages, *Airs Waters Places* was translated into Latin, but not commented on, nor used as a university text: Kibre, *Hippocrates latinus*, no. II, 25–28; cf. Siraisi, p. 287, n. 28.

21 Siraisi, *History, Medicine*, pp. 94–95. For the early Renaissance, this trend has been described by Katharine Park, "Natural Particulars: Medical Epistemology, Practice, and the Literature of Healing Springs," in Anthony Grafton and Nancy G. Siraisi (eds), *Natural Particulars: Nature and the Disciplines in Renaissance Europe* (Boston, 1999): 347–68. For some examples of this literature, see Giorgio Franciotti, *Tractatus de balneo villensi* (Lucca, 1552); Giovan Battista Donati, *De aquis lucensibus* (Lucca, 1580); Giovan Battista Cartegni, *Trattato de'venti, in quanto si appartiene al medico, e del sito della città di Pisa* (Pisa, 1628); Domenico Panaroli, *Aerologia, ovvero discorso dell'aria* (Rome, 1642), on the winds of Rome. See Cavallo and Storey, *Healthy Living*, p. 80. See also the debate on the quality of the Tiber water in sixteenth-century Rome in Siraisi, *History, Medicine*, pp. 177–86.

22 Marsilio Cagnati, *De Romani aeris salubritate commentarius* (Rome, 1599). See Siraisi, *History, Medicine*, p. 181.

23 Marsilio Cagnati, *De Tiberis inundatione medica disputatio … Epidemia Romana, disputatio, de illa populari aegritudine, quae anno 1591, et de altera, quae anno 1593, in urbem Romam invasit* (Rome, 1599).

24 Girolamo Mercuriale, *De peste in universum, praesertim vero de Venetia et Patavina*, in Idem, *Tractatus varii de re medica* (Lyon, 1618). See Siraisi, *History, Medicine*, p. 91.

25 Marilyn Nicoud, *Les régimes de santé au moyen âge: Naissance et diffusion d'une écriture médicale (XIIIe-XVe siècle)*, 2 vols. (Rome, 2007).

26 Tommaso Giannotti Rangoni, *Come il serenissimo doge di Venezia il signor Sebastian Veniero e li Veneziani possano viver sempre sani consiglio* (Venice, 1577). This text was first published in Latin: *De vita principis et Venetorum commoda semper consilium* (Venice, 1558), then translated into the vernacular by a pupil of Rangoni's (*Consiglio come i Veneziani possano vivere sempre sani tradotto nuovamente da Giacomo Pratello Montefiore medico*, Venice, 1565) and by the author himself in the 1577 edition cited above. See Cavallo and Storey, *Healthy Living*, p. 79, who also cite other city-specific regimens from the same period (for Rome by Alessandro Petroni, for Genoa by Bartolomeo Paschetti). On Tommaso Giannotti Rangoni, see the entry by Franco Bacchelli in *Dizionario Biografico degli Italiani*, vol. 54 (Rome, 2000), s. v.

27 Cavallo and Storey, *Healthy Living*, p. 79. On the localization of *regimina*, see also Siraisi, *History, Medicine*, p. 182 on Alessandro Petroni's *De victu romanorum et sanitate tuenda* (Rome, 1581).

28 Siraisi, *History, Medicine*, p. 66.

29 Tommaso Somenzi, *De morbis qui per finitimos populos adhuc grassantur* (Cremona, 1576). On these "plague disputes," see Samuel K. Cohn, Jr., *Cultures of Plague: Medical Thinking at the End of the Renaissance* (Oxford, 2010): ch. 6. The earliest European examples of disease maps relate to a plague epidemic that took place in Bari and Naples in 1690–92: see Tom Koch, *Disease Maps: Epidemics on the Ground* (Chicago, 2011), pp. 51–57.

30 Gian Battista Codronchi, *De morbis qui Imolae et alibi hoc anno 1602 vagati sunt commentariolus* (Bologna, 1603). On Codronchi, see the entry by Carlo Colombero in *Dizionario Biografico degli Italiani*, vol. 26 (Rome, 1982), s. v.

31 *Epidemics 6, 7, 1.*

32 Amatus Lusitanus, *Curationum medicinalium centuriae septem* (Barcelona, 1628: originally published 1551–1566). On his peregrinations as a converso Jew, sometimes feted and more often persecuted by the Christian authorities, see George H. Tucker, *Homo Viator: Itineraries of Exile, Displacement and Writing in Renaissance Europe* (Geneva, 2003), pp. 195–238.

33 Amatus, *Centuriae septem*, Centuria 6, curatio 68, cols. 1105–06; cf. Centuria 7, curatio 93, col. 1371: "De intestinorum affectionibus, pubblice grassantibus." "Maio mense, sicco, & calido, plures intestinorum morbis correpti sunt, scilicet, colico, cholera, ileo, dysenteria, & similibus: vagabantur autem morbi ii, & epidemiales erant."

34 In all likelihood, the index was not compiled by Amatus himself. A notice on the frontispiece states that the Index was found "in Bibliotheca Iohannis Francisci Rosselli Catalani." The Catalan physician Johannes Franciscus Rossellus, active in the 1620s, was the author of a commentary on Galen's *De differentiis et causis morborum*.

35 Amatus, *Centuriae septem*, Centuria 7, curatio 25, cols. 1257–58.

36 In previously published collections, such as that by Ruland the Elder, place is often mentioned but is not very significant from a nosological or therapeutic viewpoint. In Ruland's *Curationes*, the place of each patient is mentioned so precisely that one can literally reconstruct a map of his practice in the territory around Lauingen, but it does not seem to affect diagnosis and therapy.

37 Pieter van Foreest, *Observationum et curationum medicinalium, de febribus publice grassantibus, cum morbis epidemiis* (Leiden, 1588), republished in Pieter Van Foreest, *Observationum et curationum medicinalium ac chirurgicarum opera omnia* (Rouen, 1653): 188–259, from which I quote. See Vivian Nutton, "Pieter van Foreest and the Plagues of Europe: Some Observations on the *Observationes*," in H. L. Houtzager (ed.), *Pieter van Foreest: Een Hollands Medicus in de zestiende Eew* (Amsterdam, 1989): 25–39. On epidemic diseases in a later case collection by Gregor Horst, see Ulf Eisenreich, *Die "contagiösen" Krankheiten im Werk des Gregor Horstius (1578–1636)*, Dissertation (Giessen, 1995).

38 Alkmaar: *variolae* and *morbilli*, 1551 (*observationes* 41–43); catarrhal fevers, 1553 (*observationes* 4–6) and 1577 (*observationes* 1–2). Delft: plague in 1557–58 (*observationes* 9–25); *variolae* and *morbilli* from "universalis et coelestis origo," 1561 and 1563 (*observationes* 44–61); throat and respiratory condition, also spread in Belgium, Germany and France, 1580 (*observatio* 3). Harlem: plague of 1573 (*observationes* 27–40).

39 *Observatio* 8. As far as I know, no published text by Tyengius on this epidemic is extant. Forestus may have consulted a manuscript that has not survived: see *Scriptores de sudore anglico superstites*, ed. Christianus Gottfridus Gruner (Jena, 1847), p. 501, n. 3. Tertius Damianus' work, *Peri tou hidronousou*, published in his *Theorica medicinae* (Antwerp, 1541), is reprinted in *Scriptores de sudore anglico superstites*, cited above, pp. 19–38.

40 Thomas Jordan, *Pestis phenomena* (Frankfurt, 1576). See Joseph Janvier Woodward, "Typho-Malarial Fever: Is It a Special Type of Fever?" *Transactions of the International Medical Congress of Philadelphia*, ed. John Ashhurst (Philadelphia, 1877): 314–18.

41 Jordan, *Pestis*, ch. 19, p. 217.

42 Tobias Cober, *Observationum castrensium et Ungaricarum decades tres. Austriaca, Silesiaca, Svevica* (Frankfurt 1606): *decas* 1, *observationes* 5–6, pp. 53–59; on *Languor Pannonicus* caused by sleeping on the ground, *observatio* 10, p. 108, or by rotten beer, *decas* 2, *observatio* 1.

43 Martin Ruland the Younger, *De perniciosae luis ungaricae tecmarsi et curatione* (Frankfurt, 1600), p. 14: "morbus epidemius est, quod plures, etiam temperamento dissimiles, uno & eodem tempore invadat, ab epidemio, id est, communi causa ortus, sive ea sit aer, sive victus communis plurimis." Like his father, Martin Ruland the Younger was town physician in Lauingen and, after his father's death, personal physician of the Emperor Rudolph II. See Felicitas Söhner, *Vom Lauinger Stadtphysikus zum kaiserlichen Leibarzt: Der Alchimist Martin Ruland der Jüngere* (Munich, 2011).

44 Heinrich Meibom, unpaginated preface, in Tobias Cober, *Observationum medicarum castrensium hungaricarum, decades tres* (Helmstedt, 1685). Cober had done his medical studies in Helmstedt, where Meibom was professor of medicine.

45 Epifanio Ferdinando the Elder, *Centum historiae, seu observationes, et casus medici* (Venice, 1621; photostatic reprint, Bologna, 2001).

46 Domenico Urgesi, "Alle origini della letteratura storica mesagnese: la famiglia Ferdinando," *Studi salentini*, 70 (1993): 133–43.

47 For biographical information, I draw on Enzo Poci, "Epifanio Ferdinando: la vita, le opere e altre notizie storiche e di costume," in Mario Monti and Domenico D. Urgesi (eds), *Epifanio Ferdinando, medico e storico del Seicento* (Nardò, 2001): 219–50; and the Introduction in Maria Luisa Portulano Scoditti, *Epifanio Ferdinando medico, storico, filosofo (Mesagne 1569–1638): la vita e i brani scelti dalle sue Centum historiae* (Mesagne, 1999); Maria Luisa

Portulano Scoditti and Amedeo Elio Distante, *Epifanio Ferdinando – Le centum historiae e la medicina del suo tempo* (Mesagne, 2000).

48 An eighteenth-century biographer of Ferdinando, Domenico De Angelis, claimed that in 1616 the Venetian ambassador in Rome offered Ferdinando a medical chair in Padua: see Domenico De Angelis, *Vite de' letterati salentini* (Florence, 1710), pp. 217–30. So far, however, no documentation has been found in the Padua archives to support this claim: see Raffaele Colonna, "Epifanio Ferdinando e lo studio di Padova agli inizi del Seicento," in Mario Monti and Domenico D. Urgesi (eds), *Epifanio Ferdinando, medico e storico del Seicento* (Nardò, 2001): 66–73. Ferdinando corresponded with prominent Italian physicians and philosophers, like Cesare Cremonini and Marco Aurelio Severino.

49 The work was never published. It is extant in an eighteenth-century manuscript copy in BABr (BABr = Biblioteca Arcivescovile "Annibale De Leo," Brindisi). For a list of Ferdinando's manuscripts, see Antonio Profilo, *Vie, piazze, vichi e corti di Mesagne* (Ostuni 1894; photostatic reprint, ed. Domenico D. Urgesi, Fasano, 1993), pp. 242–56. Some of Ferdinando's printed works have been published recently in Italian translation: see Ferdinando, *La peste*, translated by Maria Luisa Portulano Scoditti and Amedeo Elio Distante (Mesagne, 2001; Italian transl. of *De peste aureus libellus*, Naples, 1626); *Epifanio Ferdinando – De Vita Proroganda*, translated by Maria Luisa Portulano Scoditti and Amedeo Elio Distante (Mesagne, 2004: Italian transl. of *De Vita Proroganda seu juventute conservanda…*, Naples, 1612).

50 As amply shown by Siraisi, *History, Medicine*.

51 BABr, Giovanni Maria Moricino, *Dell'antiquità e vicissitudine della città di Brindisi, descritta dalla di lei origine fino all'anno 1604*. MS.

52 This work was written between 1653 and 1662. It is extant in a later transcription in BABr.

53 Epifanio Ferdinando Junior (d. 1717), *Libro delle famiglie di Mesagne*, MS in four tomes dating from the early eighteenth century, in the private collection of the family Cavaliere, Mesagne. The manuscript includes genealogies of all the families living in Mesagne at the time of the author, plus those that had died out. It highlights alliance strategies, and the rising or declining fortunes of different families.

54 Annastella Carrino, "Gruppi sociali e mestiere nel Mezzogiorno di età moderna: I 'massari' in un centro cerealicolo di Terra d'Otranto (Mesagne, secoli XVI–XVIII)," *Società e storia*, 16/60 (1993): 231–78; and especially Annastella Carrino, *Parentela, mestiere, potere: Gruppi sociali in un borgo meridionale di antico regime (Mesagne: secoli XVI–XVIII)* (Bari, 1995). For her use of Ferdinando the Younger's text as a source, see, for instance, *Parentela*, pp. 12–13, 140.

55 Ferdinando the Elder, *Centum historiae*, fol. 8: "ne tantum videamur esse historici." The same remark is repeated often, for instance, on fol. 22: "Quoniam non decet medicum dogmaticum, rationalem, generosum, atque arte Hippocratica dignum tantum historias, et cantilenas decantare."

56 Ferdinando the Elder, *Centum historiae*, fol. 1: "Quantum ad primum, per res non naturales, caeteris derelictis, scilicet motu, & quiete, cibo, & potu, somno, & vigilia, excretis, & retentis, & animi perturbationibus, tantum aerem intelligo, scilicet eius qualitatem, constitutionem, anni tempus, regionem. Multum enim refert, atque conducit huiusmodi aeris cognitio ad res naturales, & praeter naturam."

57 Epifanio Ferdinando the Elder, *Theoremata medica et philosophica* (Venice, 1611), lib. 2, theorema 3, pp. 146–47. Chapter 3 of *De Vita Proroganda seu*

juventute conservanda... (Naples, 1612) is entirely devoted to the issue of air. The *Libellus de bonitate aquae cisternae* was never published.

58 BABr: Epifanio Ferdinando Senior, *De Coelo Messapiensi*, 1616, MS. (hereafter: *De Coelo*). I would like to thank Annastella Carrino and Katiuscia Di Rocco for helping me gain access to this manuscript.

59 Ibid., cc. 1–3. A later example of this subgenre in the *regimina* literature would be *L'aria celimontana* (*The Air on the Caelian Hill*) by the Roman physician Domenico Panaroli. The author of an important case collection, Panaroli defended the air of the Caelian Hill, one of Rome's seven hills, as an eligible place of residence. See Cavallo and Storey, *Healthy Living*, p. 80.

60 *De Coelo*, cc. 50–61, c. 56 on the Roman air.

61 Ibid., c. 29: "situs aliquantum altus et elevatus in semi collina, statius diffluunt aquae pluviales."

62 Ibid., c. 36. Cf. *Collectio Salernitana*, ed. Salvatore De Renzi (Naples, 1859), vol. 5, p. 7.

63 *De Coelo*, cc. 38–39: "hic enim fumus purificat sua sicca qualitate, et non insuavi odore aerem Austrinum: nam fere nulla die est in qua hujusmodi fornaces non ardeant ... et hic assiduus fumus ... maxime perficit Messapiense coelum, ita ut iure iurando affirmare ausim ob huiusmodi assiduam aeris purificatione, quae in estate fieri solet de nocte, et in hyeme de die, Messapiae de raro epidemijs tentantur."

64 Ibid., c. 41: "prestantissimus signus aeris vel tenuis et temperati, vel paulum ad siccum vergentis."

65 Ibid., c. 34: "Patruus, Avunculus and Avuncula centenarii."

66 Ibid., cc. 44–45: "Temperiem histius Arcis conservant et augent sexcenta pommaria, quae per plura stadia circum oppidum gratum spirant odorem in diversis temporibus."

67 Ibid., c. 49: "In hoc aere Patres Carmelitae non senescunt, semper eis est appetentia, numquam eos scio infirmos."

68 Ibid., c. 47.

69 Ferdinando, *Centum historiae*, fol. 93 (*historia* 30) and fol. 306 (*historia* 90).

70 *De Coelo*, cc. 20–21.

71 Ibid., c. 17: "Non solum aquam sed terram et aerem sexcenties diversificari, et vulgo dicitur La terra, l'acqua, e l'aria vanno a palmi" (c. 17). *Sexcenties*, lit. "six hundred times," is regularly used by Ferdinando to indicate an immense number. The palm was a unit of measure for length.

72 Ibid., c. 18: "ob varietatem anni temporum, ob situm et varietatem regionum et ob particulares coeli constitutiones." On the significance of *varietas* as a cognitive category in early modern medicine, see Pomata, "Observation Rising," p. 58.

73 Ferdinando, *Centum historiae*, fols. 248–68. Ferdinando also left a manuscript on this issue, *Libellus de morsu tarantulae* (1612), which I have not been able to access. On the reception of Ferdinando's views on tarantism among European physicians, see Gino Di Mitri, *Fortuna critica di Epifanio Ferdinando nella letteratura accademica settecentesca svedese sul tarantismo* (Nardò, 2001). On Baglivi see Andrea Carlino, "Il tarantismo di Giorgio Baglivi: medicina pratica, historia naturalis e scrittura etnografica," introduction to Giorgio Baglivi, *Della tarantola* (Rome, 2014): 7–33.

74 The Italian anthropologist Ernesto De Martino made extensive use of Ferdinando's description of tarantism. See below, n. 99.

75 Ferdinando, *Centum historiae*, fol. 248. Besides Simeone's case, Ferdinando also mentions a few other patients. He reports, for instance, the case of a 94-

year-old man "who could not move without crutches, but once bitten by the tarantula and after hearing the music, he started to leap and dance, beating the ground with his feet, like a wild goat" (fol. 254).

76 Ferdinando, *Centum historiae*, fol. 254, fol. 261.
77 Ibid., fol. 249, fol. 254.
78 Ibid., fol. 260.
79 Ibid., fols. 254–55.
80 Ibid., fol. 254.
81 Ibid., fol. 254: he notes that if the music therapy did not work, people would not be so stupid as to spend all their money on it: "Non essent adeo bestiales quidam pauperes, et paupercula mulieres, ut totam eorum fere substantiam erogent in musicos, tibicines et sonatores."
82 Ferdinando, *Centum historiae*, fols. 264–66. Diet, the sovereign remedy in Hippocratic medicine, does not apply to the case of the *tarantati* because they don't eat. Ferdinando lists some pharmaceutical remedies that he has found helpful: *aqua vitae*, essence of rosemary, his own distilled water, and his own *antiphalangius* (=antitarantula) electuary, of which he gives the recipe (fol. 266).
83 Ferdinando, *Centum historiae*, fol. 265: music as "exactissimum remedium."
84 Ibid., fols. 259–60.
85 The varieties of the music depend on the varieties of the temperament of the tarantulas. So in Pietro Simeone's case, for instance, it was the variant of *tarantella* called *Catena* that was effective.
86 Ferdinando, *Centum historiae*, fol. 255.
87 Ibid., fol. 261.
88 Ibid., fols. 255–62.
89 Ibid., fol. 250. In spite of these negative qualities, Ferdinando notes, the tarantula has its own utility for eliminating *bruchi* (a kind of locust without wings), which infest Apulia.
90 So, for instance, if the person bitten is of sanguine temperament, he or she will love the colour red; if he is bilious, he will love yellow, if he is melancholic, he will love a dark cloth, and so on (fols. 258–59).
91 Ferdinando, *Centum historiae*, fols. 258, 260.
92 Ibid., fol. 260.
93 Ibid., fol. 258.
94 Ibid., fol. 261: "omnes enim constamus ex quatuor elementis, & ex quatuor humoribus."
95 Ibid., fol. 262.
96 Ibid., fols. 262–62.
97 See Linda Deer Richardson, "The Generation of Disease: Occult Causes and Diseases of the Total Substance," in Andrew Wear, Roger K. French and Iain M. Lonie (eds), *The Medical Renaissance of the Sixteenth Century* (Cambridge, 1985): 175–94.
98 Ferdinando, *Centum historiae*, fol. 255: "Ut ob id alma Natura, seu Gloriosus Deus, qui est naturae auctor, mira providentia, dotare voluit diversos locos diversis, & miris virtutibus tam in mineralibus, quam in vegetalibus, quam in viventibus, ut sexcenta exempla sileamus, nam si cuncta prosequi velimus, historicas potius partes, quam philosophicas, exerceremus."
99 Ernesto De Martino, *La terra del rimorso; Contributo a una storia religiosa del Sud* (Milan, 1961), pp. 177, 247 (on Ferdinando) and in English translation, *The Land of Remorse: A Study of Southern Italian Tarantism*, transl. Dorothy Zinn (London, 2005). Several documents related to De Martino's fieldwork in Southern Italy have been published after his death: see Ernesto De Martino, *Note di campo: Spedizione in Lucania, 30 sett.–31 ott. 1952*, ed. Clara Gallini

(Lecce, 1995); Idem, *L'opera a cui lavoro: Apparato critico e documentario alla "Spedizione etnologica" in Lucania*, ed. Clara Gallini (Lecce, 1996).

100 De Martino, *Terra del rimorso*, especially pp. 178–79, 263, 272–73 for this interpretation. The anthropological literature on tarantism is vast. Recent studies include Karen Lüdtke, *Dances with Spiders: Crisis, Celebrity and Celebration in Southern Italy* (Oxford and New York, 2009); Jerri Daboo, *Ritual, Rapture and Remorse: A Study of Tarantism and Pizzica in Salento* (Bern, 2010). None of these works approaches, for depth and breadth of research or acuity of interpretation, the quality level of De Martino's classic. They follow De Martino in attributing to Ferdinando a narrow, "naturalist and positivist" view of the phenomenon (see Lüdtke, *Dances with Spiders*, p. 61; Daboo, *Ritual, Rapture and Remorse*, pp. 133–34).

101 Ferdinando, *Centum historiae*, fol. 258.

102 Ibid., fol. 266. On the medieval origins of tarantism, see De Martino, *Terra del rimorso*, pp. 228–41.

103 Ferdinando, *Centum historiae*, fol. 267: "Musica esse animae nostrae exercitium, veluti motum esse exercitium corporis, nam est laborum & dolorum levamen ac refrigerium humanarum calamitatum, quibus vita hominum undique septa est, oblivionem inducens." See also fol. 268: "Nam clarum est musicam sanare tarantatos, sive sit causa incitans, sive aliud … , sat[is] est ratione musicae incitantis tripudiare & saltare, unde ob tanta corporis agitationes veneni consopitae vires delitescentes, ac conquiescentes moventur, & foras sudoribus pelluntur, solata enim natura ob musicam in tanto duello vincit."

104 As far as I know, this has not been recognized by the historians who have written on tarantism and Ferdinando from a medical historical perspective, as for instance Henry Sigerist, "The Story of Tarantism," in Dorothy Schullian and Max Schoen (eds), *Music and Medicine* (New York, 1948): 96–116, and more recently, Maria Luisa Portulano Scoditti and Amedeo Elio Distante, *Epifanio Ferdinando – Le centum historiae e la medicina del suo tempo* (Città di Mesagne, 2000); David Gentilcore, "'Fu guarito, e perfettamente, dalla musica': Epifanio Ferdinando e il tarantismo pugliese," in Mario Marti and Domenico D. Urgesi (eds), *Epifanio Ferdinando, medico e storico del Seicento* (Nardò, 2001): 134–48; Silvana Arcuti, *Epifanio Ferdinando e il morso della tarantola* (Lecce, 2002); Gino Di Mitri, *Storia biomedica del tarantismo nel XVIII secolo* (Florence, 2006).

9 Physical City

A Royal Physician's Warsaw

Ruth Schilling

Christian Heinrich Erndtel (1676–1734) lived for 20 years in Warsaw, capital of the Kingdom of Poland, where he served as Royal Physician to the Polish king and Saxon Electoral Duke Frederick August I (1670–1733), or August II as he became known after assuming the Polish throne.[1] Every morning and evening for several years in the 1720s, Erndtel scrutinized a barometer to measure the air pressure. He also noted the wind direction and issued monthly bulletins on the quality of the water of the River Vistula and its height and temperature. Charts of this information make up 47 of 415 pages of a voluminous book he published under the title *Warsavia physice illustrata* ("Warsaw Physically Illustrated"). These charts were integral to a specific city description Erndtel projected: a description that combined elements of traditional urban panegyric in lauding the beauty and order of Varsovian architecture,[2] annalistic history,[3] city chronicle,[4] Hippocratic description, and natural history.[5] The result was an intriguing, layered mixture of city representations, sometimes closely and sometimes loosely intertwined.[6]

This paper explores how a physician occupying a high social and administrative position strove to guide readers through a city in which he lived for more than "4 lustra" (20 years), as he never tired of explaining,[7] at the close of the political era that had given him his prominence, the reign of the first Saxon-Polish ruler.[8] The purposiveness of Erndtel's description helps us, centuries later, to see Warsaw through the lens he offered to his contemporary readers. This provides one perspective on the research question from which this collective volume sprang: how were a physician's public and administrative activity, political and civic purposes, and forms of writing related to each other?[9] We will explore the Warsaw depicted by Erndtel as though we are reading his book: beginning with the title he chose for it and the book's material character; then reading its preface in comparison to the preface to a book written by another, contemporary Saxon royal physician; and finally moving chapter by chapter through *Warsavia*. Erndtel's written Warsaw can be understood on two levels: first, by asking how he communicated *about* the city; second, by asking how he communicated *in* the city as well as how he wanted his readers to perceive

DOI: 10.4324/9781315554693-13

him communicating. Both levels of communication characterized the relationship of an officially appointed royal physician with his urban surroundings. *Warsavia* reveals which facets of the city Erndtel knew best and thought most worth reporting to the Saxon and wider European public. The way he moved and talked in Warsaw reveals social and cultural borders not highlighted in his published portrait of the city.

The Book as an Object

Quarto format, bound in red leather with gold lettering, *Warsavia physice illustrata* is situated between cultural display and practical utility. It does not take the form of a richly illustrated book in folio format, which would more or less serve as a means of cultural display rather than a source of information.[10] Nor does it take the form of a cheaply priced octavo handbook, meant to be taken on field trips or excursions.[11] The format alone reveals something about the book's purpose: possessing it was meant partly to represent the owner. But it was also intended as a source of information, a book to be read and used and not only exchanged as a valuable gift. The fact that *Warsavia* is still to be found in the collections of the European national libraries and in nearly every major public and scientific library in Poland and Saxony, confirms this double nature.[12] The book belonged to library collections deemed representative of the Polish kingdom under Saxon rule[13] and, at the same time, was esteemed for its wider scientific interest, not least because it contained the first systematic weather observations undertaken in the Polish capital.[14]

The fact that Erndtel aimed at a specific erudite audience is underlined by his choice of book title. Both before and after Erndtel, the title "illustrata" was not used for city descriptions but, since the Italian Humanist Flavio Biondo (1392–1463) published *Italia illustrata* in 1474, for accounts of lands and territories.[15] Erndtel may also have been familiar with and alluding to two more recent titles. The earlier of these is the description of an air pump by the Saxon *mechanicus* Jacob Leupold (1674–1727):[16] *Antlia pneumatica illustrata. Oder/deutliche Beschreibung der so genandten Lufft-Pumpe* ("clear description of the so-called air-pump"),[17] published in 1707. The other is the *Saxonia Monumentis Viarum Illustrata* ("Saxony Illustrated by its Road Marks"), published in 1726.[18] This was the elaborate dissertation of Carl Christian Schramm (b. 1703), an *actuarius* (clerk) employed at the time in the Saxon administration.[19] Both works deal with topics that form a *basso continuo* in *Warsavia physice illustrata*: experimental observation and geographical description. Further research could help to discern the subtle implications of Erndtel's choice of his book title: did he take part in a discourse on the value of experiments, spurred by the publication of Leupold's mechanical inventions? Or did he assume that the close affinity of his description of a Polish city with a work listing all of the road and path marks in Saxony could help to enhance his book's political importance? Publications in which geographical description and political ambitions were mixed were especially prone to severe censorship.[20] It may therefore also be the case that Erndtel aimed to smooth the path of his most important monograph through this process by bestowing this specific title on it.

Weather Prognosis and Imperial Panegyric

Much has already been written about the cosmological aspect of monarchical rule in premodern times,[21] yet there is another facet of the congruence of sky and monarchy: weather observations and political rule. Erndtel explicitly underlined that he was acquainted with the minute weather observations undertaken by another royal physician, in Wroclaw (Breslau) in the period 1692–1712. In the preface to the publication of these weather charts,[22] David de Grebner (1655–1737) transformed his documentation into a celebration of the eternal character of his master's rule (Habsburg Emperor Leopold I).[23] The passage is quoted at length because it is significant for the political program within which Grebner wanted his weather observations to be seen:

> Likewise, I will add the following solemn prayers: May you have, most gracious Caesar, the favorable sight of the sky and stars and auspicious breaths of air, and may your most glorious house of Austria have manifold increase, so that either sons or no one may succeed your august Majesty. May you be the claimant of enemies' loot and spoils and the victor of all wars. In a word: When you have completed your sixty-third year and as soon as you triumph over your climacteric year, may the Godhead add a longer time of life and everlasting years in the kingdom of Philip, in which the sun never, day or night, sees a setting—years that will have an end only when the world ends.[24]

To observe the weather daily in this respect meant not only to explore, but also to adore the well-ordered course of events that godly and earthly majesty maintained. The "space of life" (*vitae spacium*) is a tiny part of the infinite universe of a godly sanctioned Habsburg Empire, in which the sun never sets, and the stars and the winds express the parallel nature of the Emperor's rule and the message of Jesus Christ. The political meaning of Grebner's daily meteorological activity could not have been made more explicit. In another preface, dedicated to the Senate of Wroclaw, Grebner juxtaposed physical exploration and panegyrical praise of the city's qualities:

> To be sure, if you look at the nature of the place, the decoration of the royal and holy buildings, the strength of the walls, the city walls decorated with lofty pyramids, the ramparts fortified by waves, the towers whose lofty peaks penetrate the clouds in the sky, the spacious

roads, running without winding, the fertility of the fields and the healthfulness of the sky [...] if you consider moreover the natural talent of human beings, their inborn skill, power, and the other excellent endowments of nature and human counsel, you would say that it was a dwelling place for heroes.[25]

The well-ordered state of a city, her fortifications, and her wide and straight streets are depicted in parallel with the fertility of the lands and the sky. The natural and cultural shape of the city expresses God's benevolence and the ruler's ability to behave according to that will. Closely describing the air and clouds in this sense means also describing the good order of governance and the wish to participate in the shaping of this governance by implying how the course of events will be, thus providing a prognostic tool for decision-makers.

In this prognostic sense, Erndtel depicted a similar program to that of Grebner, in the preface to *Warsavia*:

> I wanted therefore to illustrate this city, which has been enriched with so great a splendor by your auspices, most tranquil king, with my own observations, not just as pertains to the buildings and monuments, which have already been enumerated, or to the political state, but even the citizens, as it is relevant, and inhabitants, and their well-being and safety and those of foreigners whose number over the past thirty years has made all the greater an increase because during the reign of your holy Majesty the political state as well as trade have thrived more prosperously. I have also been led to these very undertakings by a knowledge about Warsaw's make-up and its soil, air and waters that I have put together for myself over almost twenty years, but chiefly by that bond by which I am devoted to your most august Majesty, not just as a citizen and subject, but also an employee [*stipendarius*].[26]

Looking at the date of publication, we can see that Erndtel's panegyric had a probably unintentional twist: in September 1733, Warsaw had once again been occupied by Russian soldiers, who not only guaranteed the election of August II's son as successor, but also evoked, by their marauding behavior, the devastating destruction wreaked by Swedish and Russian troops during the so-called Great Nordic War (1700–1721).[27] But Erndtel did not stop at admiring the city itself. He explored the "constitution" of her inhabitants and compared the state of the air and water, being obliged to do so "non ut civis saltem & subditus, sed & uti Stipendiarius" ("not only as citizen and subject, but also as an employee"). Following the Hippocratic program of investigation belonged to Erndtel's duties as an officially appointed physician. Let us see how he fulfilled it in print, by following him around the streets, houses, rivers, and gardens of the Polish capital.

Investigating the City

Following the dedication and the preface, Erndtel led the reader through palaces, libraries, and important sights of this Polish city. The second of the book's six chapters concerns the "Warsavian Air." It is the longest text of the main part including the aforementioned 47 pages of daily weather observations. Erndtel then discusses the water and the inhabitants. Subsequently he concentrates on illnesses, following a threefold pattern: first by informing the reader which illnesses in his opinion were most typical of the inhabitants of Warsaw ("De Morbis Warsaviensium"), then suggesting suitable therapies for them ("De Ingressu ad Infirmos Warsaviensium"). In the last chapter on illnesses, he published a substantial part of his medical journal, though, interestingly enough, not the part which was chronologically concordant with the weather charts, under the title: "Relatio specialis Morborum Warsaviensium Anni 1720. Cum Methodo Medendi."[28] This shows that he has not yet conceptualized an integrated tool for displaying weather and illness observations "on a page."[29] These three parts are equivalent in length, containing about 30 pages each. Much longer than any of the chapters of the main part of the book is a detailed catalog of plants Erndtel had found in the surroundings of Warsaw. This *viridarium* reads like a herbarium, imparting plant names, their appearance and characteristics, and the place where Erndtel had seen them.[30]

The outline of the book reveals a close reading of the Hippocratic work "on airs, waters, and places," in which the duty of a physician is described as follows:

> Whoever wishes to pursue properly the science of medicine must proceed thus. First, he ought to consider what effects each season of the year can produce; for the seasons are not all alike, but differ widely both in themselves and at their changes. The next point is the hot winds and the cold, especially those that are universal but also those that are peculiar to each particular region. He must also consider the properties of the waters; for as these differ in taste and in weight, so the property of each is far different from that of any other. Therefore, on arrival at a town with which he is unfamiliar, a physician should examine its position with respect to the winds and to the risings of the sun. For a northern, a southern, an eastern, and a western aspect have each its own individual property. He must consider with the greatest care both these things and how the natives are off for water, whether they use marshy, soft waters, or such as are hard and come from rocky heights, or brackish and harsh. The soil too, whether bare and dry, or wooded and watered, hollow and hot or high and cold. The mode of life also of the inhabitants that is pleasing to them, whether they are heavy drinkers, taking lunch, and inactive, or athletic, industrious, eating much and drinking little. That is, taking more than one full meal every day.[31]

That Erndtel knew and followed this "work program" becomes obvious in *Warsavia physice illustrata*. Erndtel fulfilled and went beyond the Hippocratic program in three ways: keeping meteorological charts, making a "relatio specialis" on illnesses in a given year, and compiling a "viridarium." These elaborations transformed a Hippocratic description of Warsaw into a description that paved the way to understanding the city and its inhabitants as part of a territory to be represented in numbers and tables.[32]

Warsavia physice illustrata announced both natural history and political purpose.[33] Erndtel stressed the fact that he was the first to give a description of Warsaw in the manner he did.[34] The closest precedent was not very close: a natural history of Poland that included no political and cultural history and consisted mainly of alphabetically arranged entries on "natural things."[35] Also going beyond traditions of political and cultural history based on archival documents, Erndtel added measurements of "airs" and "waters" and descriptions of natural objects like fossils, plants, and animals in order to make the city physically understandable. He thus displayed new tools of civic history. The novelty of his endeavor produced a double effect: the reader had to rely on Erndtel because there was no other readily available source for comparison; yet tables and lists also distanced both author and reader from what the book purported to illustrate. To describe as someone uninvolved in the object of description can empower the describer. Erndtel styled himself an explorer of an unknown world. To render a capital city "physically illustrated" was to build on early modern projects of creating the space of governance by mapping territory and by collecting and describing its contents, as Alix Cooper has shown for local botany and mineralogy in the Holy Roman Empire.[36] The distancing most evident in the book's passages on architecture, geography, and meteorology carried over into the chapters dealing with the habits of the Varsovian people.[37] Warsaw and her Polish populace were thus indigenized.

The novelty Erndtel claimed for himself also obliged him to forge new ways of establishing authenticity. As readers had to rely so heavily on his book in the absence of others like it, the tools with which Erndtel legitimized the truthfulness of his observations gained great importance. He juxtaposed variety: his own experiments, measurements, and observations; architecture and topography; verbal information from his oral interactions with other people in Warsaw; information extracted from printed works and historical testimonies. Erndtel treated natural objects such as fossils in the same way he made evident the information value of written historical documents. One good example of this way of proving the truthfulness of his observations and findings is the way he treated the legendary *basilisci* (dragons), which were said to live in the fields around Warsaw.[38] He traced the story back to the physician Johannes P. Pincier (1556–1607),[39] who apparently had observed them in 1587. This information had been handed down a chain of medical, theological, and historical writers to the jurist Nicolaus of Chwalkow,[40] who included the *basilisci* in his work on Polish public law published in 1685.[41] Erndtel hunted for the basilisk in Warsaw's royal and episcopal archives and wondered why he came up empty-handed.[42] His next step was to figure out which locally found serpent could have served as a model for what he now regarded as the mythological figure of the *basiliscus*. He had gained knowledge of local snakes from field trips to the Vistula region and familiarity with the ingredients of the royal pharmacy and compared what he knew to references to serpents in both erudite publications and conversation.[43]

Erndtel's city is a *phénomène total*[44] fathomed by all available means. It consists not only of the stone buildings and houses that expressed the urban renewal program of his patron, August II. It also consists of rivers, plants, and animals. It is not only a city where Polish nobility and commoners lived, and Saxons ruled, but also a place of particular customs across such groups, of eating and drinking, for example, and it was eventually a place where specific illnesses could be observed. Erndtel became Warsaw's physician, cicerone, historian, ethnographer, and meteorologist all in one.

This entanglement of natural and civic history produced one puzzling effect: the boundaries between the city of Warsaw, its surroundings, and the Polish territories became blurred. Erndtel vacillated between identifying things as "Warsaviense" or as "Polonicum," and he did not explain a difference. And he characterized the population by "number" and "nation" instead of by corporations, offices, and their holders, as would have been the case had he stuck to the more traditional form of city description with which the book began[45]:

> Moreover, just as it is customary in nearly all the seats of kings and princes and in metropolitan cities that the body politic [*civitates*] comprise not a single kind of nation, so too it should be known that not just Polish people, but men flowing together from almost every region, from Europe chiefly as well as Asia, make up the number of citizens and inhabitants in Warsaw.[46]

By representing the city population not only as an ensemble of corporations and institutions, but also as a mixture of national groups, Erndtel both universalized Warsaw as part of Europe and the world—nations "flowing together" (*confluentes*) like rivers—and territorialized it as part of a kingdom.

Another good example of structuring the representation of the city this way may be found in the chapter on birds. Erndtel starts by discussing wild and tame types of birds in Warsaw. He ends with a lengthy passage on the different colors and dissemination of species in Poland in general:

> It will become clear from the following chapter, wherein we discuss food in Warsaw, that the region of Warsaw is teeming with wild as well as tame birds: here, though, if it may be permitted to cite

a remarkable species from among the innumerable others that Warsaw has in common with other regions, the *Aves Nivales of Worm & Gessner*,[47] called by others winter sparrows, *Snieguli* or *Sniegulki* in Polish.[48]

Blurring city and territory resulted from looking at the city not only as an entity formed by architecture and political history, but also as an object of natural description.

What does this blurring of boundaries between city and territory tell us about the relevance of the urban sphere for Erndtel's activities as a court physician? Warsaw, natural and social, was his gateway to the world beyond the court—and the city. As court physician, Erndtel's sphere of responsibility could have been limited to that of caring for the royal family or courtiers or both. His book documented and displayed the ways in which he instead expanded his sphere far beyond the court to include a place and its population, past and present. Yet at the same time, as Erndtel hinted in his book, as court physician he oversaw not only the health of the king and royal family, but also the wellbeing of the whole administrative and military personnel. This made it a small step from describing Warsaw to describing a territory.

Communicating in and about Warsaw

The urban sphere was important to Erndtel's undertaking in another sense: as a space in which communication about natural observation and its problems as well as the exchange of curiosities could take place. In *Warsavia*, Erndtel often delivers information with statements like "I have observed" or "I have seen," often together with the assuring remark "I have remembered" or "I have kept in my memory." His own testimony is combined with that of others with whom Erndtel either observed together or shared first-hand observations. These discussions and encounters always took place in Warsaw—or at least those Erndtel found worth writing about. Being both object of interest and place of meeting made Warsaw an environment of regular exchange. Conversation, as we saw, informed him about local fauna. Weather observations were made together with state geometrician Gottfried Rautenberg as well as two lower civil servants who handled the barometer.[49] Another example of the sociability of Erndtel's scientific activities is the data concerning the weight and temperature of the Vistula, for which he cited the exact date and place and the name and occupation of the chemist carrying out the measurements with him.[50]

These urban, locally bound activities are linked to a wider European sphere by comparing the results Erndtel and his Varsovian companions achieved with findings from historical cases reconstructed from classical authors or historical treatises or advertised by scientific journals. The observations he undertook, though, needed an object of research that he

had to see for himself and accompanied by other men of scientific authority. In this sense as well, then, the city became "naturalized," an entity
defined even by the types of snakes and birds living in it. Erndtel inserted
these findings into networks of scientific exchange, which were not only
oral, but also relied on printed works. These networks were supra-
municipal and also supra-national, as he did not consider any political
boundaries in grasping all examples that were, in his eyes, relevant to the
phenomena he wanted to describe.

The "doing" of natural history in the sense of collecting and making
field observations, Bettina Dietz has argued, caused a social expansion of
the agents involved in the process.[51] The aim to document the whole
world's natural objects could only be pursued if many supporters could be
found to accomplish it. In Dietz's view, this broadened the project of natural history from being initially an activity reserved to a few people into
a project that involved many agents from various social and academic
backgrounds, thus giving the practices of natural history a specific flavor
of political and social enlightenment. In Erndtel's printed Varsovian world,
however, this social expansion had not taken place, although the practices
used there in pursuing natural history are exactly those Dietz describes.

To understand the social background of these social boundaries, it is
important to consider the implications of the official medical function
Erndtel fulfilled. He was the grandson and son of personal physicians (*Leibärzte*) of the Saxon Electors.[52] In the collection of printed funeral poems
for his deceased father, the not yet 20-year-old Erndtel was accepted by his
fathers' colleagues and friends as their equal. Not only was he mentioned
and praised in some of the poems, he was also allowed some space to compose a eulogy of his own.[53] His family background prepared Erndtel for
the social, cultural and political practices that characterized the involvement of a physician in the monarchical administrative structures of early
modern Saxony.[54]

The activity by which Erndtel was granted his *entrée* into administration
and the erudite world (and its documentation in print) was a voyage to
sights of interest in the Holy Roman Empire, the Netherlands and England
in 1706.[55] To travel and to write about these travels was something undertaken by noble persons and those who wanted to achieve or preserve
a high social and cultural status.[56] Erndtel thus followed a practice probably shared by many of his colleagues and friends. The account of this trip
was published not only in Latin, but also in English.[57] This meant that it
gained him European attention and not only a reputation in Saxony and
the Holy Roman Empire.[58] In this record of his travels, Erndtel did not
seem to consider the national or social standing of his informant as long as
the information he collected was, in his eyes, worth reporting.[59] About 25
years later, this had drastically changed: in *Warsavia physice illustrate*,
there is a notable difference between the way Erndtel treated written testimonies and the way he treated the face-to-face social relationships that he

chose to write about. In presenting written testimonies, Erndtel only discerned between the value he attached to the information given in the book or manuscript he consulted. As we have seen in the example of the *basilicus*, this means that sources are juxtaposed from different origins: medical writings from Marburg or the archive of a Polish bishop. In describing the content rather than the social context of his scientific endeavors, Erndtel mentioned only his personal relationship to the *collegium* of personal physicians to the nobility,[60] the experiences and connections he had made while accompanying parts of the Saxon army in Poland,[61] and two persons with whom he had undertaken his experiments: the geometrician Gottfried Rautenberg [62] and the chemist and apothecary Georg Lebmann.[63]

Honoring the other personal physicians in the preface probably served as a *captatio benevolentiae* in a concrete sense: to prevent criticism and envy by his professional and social peers.[64] His book might also have been an attempt to reconnect him to Saxon circles. Looking at the ranks named in the Saxon court calendar, Erndtel's career as a personal physician was not so successful: in contrast to most of his colleagues, he was never appointed Privy Counsellor at court.[65] This may have had something to do with the distance between Warsaw and Dresden, a hypothesis that would need to be verified or negated by future research.

As part of the group of personal physicians, Erndtel nevertheless performed a key function in the medical administration: he was responsible not only for the king's health, his household's medical care and privileged members of the court, but also for legal proposals concerning medical matters.[66] Moreover, he fulfilled supervisory functions at examinations of non-academic physicians, inspection of apothecaries, and prevention of epidemics in the Saxon military in Poland.[67] If and how his activities differed from those of his colleagues residing in Dresden is an open question.[68] Little to nothing is known about the concrete interaction of personal physicians in Warsaw. It is not even altogether clear how many personal physicians were installed permanently in the Polish capital.[69] We learn from Erndtel's *Warsavia* that his official functions allowed him to lead a private practice, though we do not know if this overlapped in parts with certain duties he had to fulfil as an officially appointed physician. It might have been the case that in this respect he was treated like a town physician of Warsaw who was obliged to treat patients in need, though he did not mention this in his book.

The picture of the city's patients drawn by Erndtel contradicts his parallelization of Warsaw to a *theatrum mundi* of "men flowing together from almost every region," quoted above. Without exception, these patients are all Polish, which suggests an ethnic dimension to this doctor–patient relationship.[70] The patients Erndtel treated at the Varsovian Court apparently required him to treat them discreetly, whereas the patients from his private practice in town probably had no influence on his publication activities. This also shows the effect of how Erndtel understood the power of the place in which he worked. Warsaw, although a meeting place of all kinds of people, was formed and produced by the specificity of her character as a city with certain kinds of illnesses, which, for Erndtel, was probably evident most clearly in groups that had already lived there for generations. He elaborated this specificity by comparing Warsaw with other European capitals and their illnesses.[71] Erndtel could have asked whether the power of place also expressed itself in the health of people who had arrived recently, such as Saxon administrative personnel. Yet he does not seem to have considered this. His behavior reveals cultural and social divisions among Saxons and Poles in Warsaw at this time.[72] These divisions were expressed not only in the contrast Erndtel drew between Saxon and Polish social circles, but also in his treatment of the members of the Saxon administration. He referred to other court physicians as colleagues with whose works he wished to be associated. In making observations as we saw, on the other hand, he was assisted by civil servants who fulfilled manual tasks, such as handling the barometer, which Erndtel did not wish to undertake (or did not have the knowledge to do), a division of labor which confirmed his social standing.

Garden City

Warsavia physice illustrata ends with a catalog of plants. Though separately paginated as an appendix, it can be read as the book's splendid culmination, a veritable "garden" of knowledge. In this "Garden or Catalog of Plants which grow around Warsaw,"[73] Erndtel gave a description of Warsaw's flora that was unprecedented in the variety of plants listed and in the citing of different names for each, together with the authorities who used them.[74] Erndtel stuck to the alphabetical order characteristic of pre-Linnean plant catalogs. His method of classification was influenced by Augustus Quirinus Rivinus (1652–1723),[75] who had been director of the botanic garden of the University of Leipzig and who was one of Erndtel's academic teachers during his university studies. Rivinus promoted the idea of plants being classifiable by their petals, an idea Erndtel followed in the "viridarium." In describing specimens, he was careful to mention exceptions to the usual number of petals.[76]

As with his weather charts, Erndtel documented Warsaw's natural history at the most advanced level of knowing with which he was familiar. This rendered the "viridarium" a summing up of the whole book rather than a mere appendix. Each kind of plant is framed not only in the local context and circumstances in which Erndtel found it, but also in relation to what Erndtel could glean from recent literature on botany in general and on local situations in other countries and cities and even particular *horti medici* or *botanici*. The description of hemp (*cannabis spuria*) thus begins with a specimen found locally by a Polish knight and ends with the statement that the same type of plant was found in Parisian forests and gardens.[77] As throughout *Warsavia*, Erndtel's local botanical findings are authenticated by reference to date, place, and accompaniment:

> I saw this little plant for the first time in Warsaw growing on Mt. Mary on a steep spot on 15 May 1714. There, together with an associate at the time in botanical excursions, the illustrious Lord Heucher, I examined it more closely on account of the singular elegance and verdant pleasantness of the plant.[78]

As throughout *Warsavia*, the sociability of observing was limited to the intellectual and officeholding Saxon elite, in this case Johann Heinrich von Heucher (1677–1747), personal physician to the same ruler in his capacity as Saxon Electoral Duke Frederick August I.[79] Mentioning von Heucher related Erndtel's activity in Warsaw to the Dresden court and its intellectual life.

Erndtel's catalog announced that it concerned plants growing "around" (*circa*) Warsaw. "Circa" is used broadly here. As in the main part of the book, the boundary between city and territory is stretched to the point that one forgets Erndtel did not aim explicitly to depict the flora of the Polish kingdom as a whole, but only of its capital. In addition, medical properties of plants are given as specific less to Warsaw than to curing "Polish" illnesses.[80] Documenting a kind of plant known to grow in other places as growing at the eastern wall of a Warsavian orphanage in August 1729 localized the plant within the city yet also delocalized the city. Warsaw, in this sense, was everywhere. A city "physically illustrated" was a city at once naturally and politically beyond itself.

A Culture of Place

Being the descendant of a line of official court and town physicians made Erndtel especially aware of the importance of the social, natural, and cultural environment in which—and about which—he acted. This awareness can be seen as a culture of place, because it represents a specific knowledge of everyday surroundings gained not by one person, but probably grown over several generations. Not only was this knowledge fundamental for daily interactions at court, it was also crucial for Erndtel's ability to treat his patients successfully, as he emphasized in *Warsavia*.[81] Knowledge of local environment also belonged to a wider pattern, the Hippocratic investigation of airs, waters, places, on which Erndtel built a splendid elaboration of the city as a *phénomène total*, a work of both art and nature whose good order celebrated the king he served. Erndtel's Warsaw contained several sparkling and not always consistent facets: the parallelization of the natural and cultural history of the city territorialized it and, at the same time, enlivened it as a meeting place of living things, including animals and plants as well as people. Enlightened inquiry into the city also equated everything "Varsovian" with comparable phenomenon of the known urban world. The respect Erndtel showed toward Polish historical sources did not modify his social behavior, which restricted him to move in relatively closed circles even though he lived for two decades in Warsaw.

What it meant to be an officially appointed physician went without saying for Erndtel, his projected readers, and the persons with whom he interacted. Yet he creatively reworked the culture of place he shared with his predecessors into an empirical, scholarly, and sociable inquiry into place and health. Erndtel's acute awareness of these possibilities was enhanced by the fact that he lived and worked during the coming together of two political realms, two territories, through the personal union of Saxony and Poland. *Warsavia physice illustrata* can thus be deciphered as a long and elaborate meditation on and writing of the interdependence of office, cultural place, and environment of health, at once corporeal and political, inspired by the holding of public office yet also both enabled and limited by the ways in which office—especially high office of expansive scope—could distance a physician from his surroundings.

Notes

Acknowledgments: This chapter was researched during my participation in the ERC-funded project "Ways of Writing: How Physicians Know 1550–1950," headed by Volker Hess and Andrew Mendelsohn, and benefited much from a commentary by Alexander Kästner at a workshop for this volume. I thank Marion Mücke, Roland Helms, and Thomas Schnalke for ideas and information.

1 Erndtel's biography is not mentioned in any of the main relevant biographical dictionaries of this time, neither in Friedrich A. Weitz, *Das gelehrte Sachsen oder Verzeichniß derer in den Churfürstl. Sächs. und incorporirten Ländern jetztlebenden Schriftsteller und ihrer Schriften* (Leipzig 1780), nor in Johann Christoph Adelung, Christian Gottlieb Jöcher, Heinrich Rotermund, *Allgemeines Gelehrten-Lexicon: darinne die Gelehrten aller Stände sowohl männ-als auch weiblichen Geschlechts, welche vom Anfange der Welt bis auf ietzige Zeit gelebt* (Leipzig 1750), vol. 2: D-L, or Johann Heinrich Zedler, *Großes vollständiges Universal-Lexikon* (Leipzig 1734), vol. 8: E, www.zedler-lexikon.de (last consulted 30 December 2013). The archive of the Leopoldina contains no biographical material. The information we have is provided by Erndtel himself in his publications: see http://thesauraus.cerl.org/cgi-bin/record.pl?rid=cnp00439556 (last consulted 15 December 2013). There are different spellings of his name during his lifetime: Ernd(e)l or Erndt(e)l and Ernd(t)elius.
2 Christian Heinrich Erndtel, *Warsavia physice illustrata, sive de aere, aquis, locis et incolis Warsaviae, eorundemque Moribus et Morbis Tractatus. Cui Annexum est Viridarium, vel Catalogus Plantarum circa Warsavia nascentium* (Dresden, 1730), pp. 8–29.
3 Ibid. et passim.
4 Ibid. et passim.

5 Erndtel, *Warsavia*, passim. For similar entanglement of a physician's urban activities and chronicle writing, see Pomata, "A Sense of Place," Chapter 8 of this volume.

6 For the image of the city as a field of research, see Peter Johanek, "Bild und Wahrnehmung der Stadt: Annäherung an ein Forschungsproblem," in idem (ed.), *Bild und Wahrnehmung der Stadt* (Vienna, 2012): 1–23; for the image of cities in the eighteenth century, see Mascha Bisping, "Die ganze Stadt dem ganzen Menschen? Zur Anthropologie der Stadt im 18. Jahrhundert: Stadtbaukunst, Architektur, Ästhetik, Medizin, Literatur und Staatstheorie," in Maximilian Bergengruen (ed.), *Die Grenzen des Menschen: Anthropologie und Ästhetik um 1800* (Würzburg, 2001): 183–203; Gudrun Schwibbe, *Wahrgenommen: Die sinnliche Erfahrung der Stadt* (Münster, 2002).

7 Erndtel, *Warsavia*, p. 3.

8 See with further references Norman Davies, *God's Playground: A History of Poland*, vol. 1: *The Origins to 1795* (New York, 2005), pp. 371–85.

9 See Dross, "'De Officiis'," Chapter 4 of this volume; Di Giammatteo and Mendelsohn, "Reporting for Action," Chapter 5 of this volume.

10 For the relationship between print format and representational use, see Volker Bauer, "Strukturwandel der höfischen Öffentlichkeit: Zur Medialisierung des Hoflebens vom 16. bis zum 18. Jahrhundert," in *Zeitschrift für Historische Forschung*, 38 (2011): 585–620.

11 See Alix Cooper, *Inventing the Indigenous: Local Knowledge and Natural History in Early Modern Europe* (Cambridge, 2007), pp. 51–86.

12 This is the result of research undertaken in the online-accessible catalogues of the national libraries and other major libraries in Poland and Germany.

13 See Ewa Tomicka-Krumrey, *Das Buch und die sächsisch-polnischen Beziehungen im 18. Jahrhundert*, exhibition catalogue (Warsaw, 1998); Tomicka-Krumrey, "Die Gelehrsamkeit und das Buchwesen," in *Polen und Sachsen: Zwischen Nähe und Distanz*, issue of *Dresdner Hefte*, 50.2 (1997): 27–35.

14 See Gustav Hellmann, *Die Entwicklung der meteorologischen Beobachtungen bis zum Ende des XVIII. Jahrhunderts* (Berlin, 1927), p. 30.

15 Flavius Blondus, *Italia illustrata*, vol. 4 of the Edizione Nazionale delle Opere di Biondo Flavio, ed. by Paolo Pontari (Rome, 2011); see also Ottavio Clavuot, "Flavio Biondos Italia illustrata: Porträt und historisch-geographische Legitimation der humanistischen Elite Italiens," in Johannes Helmrath and Ulrich Muhlack (eds), *Diffusion des Humanismus* (Göttingen, 2002): 55–76.

16 He lived from 1674–1727. Following his unfinished university studies he founded a workshop where he taught students and artisans in the *artes mechanicae*. From 1720 he worked on a great compendium of technical instruments and mechanical procedures, *Theatrum Machinarum Generale oder Schauplatz des Grundes mechanischer Wissenschaften* (Leipzig, 1724 ff).

17 Jacob Leupold, *Antlia Pneumatica Illustrata. Oder/deutliche Beschreibung der so genandten Lufft-Pumpe/Darinnen ausführlich gezeiget wird/was solche sey/ und wie sie nebst denen zugehörigen/so wohl alten als gantz neu-inventirten Machinen zu gebrauchen/Alles in vielen deutlichen und accuraten Figuren entworfen/und zum andern mahl/nebst der ersten Continuation, und einem Verzeichniß unterschiedl. Mathematischen und Physicalischen Instrumenten heraus gegeben* (Leipzig, n.d.).

18 Carl Christian Schramm, *Saxonia Monumentis Viarum Illustrata. Hoc est De Statuis Mercurialibus Columnis Brachiatis ac Milliaribus Von denen Wege-Weisern, Armen- und Meilen-Säulen Una Cum affinibus de Angariis et Parangariis, Postarum Origine, Viis Publicis Milliaribus in Genere et Juribus Eorum*

Tractatio Historico-Juridico-Politica, accedentibus Praeter Rescriptor. Responsor. Documentorum Appendicem (Wittenberg, 1726).

19 For his career, see the indications given in "Schramm, Carl Christian," in Carl Günther Ludovici, *Großes Universal Lexicon aller wissenschaftlichen Künste, welche bishero durch den menschlichen Verstand und Witz erfunden worden* (Leipzig and Halle, 1743), vol. 35: cols. 1081–84.

20 Agatha Kobuch, *Zensur und Aufklärung in Kursachen: Ideologische Strömungen und politische Meinungen zur Zeit der sächsisch-polnischen Union* (Weimar, 1988), pp. 20, 140.

21 The literature concerns either astrological or religious-sacral components: Monica Azzolini, *The Duke and the Stars: Astrology and Politics in Renaissance Milan* (Berlin, 2013); Paul Kléber Monod, *The Power of Kings: Monarchy and Religion in Europe, 1589–1715* (New Haven, 1999); Benjamin Kram, "Astrologie und politische Autorität: Das Horoskop des württembergischen Herzogs Johann Friedrich (1582–1628) im Kontext historischer Astrologie in der Frühen Neuzeit," in *Von Goldmachern und Schatzsuchern: Alchemie und Aberglaube in Württemberg*, exhibition catalogue (Stuttgart, 2013): 23–26; Alfred Schmid, *Augustus und die Macht der Sterne: Antike Astrologie und die Etablierung der Monarchie in Rom* (Cologne, Weimar, Vienna, 2005).

22 David de Grebner, *Tractatus septem, quorum I. Ephemerides Meteorologicae Vratislavienses ab Anno 1692 ad 1712. II. Animadversiones in Histor. Morborum, qui Anno praeteriti Seculi LXXXXIXII0 Vratislaviae grassati sunt, adornatam à Leopold. Acad. N.C. Collegis Vrat. IIII. De Plagio Medico. IV. Theatrum Medicum Antagonisticum. V. Additamentum in Paragraphen Hippocrat. Galenicam in Theodori Craanen Tractatum Physico-Medicum de Homine. VI. Specimen Medicinae Practicae Veterum restitutae. VII. Numismata quatuor argentea Notis illustrata; Cum Indice Rerum & Verborum memorabilium* (Leipzig, 1714).

23 Court physician under Emperor Leopold I. Other ways of writing his names are: David von Graebner and David von Grabner. He lived from 1655–1737. See http://thesaurus.cerl.org/cgi-bin/record.pl?rid=cnp00109582 (last consulted 7 April 2014).

24 Grebner, *Tractatus*, unpaginated preface: "pariter subjuncturus haec Vota solemnia. Sint TIBI, INDULGENTISSIME CAESAR, Caeli Astrorumque Aspectus benefici, Aërisque; Flatus propitii, & Gloriosissimae DOMUI AUSTRIACAE Incrementa magna, ut AUGUSTISSIMAE MAJESTATI aut FILII succedunt aut nemo. Sis Vindex Hostium Praedae & spolii, omniumque; Bellorum Victor. Verbo: Addat Numen Divinum Anno ex septies novem confecto & Climacterico jam jam superato, longius Vitae Spacium, Annosque; Philippico Regno, in quo Sol ille noctuque; nunquam cernit Occasum, perennes, nec nisi cum Mundi Fine finituros."

25 Grebner, *Tractatus*, unpaginated preface: "Certe si loci naturam, si aedium regiarum atque; sacrarum Ornatum, si Murorum fortitudinem, si Moenia celsis ornata Pyramidibus, si munita fluctibus Propagnucula, si Turres, ardua quae aërias intrant fastigia nubes, si Plateas spatiosissimas & sine anfractu excurrentes, si Agrorum Fertilitatem, Caelique; Salubritatem spectes, …: si insuper Hominum Indolem perpendas, Ingenium, virtutem, aliasque; Naturae & humanii Consilii Dotes eximias, Heroum esse Domicilium dixeris."

26 Erndtel, *Warsavia*, unpaginated preface: "Hanc igitur urbem tanto splendore sub Auspiciis TUIS, REX SERENISSIME, auctam, illustrare volui meis observationibus, non quidem quoad aedificia & monumenta jam recensita, vel

Politicum statum, sed saltem cives quod attinet & incolas, eorumque & advenarum salutem & incolumitatem, quorum numerus ab his triginta annis eo majus sumpsit incrementum, quo felicius regnante SACRA TUA MAJESTATE, status Politicus aeque atque commercia floruerunt. Induxit me ad hos ipsos ausus, & cognitio, quam de Warsaviae constitutione atque ipsius solo, aëre & aquis comparavi mihi per quatuor fere lustra, praecipue autem obligatio illa, qua Majestati Tuae AUGUSTISSIMAE, non ut civis saltem &subditus, sed & uti Stipendiarius sum devotus."

27 Davies, *God's Playground*, p. 380.
28 There is a shift from linking meteorological and astronomical calculations to combining meteorological and medical observations, which would be worth investigating in its own right. See the rich source material gathered in Hellmann, *Entwicklung*; for combining epidemiological and meteorological data in the second half of the eighteenth century, see J. Andrew Mendelsohn, "The World on a Page: Making a General Observation in the Eighteenth Century," in Lorraine Daston and Elizabeth Lunbeck (eds), *Histories of Scientific Observation* (Chicago, 2011): 396–420.
29 See Mendelsohn, "World on a Page."
30 Erndtel, *Warsavia*, viridarium, for example, p. 12.
31 Hippocrates, *peri aeron*, 1. The translation is by W.H.S. Jones (1923), consulted online at www.perseus.tufts.edu/hopper/text (last consulted 1 August 2013).
32 See Jan Brügelmann, "Observations on the Process of Medicalisation in Germany, 1770–1830, Based on Medical Topographies," in *Historical Reflections/ Réfléxions historiques*, 1 (1982): 131–49; Richard Wrigley (ed.), *Pathologies of Travel* (Amsterdam, 2000); Tanja Zwingelberg, *Medizinische Topographien, städtebauliche Entwicklungen und die Gesundheit der Einwohner urbaner Räume im 18. und 19. Jahrhundert* (Göttingen, 2013).
33 Erndtel, *Warsavia*, unpaginated preface.
34 Erndtel, *Warsavia*, pp. 2–3.
35 Erndtel did not mention this work by Polish Jesuit Gabriel Rzauczynski, *Historia Naturalis Curiosa Regni Poloniae: Magni Ducatus Lituaniae, Annexarumque Provinciarum, In Tractatus XX Divisa: Ex Scriptoris probatis, servata primigenia eorum phrasi in locis plurimis, ex M.S.S. variis, Testibus oculatis, relationibus fide dignis, experimentis, desumpta* (Sandomir, 1721), in which "natural things" included fossils, stones, plants, animals, waters, mountains, soils and parts of the human anatomy. Although the title mentions experiments, the author did not indicate if and when his knowledge derived from such a source. Many pages include examples from all other Europe, not only Poland.
36 Cooper, *Inventing the Indigenous*, pp. 173–86.
37 Erndtel, *Warsavia*, pp. 133–213.
38 For the mythology which evolved around the *basiliscus*, see Hermann Güntert, "Basilisk," in Hanns Bächtold-Stäubli and Eduard Hoffmann-Krayer (eds), *Handwörterbuch des deutschen Aberglaubens* (Berlin and New York, 2000), vol. 1: cols. 935–37.
39 Pincier travelled to Silesia and Poland in 1577–1581. After his graduation he taught medicine at the "Hohe Schule" zu Herborn and became its Pro-Rector in 1591, 1594, 1603. See Friedrich Otto, "Pincier, Johannes," in *Allgemeine Deutsche Biographie* (1888), Online Version: URL: www.deutsche-biographie. de/pnd116186232.html?anchor=adb (last consulted 7 April 2014); Dieter Wessinghage, *Die Hohe Schule zu Herborn und ihre Medizinische Fakultät, 1584–1817-1984* (Stuttgart, 1984), p. 25.

40 Nicolaus De Chwalkow a Chwalkowski, *Regni Poloniae Ius Publicum* (Königsberg, 1684).
41 Erndtel, *Warsavia*, p. 61.
42 Erndtel, *Warsavia*, p. 62.
43 Erndtel, *Warsavia*, pp. 62–63.
44 I adapt this expression from the *Annales*-school program of *histoire totale*, uniting cultural, economic, natural, and social history; see Lucien Febvre, *Combats pour l'histoire* (Paris, 1953), p. 20; Axel Rüth, *Erzählte Geschichte: Narrative Strukturen in der französischen Annales-Geschichtsschreibung* (Berlin, 2005), pp. 89–94.
45 On the city as bundle of different corporations, see Klaus Friedland (ed.), *Gilde und Korporation in den nordeuropäischen Städten des Mittelalters* (Cologne, 1984).
46 Erndtel, *Warsavia*, p. 135, "Sicuti autem in omnibus fere Regum & Principium sedibus & Metropolitanis Urbibus fieri solet, ut non ex uno nationum genere componantur civitates, ita & Warsaviae non Polonos saltem, sed ex omnibus fere, Europae praesertim & Asiae etiam partibus confluentes homines, civium atquae incolarum numerum constituere, sciendum est."
47 This refers to Conrad Gesner, *Historia animalium liber III, qui est de avium natura* (Zurich, 1555), and Ole Worm (1588–1654), physician, antiquarian, and intellectual figure in Copenhagen and the Danish Court.
48 Erndtel, *Warsavia*, p. 64, "Quod Avium ferarum aeque ac domesticarum Warsaviensis tractus sit feracissimus, ex capite sequenti constabit, ubi de alimentis Warsaviensium verba facimus: hic saltem, ut singularem speciem allegare ex innumeris fere aliis, quas cum caeteris regionibus Warsavienses habent communes liceat *Aves Nivales Wormii & Gesn.* aliis Passeres hyberni, Polonis *Snieguli* vel *Sniegulki* appellati."
49 Erndtel, *Warsavia*, p. 66.
50 Erndtel, *Warsavia*, p. 133.
51 Bettina Dietz, "Aufklärung als Praxis: Naturgeschichte im 18. Jahrhundert," *Zeitschrift für Historische Forschung*, 36.2 (2009): 235–57.
52 See Eugen Sachs, "Dr. med. Heinrich Erndel: Stadtphysikus zu Dresden," in *Neues Archiv für Sächsische Geschichte*, 16 (1895): 292–306.
53 *Schuldiges Ehren-Gedächtnüß/Welches Den weiland Hoch-Edlen/best- und Hochgelahrten Herrn Heinrich Erndteln/uff Bereuth und Mulda/Der Medicin weitberühmten Doctori, wie auch zweyer Durchläuchtigster Chur-Häupter zu Sachsen, nehmlich Joh. Georgi III. Glorwürdigsten Andenckens/und Joh. Georgi IV. hochbestallt-gewesenen Leib-Medico, seel. Am Tage Seiner Christl. angestellten Leich-Begängnüß/war der 21. September 1693 aus hertzlichen Mitleiden und zum Trost der hochbetrübten Hinterlassenen Stifften. wolten Drey nachgesetzte Gönner und Freunde* (Dresden, n.d.) The print does not contain page numbers.
54 There is a significant lack of in-depth research on the personal physicians of August II. See the anecdotal essay by Hans Beschorner, "Augusts des Starken Leiden und Sterben," *Neues Archiv für Sächsische Geschichte* 58 (1937): 48–84; this lack of research does not coincide with a remarkable wealth of archival sources: see, for example, Dresden, Sächsisches Haupt- und Staatsarchiv, 10024 Geheimes Kabinett, Loc. 7169/11 Bestallungen med. Hofpersonal, 10026 Geheimes Kabinett Loc. 529/1 Die Einrichtung des Collegii sanitatis oder Medici universalis betr. 1710–1761, 10026 Geheimes Kabinett, Loc. 528/7, fol. 1–111, Medicinalia 1734–1750; for the political institutions during the personal union see Mariusz Markiewicz, "Politische Institutionen und Prozeduren der Sächsisch-Polnischen Personalunion: Das Geheime

Kabinett in Sachsen und die zentralen Ämter der Rzeczpospolita in den
Jahren 1717 bis 1733," in Rex Rexheuser (ed.), *Die Personalunionen von
Sachsen-Polen 1697–1763 und Hannover-England 1714–1837: Ein Vergleich*
(Wiesbaden, 2005): 51–65.

55 Erndtel probably deliberately only concentrated on protestant sights.

56 Laetitia Boehm, "Studium, Büchersammlung, Bildungsreise: Elemente gelehrter
Allgemeinbildung und individueller Ausprägung historisch-politischer Weltan-
schauung im konfessionellen Zeitalter," in Menso Folkerts (ed.), *Die Bausch-
Bibliothek in Schweinfurt: Wissenschaft und Buch in der Frühen Neuzeit*
(Halle, 2000): 117–51; Thomas Freller, *Adlige auf Tour: Die Erfindung der Bil-
dungsreise* (Stuttgart, 2007); Thomas Grosser, "Reisen und soziale Eliten:
Kavalierstour, Patrizierreise, bürgerliche Bildungsreise," in Michael Maurer
(ed.), *Neue Impulse der Reiseforschung* (Berlin, 1999): 135–76; Michael
Maurer, "Kulturmuster Bildungsreise," in Daniel Fulda (ed.), *Kulturmuster der
Aufklärung* (Halle, 2010): 81–99.

57 Christian Heinrich Erndtel, *De itinere suo Anglicano et Batavo annis 1706 et
1707 facto* (Amsterdam, 1711); the same, *The relation of a journey into England and Holland: in the years, 1706, and 1707. By a Saxon Physician, in
a letter to his friend at Dresden, wherein are contain'd many Passages and curious Observations in Anatomy, Surgery, Physick, and Philosophy* (London,
1711).

58 See Frederic Ruysch, *Thesaurus anatomicus nonus, in quo varia, circa corpus
humanum notatu digna occurrunt*, vol. 9 (Amsterdam, 1714), pp. 7–8. I thank
Roland Helms for this information.

59 Erndtel, *De itinere*, passim.

60 Erndtel, *Warsavia*, unpaginated preface.

61 Erndtel, *Warsavia*, pp. 58–59.

62 Erndtel, *Warsavia*, pp. 66–67.

63 Erndtel, *Warsavia*, p. 133.

64 Erndtel, *Warsavia*, unpaginated preface, and pp. 2–3.

65 *Churfürstlich-Sächsischer Hof- und Staatskalender* (Leipzig, 1728), fol. Br;
(Leipzig 1729), fol. B2r; (Leipzig 1731), fol. B3r; (Leipzig 1732), fol. Ir; (Leipzig 1733), fol. B3v. I thank Alexander Kästner for this information.

66 Dresden, Sächsisches Haupt- und Staatsarchiv 10026 Geheimes Kabinett Loc.
529/1 Die Einrichtung des Collegii sanitatis oder Medici universalis betr.
1710–1761.

67 Ibid. and 10026 Geheimes Kabinett, Loc. 528/7, fol. 1–111, Medicinalia
1734–1750.

68 This should be treated as a part of the communication history between the
courts at Dresden and Warsaw, hitherto analysed mainly with a focus on cultural production: Katrin Keller, "Personalunion und Kulturkontakt: der Dresdner
Hof im Zeitalter der sächsisch-polnischen Union," in Rexheuser, *Personalunionen*: 153–76.

69 Erndtel, *Warsavia*, unpaginated preface, and pp. 2–3.

70 Erndtel, *Warsavia*, p. 183.

71 Erndtel, *Warsavia*, pp. 145–76.

72 Divisions are underlined in Karlheinz Blaschke, "Sachsens Interessen und Ziele in
der sächsisch-polnischen Personalunion," in Rexheuser, *Personalunionen*: 67–86.

73 "Viridarium vel catalogus plantarum circa Warsaviam nascentium." I am
indebted to Alexander Kästner for pointing out that this *viridarium* should be
read as an essential part of Erndtel's book.

74 See the book review in the *Commercium litterarium: Norimbergae Sumptibus
Societatis, Commercium litterarium ad rei medicae et scientiae naturalis*

incrementum institutum quo quicquid novissime observatum agitatum scriptum vel peractum est succinte dilucideque exponitur (Nuremberg, 1731), unpaginated. I thank Annemarie Kinzelbach for referring me to this review. On the *Commercium litterarium*, see Kinzelbach and Ruisinger, "Trading Information," Chapter 11 of this volume.

75 Augustus Quirinus Rivinus, *Ordo plantarum, quae sunt flore irregulari hexapetalo* (n.p., 1720).

76 Erndtel, *Warsavia physice illustrata*, Viridarium, p. 8.

77 Erndtel, *Warsavia*, Viridarium, p. 27.

78 Erndtel, *Warsavia*, Viridarium, p. 14. "Vidi hanc plantulam prima vice Warsaviae circa Mariae montem in acclivi loco crescentem d. 15 Maji anni 1714. Ubi, una cum Herbationis tunc socio Ill. Dno. Heuchero, accuratius examinavi illum, propter singularem elegantiam & laeto viridem plantulae amoenitatem."

79 Heinrich W. Reichardt, "Heucher, Johann Heinrich von," in *Allgemeine Deutsche Biographie* (1880), www.deutsche–biographie.de/pnd117524034.html ?anchor=adb (last consulted 6 April 2014).

80 Erndtel, *Warsavia*, Viridarium, for example, p. 72.

81 Erndtel, *Warsavia*, pp. 135, 145–46.

Part IV
Translating, Translocating

10 Transformative Itineraries and Communities of Knowledge in Early Modern Europe

The Case of Lazare Rivière's *The Practice of Physick*

Elaine Leong

In 1655, London publisher Peter Cole stocked the shelves in his bookshop with a new medical title. *The Practice of Physick in Seventeen Several Books* offered readers information on "The Nature, Cause, Differences, and Several Sorts of Signs; Together with the Cures of all Diseases in the Body of Man."[1] According to Cole's own preface, the work was ambitiously intended to "profit many millions, not only of this Generation, but of all that shall follow, till the world become one great Bone-fire; or this Nation and Language perish together."[2] Included in the "many millions" were the "Poor of this Nation," "Sea-farers," soldiers, surgeons, apothecaries, midwives and, particularly, ladies and gentlewomen.[3] The broad target audience of the title might suggest that the book belonged to the flourishing genre of medical works written for a popular readership; yet *The Practice of Physick* was in fact a translation of the physician and professor of physic Lazare Rivière's *Praxis medica*.

The story of the *Praxis medica* begins in 1630s Montpellier where Rivière offered a series of lectures on practical medicine at the University. Unbeknownst to Rivière, one of his students shared his lecture notes with a printer-publisher, and in 1640, the lectures began a new life as a medical textbook. The book was an instant commercial success, and multiple reprints were issued in major printing centers throughout Europe. In 1655, Peter Cole and his long-time publishing partner Nicholas Culpeper brought Rivière's work to English audiences. By then, just 15 years after the first edition appeared, the publishers were able to advertise that 15,000 copies of the Latin edition had been sold. Like the Latin and French editions, *The Practice of Physick* flew off London booksellers' shelves, and ten editions appeared over the next decade or so.[4] Through *The Practice of Physick*, Rivière's *practica* lectures became one of the most read university lecture courses on medicine in late seventeenth-century England.

DOI: 10.4324/9781315554693-15

From the first edition, the English book producers oriented *The Practice of Physick* not only to the original audience of university students and practicing physicians needing a refresher course, but also to lay readers and more specifically to "ladies and gentlewomen."[5] Produced in the immediate aftermath of the English Civil War, the translation and publication of Rivière's *Praxis medica* was part of Cole and Culpeper's ongoing scheme to bring Latinate university-based medical knowledge to broader audiences. Cole and Culpeper's publishing efforts were, from the start of their partnership, framed by contemporary urban politics, and the story of transforming the *Praxis medica* into *The Practice of Physick* is no different. At the same time, early modern publishing was of course a commercial venture, and book producers such as Cole and Culpeper needed to balance their political goals with the practicalities of book sales and keeping their business afloat. As we will see below, these tensions are evident in the very materiality of *The Practice of Physick*.

In the English context, then, the work that began life as a series of lectures in one of the most established medical schools in Europe became reading material for householders and housewives. This new reading audience responded enthusiastically to Rivière's work. Surviving copies of the book abound in modern libraries, many of which contain ownership inscriptions and marginal annotations. This article traces the *Praxis medica*'s journey from university settings into early modern homes. I examine three crucial stages in this journey: first, the codification of the original *practica* lectures into print; second, the transformation from the *Praxis medica* to *The Practice of Physick*; and, finally, how readers engaged with and appropriated the knowledge offered by the book. Each of these steps, I show, left its epistemic footprint on Rivière's *practica* and together form what might be termed an epistemic itinerary. By that I mean itineraries in which bodies of knowledge (as small as a one-line recipe and as large as a multi-volume work) become entangled as they journey through the winding, convoluted processes of early modern book production and reading and writing practices.[6] Reading and note-taking practices are now recognized as knowledge codification processes.[7] The story of Rivière's *Praxis medica*, I suggest, demonstrates that there is much to be gained by paying close attention to the route (and pit stops) that knowledge takes in this process.

The epistemic itinerary of Rivière's *Praxis medica* makes a fascinating story of vernacularizing medicine in the early modern period. It is a story in which medical genres shift and merge and in which there was a myriad of different ways to read and write medicine. These various processes of knowledge transfer and production undertaken by a wide range of historical actors, I argue, worked together to construct a new vernacular medical space on paper in which physicians and university professors metaphorically rubbed shoulders with English housewives. The city of London, with its vibrant print culture and booming book trade, acted as an ideal setting and hub for these transactions.

Lazare Rivière and the *Praxis medica*

Born in Montpellier, Lazare Rivière (1589–1655), physician and professor at the University of Montpellier, spent the major part of his life in his native city. From his medical writings, Rivière emerges as a prolific author who ran a successful and busy medical practice. He authored seven major medical works. Four of these were penned during his lifetime: *Praxis medica*, *Methodus curandorum febrium*, *Observationes medicae*, and *Institutiones medicae*. Three more—*Opera medica universa*, *Arcana Lazari Riverii*, and *Riverius reformatus*—were posthumously issued collations of his works.[8] All of these works appeared in multiple editions in various European printing centers. In particular, *Praxis medica* and *Observationes medicae* enjoyed long publication histories in Latin, English, and French, with the last edition issued in the 1720s. The posthumous collations *Opera medica universa* and *Riverius reformatus* also continued to be printed into the 1730s. In *The Medical World of Early Modern France*, Laurence Brockliss and Colin Jones have argued that the popularity and long circulation of Rivière's works demonstrate his importance and impact on French medical knowledge. Rivière and the *Praxis medica* thus feature as the main example for their discussion of medical doctrine.[9] Similarly, Lester King also chose Rivière as his case study to exemplify early modern Galenic ideas.[10] Yet Rivière was more than just a conservative Galenist. He authored *Observationes medicae* and so participated in consolidating the newly developing medical epistemic genre of *observationes*. He was also an avid advocate of the use of chemical medicaments.[11] Most importantly, Rivière's writings suggest that he was an active participant in contemporary epistolary intellectual networks. Rivière himself alludes to these networks in the preface to the *Praxis medica*. In addition, his *Observationes medicae* concludes with a section of "Observationes ab aliis communicatae." According to Rivière, the section is a collation of observations from practitioners who were diligent enough to note down interesting cases but who might not yet have enough cases to fill an entire book. A number of these observations, such as those by Montpellier-based physician Simeone Jacoz, are framed with personal (often rather flattering) letters to Rivière.[12] Many of the contributors to this section worked in Montpellier and Grenoble, suggesting that local connections played a crucial role in Rivière's knowledge network.[13]

Of Rivière's many publications, *Praxis medica* emerges as his most reprinted and circulated text. In late seventeenth-century Europe, readers could access the text in Latin, French, and English in a variety of formats. Rivière conveniently gives modern readers an origin story in the 1653 expanded edition of the work. As described above, the book started life as a series of lectures on practical medicine. Rivière was careful to stress that these lectures were constructed from his own readings of the various *practicae* available at the time. Channeling the trope of the shy and humble author, he emphasized that, despite repeated request by his students, he never intended for these lectures to be published and that they had been put into print by one of his students. The work evidently met with surprising (to the modest Rivière, at least) popularity and, within two years, no less than six editions were published in various printing centers around Europe. In addition, scholars and physicians from France, Germany, Holland, and Italy all pleaded with him to augment his exposition of medicine's *practica* with *theoria*. The 1653 edition represents the fruits of Rivière's response to these requests and offers sections on the nature, differences, causes, diagnosis, prognosis, and cures for disease. It seems that Rivière was not boasting when he chronicled his contemporaries' pleas as, over the next hundred years, this new enlarged *Praxis medica* was abridged, translated, issued, and reissued from presses from Lyon to Geneva to Venice to Paris to London.

Rivière's *Praxis medica* follows the long-established medical genre *practica medicina*, which flourished in the medieval period.[14] Characterized by head-to-toe arrangement of brief chapters on signs, causes, and cures of diseases, these texts aimed to provide students and those practitioners needing a refresher course with easy to navigate, up-to-date information on practical medicine.[15] In both its structure and content, the genre draws upon and is related to lectures on practical medicine at universities. These lectures usually followed a pattern in which the professor covered the diagnosis and cures of the diseases in particular parts of the body for the first two years and fevers, which were regarded as diseases of the whole body, in the third year.[16] Indeed, Rivière's lectures on fevers were initially published separately as *Methodus curandorum febrium*.[17] They were only later combined with the chapters addressing diseases in particular parts of the body in the expanded 1653 edition of *Praxis medica*.[18]

In fact, the 1653 edition of *Praxis medica* serves as an interesting example of the kinds of epistemic change that occur to a body of knowledge when it crosses from one communication medium and knowledge-transfer context to another. Aside from completing Rivière's *practica* lecture series by the inclusion of the treatise on fevers, the 1653 edition is enriched in several other ways. Six new chapters were added to the original ten, thus providing information on diseases of the eyes, ears, nose, tongue, teeth, and the mesentery, pancreas, and omentum.[19] Additionally, as he described in his preface, Rivère also included *theoria*, by which he meant information on the signs, symptoms, and causes of each disease. The degree to which he expanded each chapter varied from disease to disease. For example, in the chapter "De syncope," the 1640 edition provided only a short introduction to disease causation, followed by possible treatments.[20] The entry in the 1653 edition, on the other hand, begins with references to discussions of the topic by classical and medieval authorities—Galen, Avicenna, and Hippocrates.[21] This is followed by a section on terminology and detailed description of causes and signs of the diseases. Readers are then offered two illustrative cases, one of which was observed by Rivière himself and the other extracted from Petrus Salius Diversus "lib. de affectibus particularibus cap.4."[22] The entry ends with a similar list of treatments and remedies as that presented in the 1640 edition.

If we believe Rivière's preface, we can consider the first Parisian edition of the *Praxis medica* as a printed version of student lecture notes.[23] In that sense, we may view the text as a record of an event located within a specific temporal and spatial context. Within the university medicine course, *practica* lectures were designed to complement and be complemented by lectures on medical doctrine. Thus, short entries like "De syncope," with only a few lines describing the causes of the disease, served the needs of most students. After all, they would receive additional instruction in other lectures. In a stand-alone book, though, the situation is much different. Here, students or practitioners expect the reference work on which they have spent their money to provide the whole picture. The aim of the printed book is to offer more generalized forms of knowledge, ideally no longer tied to specific geographical and temporal points, designed to appeal to a broad audience. The separation of the practical and theoretical elements of medicine, as conducted within university lecture courses, did not make sense within this new communication medium. If the fleeting university lecture requires listeners and note-takers to scramble to remember and record information, the printed text invites readers to ponder, compare and relate it to other works.[24] Accordingly, the expanded edition of *Praxis medica* provides full references, as seen in the example of the citation of Petrus Salius Diversus, to enable readers to delve further into the topic if desired. Hence, while the different versions of *Praxis medica* might have originated from Rivière, they fulfill quite different epistemic tasks. The transition from university lectures to printed text in the 1653 *Praxis medica* broadened the kinds of user accessing and interacting with the body of knowledge. With the widely available printed version, readers were able to converse, as it were, with Rivière on paper. These conversations might take the form of personal letters to the author requesting additions and changes to the text or, more quietly, contestations or agreements written in the book margins. As we will discover later in this chapter, long after Rivière's death in 1655, readers continued to engage with well-thumbed copies of *Praxis medica*. The transformational step from lectures to print created a new space for Rivière's *practica* lectures—one that was no longer tied to a particular place and time.

London, Urban Politics, and the Printing of *The Practice of Physick*

By the mid-seventeenth century, London printers and booksellers offered the English reading public a wide array of vernacular medical books. Readers could pick and choose from an assortment of herbals, pharmacopeias, general medical guides, surgical handbooks, midwifery manuals, regimens, and medical recipe books.[25] While many booksellers had medical books on their lists, perhaps the most influential book-producing team during this period was the author-translator Nicholas Culpeper and his partner the printer-bookseller Peter Cole. Working closely together, they crafted a whole range of texts aimed at providing English readers with the tools and knowledge to self-diagnose and self-medicate. If we stepped into Cole's bookshop at the sign of the printing press in Cornhill near the Royal Exchange in 1655, we might find shelves laden with titles such as *The English Physitian Enlarged, A Directory for Midwives, Galen's Art of Physick, The Anatomy of the Body of Man, A New Dispensatory*, and *The Practice of Physick in Seventeen Books*.[26] The last title is one of more than a dozen English translations of Latin medical texts produced by Peter Cole, Nicholas Culpeper, and others in London after the Civil War.[27] As Faye Getz and others have argued, translation played an important role in the production of medical knowledge in late medieval and early modern England, and many bestselling Tudor and Stuart medical books were in fact translations from Latin or from European vernaculars.[28] In late 1640s London, taking advantage of the lapse in print regulation and the growing English reading public's seemingly insatiable appetite for books, Cole and Culpeper began working together on a translation of the 1618 edition of *Pharmacopoeia Londinensis*. The result, *A Physicall Directory*, was published in 1649 and became an instant bestseller. With this commercial success, the working relationship between Cole and Culpeper blossomed. Over the next five years until Culpeper's death in January 1654, the two worked on more than half a dozen book projects, including *The English Physitian, The Directory for Midwives*, and the translation of *Pharmacopoeia Londinensis*.

From their first project "Englishing" the London College of Physicians' *Pharmacopoeia Londinensis*, Cole and Culpeper were motivated by political aims. In his prefaces, Culpeper proclaimed that they were acting for the good of the commonwealth and fought to end physicians' monopoly on Latin medical knowledge by opening access to English readers. For Culpeper and Cole, "the use of Latin was a scholars' conspiracy, ensuring that theology, law and medicine would be unintelligible to laymen, and accessible only to those who could afford an expensive professional education."[29] Culpeper explains in the preface to the *Physicall Directory* that he strove to supply English readers with the whole model of physic in their native language.[30] By opening access to learned medical knowledge, his aim was to "make an Industrious Diligent, Rational [English] Man a knowing Physitian."[31] Culpeper's fight to free medical knowledge from the clutches of the physicians and his critical attitude toward what he considered the physicians' base medical practice can be felt throughout the books produced in this period.[32] In medicine as in many other politically controversial areas, printed paper became a battleground.[33]

As the frontman and writer of these projects, Culpeper was the more vocal of the book production duo, but we must not underestimate Peter Cole's role. Cole, as Jonathan Sanderson and Elizabeth Lane Furdell tell us, not only kept company with figures such as the Leveller and medical practitioner William Walwyn, but also printed petitions by puritan leaders such as Lord Mayor Issac Penington (c. 1584–1661) and was the principal publisher of the works of puritan divines such as William Bridge (c. 1600–70) and Jeremiah Burroughes (1559–1646).[34] After Culpeper's death in early 1654, Cole continued the pair's endeavors to broaden access to medical knowledge. Doubtless driven partly by commercial interests, Cole was instrumental in bringing key Latin works by continental authors to the English reading public. Upon his death, Cole's stock was picked up by none other than John Streater, well known as a political pamphleteer and publisher of medical and scientific books. While Streater might have focused more on vernacularizing legal knowledge, he shared Culpeper and Cole's goal of eradicating the boundary between the learned and the vernacular.[35] The translation and publishing of learned medical works in the 1650s was thus tightly tied to contemporary urban politics and debates concerning knowledge and information access.

In 1654, perhaps spurred by the success of the *Physicall Directory*, Cole and Culpeper appeared to have grander ambitions. That year, continuing the pair's efforts to translate and open up learned medical knowledge to new audiences, Cole registered seven new medical titles with the Stationers Company at one go.[36] All of these were translations of Latin works by continental medical authors, including Rivière, Jean Riolan, Daniel Sennert, Thomas Bartholin, John Johnston, and Jean Fernel.[37] A few years later, whether by design or encouraged by market forces, Cole marketed these translations together as *The Physitian's Library*, offering English readers open access (at a price) to the writings of the who's who of learned medicine at the time. Unfortunately, Culpeper died before he was able to complete translating even one of the many tomes registered. Cole was thus forced to tender the job to two new translators, Abdiah Cole and William Rowland. Culpeper's absence is clearly felt in the tone of the translated prose. Earlier translations by the team are characterized by Culpeper's numerous interjections in the text. For example, in *The London Dispensatory*, while providing his readers with fairly faithful translations of medical formulas, Culpeper queried and offered his own opinions at the end of each entry. The printed page thus became an arena in which Cole, Culpeper, and the College of Physicians struggled over medical practice and knowledge. The new translators stepped into Culpeper's shoes to complete the assigned task of translation, but they could not or perhaps did not want to emulate Culpeper's distinctive voice. Most of the works registered in 1654, including the two works by Lazare Rivière, made it through the book production process, but they appear to be fairly straightforward translations of the Latin originals, lacking obvious additions and contestations.[38] If these later translations lack Culpeper's forceful tone, they remain significant in the duo's politically motivated plans for increasing knowledge access. The works later designated as *The Physitians Library* brought an extensive body of learned European medical discourse to a new reading public.

This was no mere repackaging of learned medicine for vernacular audiences. *The Practice of Physick* resembles *Praxis medica* in content, but as a book and a material object, they are worlds apart. Peter Cole and his team took Rivière's students' textbook or physicians' *vade mecum* and transformed it into a luxury object for wealthy lay readers. In doing so, as we will see, Cole merged epistemic genres that were largely distinct in the learned medical sphere, and he thereby cultivated new kinds of book consumer. The most obvious change is perhaps the choice of book format. In contrast to the mostly octavo-sized Latin and French editions of *Praxis medica*, Cole's volume is a weighty folio-sized tome with generous margins and ornamental borders.[39] With paper costs paramount in early modern book production, this format is revealing of Cole's projected readers. Where the Latin and French editions are designed to be inexpensive and portable, *The Practice of Physick* is designed to be slowly and (perhaps repeatedly) pored over. In producing such a book Cole was making a bold move. Certainly, the English vernacular medical book market was booming in 1650s London, but many of the volumes on the booksellers' shelves were offered at the cheaper octavo or even duodecimo formats.[40] Even Culpeper's successful *The London Dispensatory*, first issued in folio, turned to the more affordable quarto format from the second edition onwards. These tracts were directed at the urban middling sort who eagerly sought out information of all kinds and who ably mixed self-administered medical care with the wide variety of services offered on the lively medical marketplace in the city. It is unlikely that this community of readers could afford a 500-page folio-sized book. Cole's decision to publish Rivière's works in folio, thus, is suggestive of his desire to tap into or even create a new reading market. This market consisted of affluent readers with interests in health-related information and responsibility for providing medical services. Thus, while in the prefatory materials Cole and Culpeper might frame their endeavors within contemporary political discussions of knowledge access, when it came to identifying actual buyers for the work they pragmatically targeted wealthy elite readers. This tension serves as a stark reminder of the multiple political, economical, and cultural negotiations that had in a hand in shaping early modern publishing and book production.

While in his preface Cole is careful to address the work to a wide audience, he returns repeatedly to one particular group of readers—"many of the Gentry, especially of Ladies and Gentlewomen." These wealthy English women, according to Cole, could use the knowledge gleaned from the work to determine and shape their medical encounters with physicians, to provide basic medical care for their family and dependents and for their charitable works with the poor.[41] As recent studies have shown, many gentlewomen were responsible for the running of large urban households and country estates, and providing healthcare was considered merely one of their many duties.[42] Additionally, contemporary conduct book writers such as Richard Brathwaite specifically commend medical reading as a desirable trait in the ideal English gentlewoman. The extant medical notebooks of women such as Elizabeth Freke and Margaret Boscawen suggest that many women did consult contemporary medical print in order to educate themselves in medical know-how.[43] In addressing his book to this particular group, Cole places his product alongside a cluster of titles in the very successful genre of printed medical recipe collections many of which, like the contemporary bestseller *A Choice Manual of Rare and Select Secrets*, were geared toward the increasing numbers of female readers.[44]

The project of evolving a book which originated as a series of university lectures into a book for a lay female audience required more than a mere translation from Latin into the vernacular, or the repackaging of the book as a material object. Cole was well aware that he needed to provide additional explanations throughout the text. From amending the chapter titles to providing a glossary, the additions worked to ensure that their targeted audience could make the most use out of Rivière's work. The changes to the chapter headings were fairly simple—most involved merely an explication of the Latin medical term. For example, where in the 1653 Latin edition, book four, Chapter 7 is titled "De Hamorrhagianarium," in the English version, it is titled as "Of the Bleeding at the Nose, called Haemorrhagia."[45] Within the text, many of the "hard phrases" such as "mascatories" are explained in context by "more easie words" like "chewing medicines." The import of these seemingly small changes to both book producers and consumers alike is signaled by the fact that they are explicitly mentioned and painstakingly explained by Cole in his preface.[46]

Aside from parsing chapter headings and difficult words, Cole also provided a lengthy glossary at the end of the text. He explains that to aid his readers, particularly those "honorable Ladies and Gentlewomen [...] and for [...] all others unacquainted with the Greek and Latin Tongues, and consequently unable to understand divers terms of Art, and other words drawn from the said Tongues [...] [he] caused a *Physical Dictionary* to be added." Never shy to advertise other books on his shelves, he also advises that if any reader requires a fuller explanation of simple or compound medicines, they should consult Nicholas Culpeper's *The London Dispensatory*.[47] The glossary, titled "A Physical Dictionary. Expounding such words, as being terms of Art, or otherwise derived from the Greek and Latin, are dark to the English Reader" was a big undertaking. Aside from being grandly titled as a "dictionary," it had its own title page—suggesting that Cole, at some point at least, envisioned it being sold or circulated as an independent text. After all, he writes: "This Dictionary is of use in the reading of all other Books of this Nature in the English Tongue."[48]

The 13-page long dictionary contains a wealth of curious, at times random but undoubtedly helpful information including:

> Ascent: going up.
> Cupping-glass: is that which Physitians use to draw out Blood with Scarrifying of the Skin, Glasses fastened with lighted Tow or Flax.
> Hemiplegia: the Palsey possessing one side.
> Pubes: the hairy Hillock above the privities in men and women. The word signifies ripeness, because that hair being grown out, testifies the parties to be fit to engender.
> Tile tree: a Linden tree there grow two on Newington green they bear sweet blossomes.
> Zacutus Lusitanus: a famous Physitian; A Jew that practiced at Amsterdam in Helland. He has wrote divers excellent Treatises of physick, sutable to the Principles of Hippocrates and Galen.[49]

From verbs to medical technologies to Latin medical terms to contemporary medical authors, the text covers a wide range of knowledge categories and areas and is clearly aimed at a broad reading audience. Yet, the specific reference to Newington Green in the entry on the Tile Tree suggests that if Cole's ideal readers did not permanently reside in London, they were familiar with the city. As alluded to earlier in this essay, Rivière's location in Montpellier meant that his writings are strongly connected with southern France. For example, many of the observations offered in the *Observationes medicae* took place in cities such as Montpellier or Grenoble. Cole's glossary, though, is firmly located in urban London suggesting that the project to translate Rivière functioned on both a linguistic and cultural level.

Cole's commission and inclusion of such a dictionary was not in itself innovative. Earlier vernacular medical tracts such as Giovanni da Vigo's *The Most Excellent Workes of Chirurgerye* (1543) and Thomas Brugis' *The Marrow of Physicke* (1640) also provided glossaries of sorts. However, Cole's version is unusually lengthy and diverse. Brugis' glossary, for example, is only two pages long and concentrates on providing brief explanations of specialist terms like astringent and decoction.[50] The presence of these glossaries suggests that while many household medical practitioners possessed the skills to provide a range of healthcare to their dependents, when faced with a translated medical textbook, many still required a crib sheet of sorts.[51] Indeed, there was evidently a market for such books. Peter Cole never went ahead with issuing his "dictionary" as a stand-alone book. But only two years after the publication of *The Practice of Physick*, another glossary attached to a medical book, a translation of Jean de Renou's

Dispensatorium medicum (1609) was later published as a separate title, confusingly also called *A Physical Dictionary*.[52] This stand-alone medical dictionary evidently enjoyed a broad readership as it was issued in multiple editions in both folio and duodecimo formats. Although the dictionary or glossary included in *The Practice of Physick* is merely an example in a group of such texts, the diverse knowledge categories included by Cole and his cohort suggests that their aims differed slightly from Brugis' and other texts. Not only were they explaining unfamiliar vocabulary, but they were also introducing new materia medica and key medical authors. At first glance, it may seem odd that readers are introduced to the physician and medical author, Zacutus Lusitanus, in a medical dictionary. Yet, this inclusion might be partly explained by the fact that Lusitanus was one of the authors whose works Cole later published and advertised as part of his *Physitian's Library*.[53] When viewed within this context, the dictionary is in effect, much more than a crib sheet but also perhaps a sneaky way to educate and inform their potential customers of new products.[54]

Finally, Cole's enterprise to make available learned medical works to a new audience also freed him from the traditional conventions of Latinate medical publishing. Like many other vernacular medical book producers of the period, he felt comfortable in mixing up both genres and authors. Alas, for Cole, not all of his translations of learned medical works were as commercially successful as Rivière's *The Practice of Physick* and, subsequently, many were often repackaged and sold in bundles.[55] This was a practice continued by John Streater in the 1660s when he took over Cole's stock and the publication of these titles.[56]

Particularly significant for our story is that, from the 1658 edition onwards, the English versions of Rivière's *Praxis medica*, his *Observationes* and Jean Fernel's *Consilia*, all of which circulated as separate titles in Latin, were packaged as one volume. This can clearly be seen on the title pages. The 1658 title page (Figure 10.1) lists the observations as Chapters 18–21, Fernel's *Consilia* as Chapter 22 and Cole's dictionary as Chapter 24. The 1672 title page (Figure 10.2) literally presents the translated *Observationes medicae* and Fernel's *Consilia* merely as addenda. Here, the page is visually dominated by the proclamation that the book is

> chiefly a translation of THE WORKS of THAT Learned and Renowed Doctor LAZARUS RIVERIUS… To which are added Four Books containing Five Hundred and Thirteen Observations of Famous Cures. By the Same Author. And a Fifth Book of Select Medicinal Counsels. By John Fernelius.[57]

Thus, Fernel, a noted author in his own right, in both editions gets reduced to just another physician providing medical cases. The pairing together of Rivière's *Praxis medica* and *Observationes* forged a new mode of transmission for Rivière's texts in England—one distinct from the Latin and French

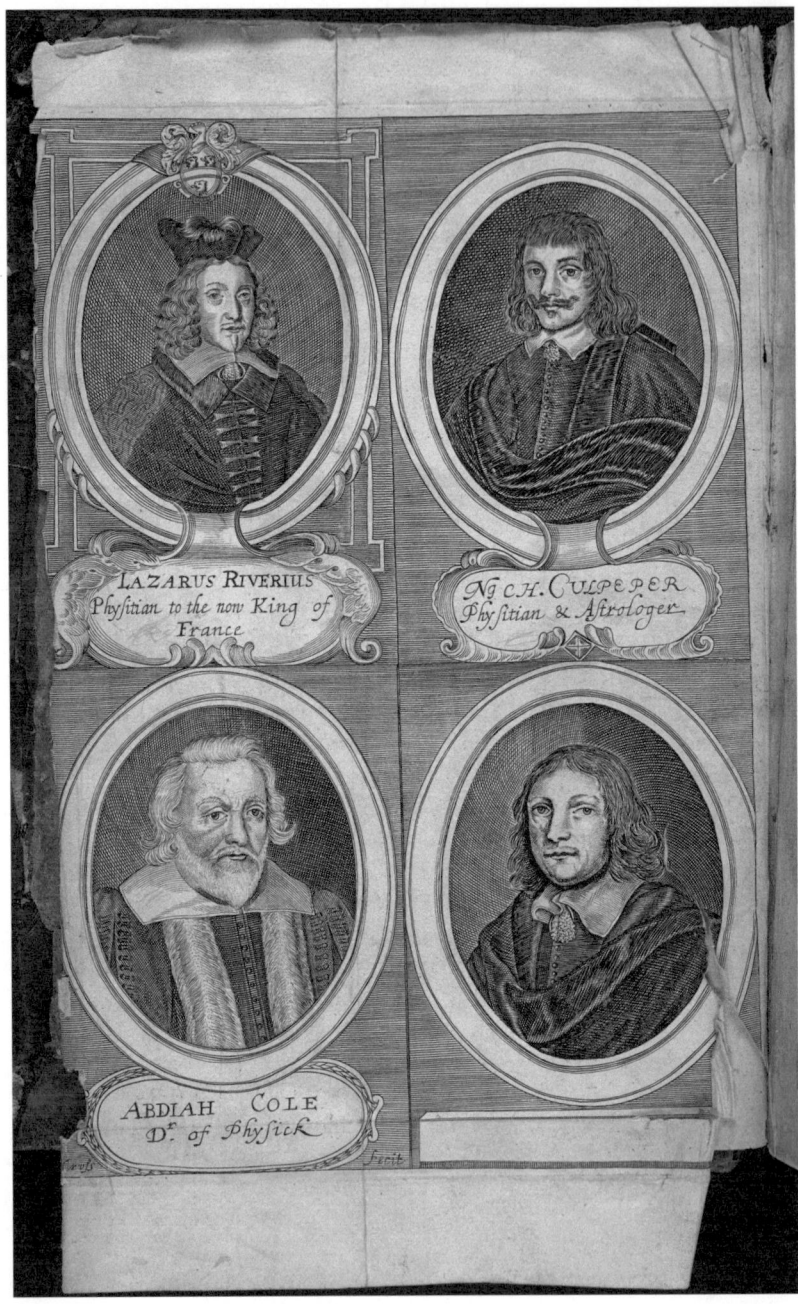

Figure 10.1 Lazare Rivière, *The Practice of Physick* (London, 1658), title page and frontispiece. © The British Library Board (1489.e.23).

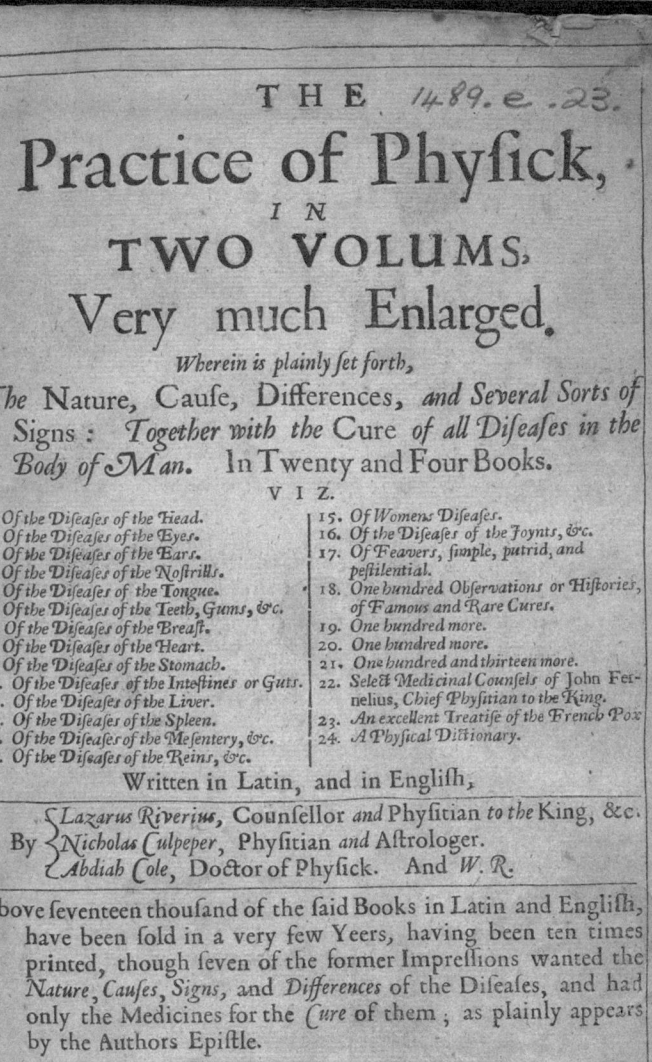

THE *1489. e. 23.*

Practice of Physick,

IN

TWO VOLUMS,

Very much Enlarged.

Wherein is plainly set forth,

The Nature, Cause, Differences, *and Several Sorts of*
Signs : *Together with the* Cure *of all Diseases in the*
Body of Man. In Twenty and Four Books.

VIZ.

1. *Of the Diseases of the* Head.
2. *Of the Diseases of the* Eyes.
3. *Of the Diseases of the* Ears.
4. *Of the Diseases of the* Nostrills.
5. *Of the Diseases of the* Tongue.
6. *Of the Diseases of the* Teeth, Gums, &c.
7. *Of the Diseases of the* Breast.
8. *Of the Diseases of the* Heart.
9. *Of the Diseases of the* Stomach.
10. *Of the Diseases of the* Intestines or Guts.
11. *Of the Diseases of the* Liver.
12. *Of the Diseases of the* Spleen.
13. *Of the Diseases of the* Mesentery, &c.
14. *Of the Diseases of the* Reins, &c.

15. *Of* Womens *Diseases.*
16. *Of the Diseases of the* Joynts, &c.
17. *Of* Feavers, *simple, putrid, and* pestilential.
18. *One hundred* Observations *or* Histories, *of* Famous *and* Rare Cures.
19. *One hundred more.*
20. *One hundred more.*
21. *One hundred and thirteen more.*
22. *Select* Medicinal Counsels *of* John Fernelius, *Chief* Physitian *to the* King.
23. *An excellent* Treatise *of the* French Pox
24. *A* Physical Dictionary.

Written in Latin, and in English,

By { Lazarus Riverius, Counsellor *and* Physitian *to the* King, &c.
{ Nicholas Culpeper, Physitian *and* Astrologer.
{ Abdiah Cole, Doctor of Physick. And W. R.

Above seventeen thousand of the said Books in Latin and English,
have been sold in a very few Yeers, having been ten times
printed, though seven of the former Impressions wanted the
Nature, Causes, Signs, and *Differences* of the Diseases, and had
only the Medicines for the *Cure* of them ; as plainly appears
by the Authors Epistle.

LONDON:

Printed by Peter Cole, Printer and Book-seller, and are to be sold at his Shop, at the
Sign of the Printing-press in Cornhil, neer the Royal Exchange. 1655.

Figure 10.1 (Cont.)

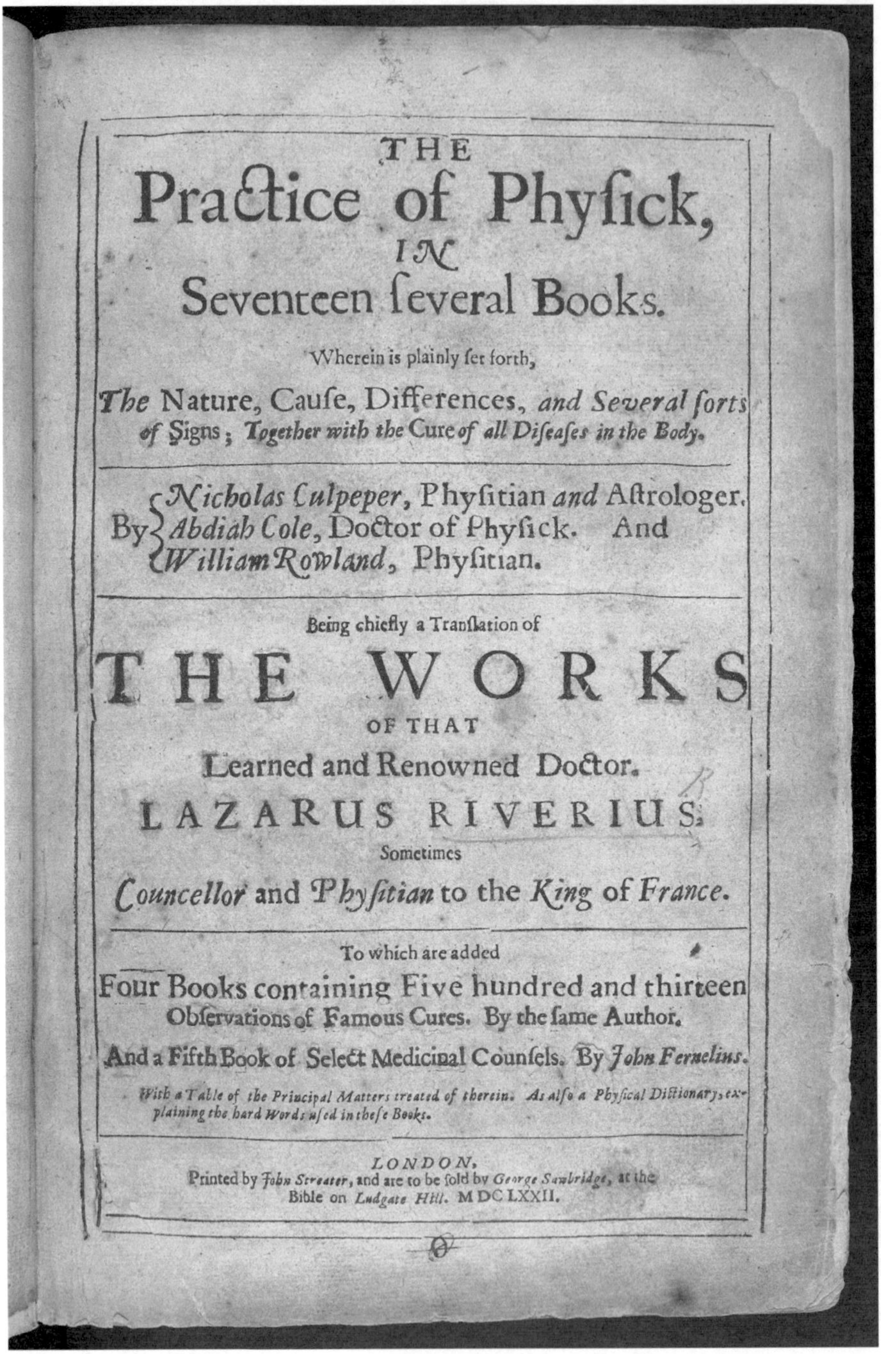

THE

Practice of Physick,

IN

Seventeen several Books.

Wherein is plainly set forth,

The Nature, Cause, Differences, *and Several sorts of* Signs ; *Together with the Cure of all Diseases in the Body.*

By { *Nicholas Culpeper*, Physitian *and* Astrologer. *Abdiah Cole*, Doctor of Physick.   And *William Rowland*, Physitian.

Being chiefly a Translation of

THE WORKS

OF THAT

Learned and Renowned Doctor.

LAZARUS RIVERIUS,

Sometimes

Councellor and *Physitian* to the *King* of *France.*

To which are added

Four Books containing Five hundred and thirteen Observations of Famous Cures. By the same Author.

And a Fifth Book of Select Medicinal Counsels. By *John Fernelius.*

With a Table of the Principal Matters treated of therein. As also a Physical Dictionary, explaining the hard Words used in these Books.

LONDON,

Printed by *John Streater*, and are to be sold by *George Sawbridge*, at the Bible on *Ludgate Hill*. MDCLXXII.

Figure 10.2 Lazare Rivière, *The Practice of Physick* (London, 1672), title page. © The British Library Board (Wing R1559A).

editions which continued to circulate as separate titles. While readers of French and Latin were encouraged to savor and appreciate the *Observationes* as a new epistemic genre, in English, readers encountered Rivière's observations and cases more as a supplement to *Praxis medica*. Yet, this offering by Cole and his team is significant as it not only brings a new epistemic genre of learned medicine to vernacular readers but through processes of writing, translation and reading, early modern English readers became part of Rivière's pan-European knowledge community.

Reading *The Practice of Physick*

Scholars of the history of reading have long argued that "reading gives meaning" and that reading is a highly individualistic and culturally conditioned activity. Each reading is seen as a construction of knowledge in particular historical settings.[58] Furthermore, reading, writing and note-taking practices are now also themselves recognized as knowledge codification processes that leave behind their own epistemic footprints.[59] Within this framework, the study of medical texts from the reader's point of view is crucial to our understanding of medical books and the transmission of medical knowledge in the early modern period. The long and complex publishing history of Lazare Rivière's works suggests that they were well regarded by book consumers and readers. Copies of the *The Practice of Physick*, in particular, often contain ownership notes and/or marginal annotations and markings revealing not only past readers' interest in and intellectual engagement with the work, but also the high value put upon the material book by previous owners.

English readers' encounters with *The Practice of Physick* can be traced through a wide range of annotations and marks.[60] Aside from marking up copies of the printed book, readers, of course, also took notes from their texts into their manuscript notebooks. As numerous historians of medicine and science have demonstrated, analyses of these kinds of notebooks reveal a wealth of information on how readers encountered and codified knowledge. While examination of reading notes in manuscript notebooks allow us to reconstruct the reading and epistemic practices of individual readers, as I will show below, analysis of a range of annotated copies enable us to make generalizations about the reception of a work within particular geographical and temporal boundaries.[61] Ownership notes written on the title page and, surprisingly often, on random pages throughout the text, provide glimpses of the identity of past readers. The Folger Shakespeare Library's copy of the 1678 edition, for example, has inscribed in the front matter three names: Mary Burbidge, Francis Young, and Thomas May.[62] Each of these owners has provided modern readers with a sliver of information. Thomas May tells us that he is from Ray. Francis Young notes that he bought the book for 8 shillings on April 25, 1684. Finally, Mary Burbidge tells us that she only came into possession of the book in 1721, nearly 50 years after the publication of the work. These three readers were in good company in their perusal of Rivière's works. Many other copies of *The Practice of Physick* contain ownership notes. James Hamilton, for example, signed his copy of a 1678 edition of the work and John Coupe and Jonathan Brereton wrote their names in a copy of 1668 edition.[63] While we have little biographical information on these readers, their ownership notes are testaments to the popularity of the work and the presence of multiple ownership notes in particular copies suggest a lively second-hand market.

Mary Burbridge's note also highlights two further points. Firstly, Peter Cole successfully reached a target reading audience of ladies and gentlewomen. Despite the fact that early modern women were more reticent in leaving traces of their reading practices, a number of copies of *The Practice of Physick* contain ownership notes written by female readers. For example, a copy of the 1672 edition has inscribed on the first page "Amey Lock her Booke." This inscription was later crossed out and a second ownership note "Amey Forster" was written onto the title page of the work suggesting that the book accompanied Amey as she moved families and households upon marriage. Other copies of *The Practice of Physick* which passed through female hands include the 1672 edition in the Huntington Library which was once owned by Eliza Boo[n?]d and the 1661 edition in the Wellcome Library which was consulted by a number of readers including Margaret Serte.[64] In many ways, we should not be surprised that Mary, Amey, Eliza and Margaret took up Peter Cole's offer of Rivière's works as early modern women were enthusiastic consumers of vernacular medical print. Culpeper, in particular, was a favored author by a number of women who have left us traces of their medical reading practices.[65] Through Culpeper and Cole's translation of Rivière's text, the women named here participated, as readers, in a vernacular knowledge community spanning beyond the confines of their households and spheres of knowledge.

Returning to the Folger copy of *The Practice of Physick*, Mary Burbridge's early eighteenth-century ownership note also alerts us to the longevity of Rivière's work. Burbridge was not the only eighteenth-century inscriber. Margaret Serte's copy of the work passed onto George Holland who signs his name in 1775. In other cases, William Douglas of Cavers signed the Wellcome Library's 1668 edition in 1743, and Robert Webbe signed a copy of the 1655 edition in 1702.[66] These numerous eighteenth-century inscriptions indicate that *The Practice of Physick* continued to be consulted by readers decades after it first appeared on the English book market. Paired with the fact that collected editions of Rivière's works continued to be printed in Latin and French well into the first quarter of the eighteenth century, it is evident that *The Practice of Physick* resonated with readers' needs and interests far beyond its original intended sphere of circulation.

Many of the owners named above also left other marks within their copies of *The Practice of Physick*. Some used common selection marks such as "+" or "*" or under-linings to mark out passages which once struck them as useful or worthy of a second read. These kinds of marks have increasingly come under the scrutiny of historians of reading who utilize them to tease out and further understand social, political and cultural continuities and changes. In terms of *The Practice of Physick*, these marks demonstrate particular readers' interests and use of the work. For example, one particular reader marked up multiple passages by pressing on the page with the edge of his or her fingernail. He or she appeared to have particular interests in the sections on "collick," scurvy, ailments of the kidney, stoppages of the liver, jaundice, stoppage of terms, immoderate fluxes and pestilential fevers.[67] Within these sections, multiple diagonal lines draw the attention of subsequent readers to the various signs of these ailments and, most frequently, to the many applicable remedies. The fingernail imprints here function as markers both to remind the annotator of their own selected passages and to alert future readers to useful information. When taken together, the marks also work to create a text within a text. That is, we can imagine the selection marks to codify a personalized collation of information geared toward the medical interests and practices of that annotator. Rivière's original knowledge schema, geared toward offering a general overview of medicine, is replaced by one concentrating on a set of ailments and diseases troubling a particular household and a collection of handpicked recipes.

A 1678 edition of *The Practice of Physick* further demonstrates that the work was not only read by contemporaries but also incorporated, to a certain extent at least, in their quotidian medical practices. Firstly, use is indicated by additions in the index of the text. Not content with the index provided by Cole and his team, a reader has inserted two entries on "sciatica" with their corresponding page numbers to the printed index and, thus, revealing not only his medical interests but also the fact that he has studied the text to locate the sought after information.[68] Further use is suggested by the three additional pages of medicinal recipes written into the back flyleaves.[69] Dating from the 1680s, these include numerous recipes for the scurvy, itches, coughs and agues. Like other contemporary collections of such recipes, many of these are supported by personal endorsements via first or second-hand observations and experiences.[70] For example, one recipe is titled "An Easy & Rare medesine which Helped mee more Agaynst the scurvy & Itching than any" and another "An Easy medesine which Cured my mayd Judah of An Ague in 1684."[71] The supplementary recipe collection acts both as an archive recording past cures and as a treasure trove of information for potential future uses. In this, it shares an epistemic function with Rivière's *Observationes*, which were included in this edition of *The Practice of Physick*. However, while Rivière's *Observationes* offers conversations and knowledge gleaned from an international epistolary network of learned men, the handwritten recipe collection is constructed from familial and friendship links now long lost alongside the identity of the compiler. Hence the physical binding together of Rivière's and the anonymous readers' knowledge collation efforts creates a work that traverses multiple boundaries. Records of cures performed by university-trained physicians now sit comfortably (for the reader at least) next to cures the reader used for family and dependents.

Conclusions

In 1721, when Mary Burbidge wrote her name on a 1678 copy of *The Practice of Physick*, Rivière's works had been in print in Latin for almost a century and in English for more than 60 years. Within this time, medical know-how that began life in university lecture halls in Montpellier ended up on the desks of early modern English householders. What was once deemed appropriate information for the perusal of learned physicians became information to be recorded, treasured, and passed on between family members. The journey that Rivière's lectures took from their first outing in the 1630s to Burbidge's readings involved a variety of different kinds of translation and numerous intermediaries. At each step, the body of knowledge once known as Rivière's *Praxis medica* morphed ever so slightly. At each turn, the distinct, clear-cut genre boundaries of academic medicine blurred. At the hands of Peter Cole and his cohort, traditional medieval genres such as the *practica* and *consilia* were physically bound with newer genres like the *observationes*. Several processes drove these transmutations. The initial combination of practical and theoretical medical knowledge was no doubt shaped by both the change of communication media and by commercial needs. The translation from Latin into English was steeped in the political ambitions and economic needs of a group of political and religious radicals acting in the turmoil of post-Civil War London. Once readers got hold of particular texts, they applied their own lenses and filters, and thus what originated as a series of university lectures on the practical side of physic became a knowledge source for household medical practitioners.

Medical books such as Rivière's *Praxis medica* have long been studied as paths for the transmission of learned medical knowledge. Yet, as demonstrated by this short study of the *fortuna* of Rivière's works in England, early modern knowledge transfer was anything but linear. Rather, knowledge followed complex epistemic itineraries. The story of Rivière's *Praxis medica* encourages us to follow these epistemic itineraries and delve further into the intricacies of book production. From Rivière gathering notes for his lectures from existing texts, to his student bringing the work to a printer/publisher, to Rivière's fellow physicians' epistolary requests to augment the 1640 edition to Peter Cole and his team's collective efforts to translate, repackage and extend the work, all of these steps were continually shaped by multiple individuals. By putting Rivière's lectures in print and on paper, the book producers collectively constructed a new medical space—one where vernacular medicine overlapped with learned discourses, and where readers and authors engaged across linguistic, temporal, spatial, and geographical boundaries. When Rivière delivered his *practica* lectures at the University of Montpellier in the 1630s, I doubt he imagined that his words would be read by an English gentlewoman nearly a century later.

Notes

Acknowledgments: Early drafts of this chapter were circulated in the "3P" working group within the ERC-funded project Ways of Writing: How Physicians Know, 1550–1950 at the Institute for the History of Medicine, Charité Berlin; the science in translation reading group at the Max Planck Institute for the History of Science; and the early modern medicine reading group at the University of Cambridge. I thank my friends and colleagues in Berlin and Cambridge for their insightful comments and suggestions. I am particularly grateful to the editors of the present volume for all their help in shaping and framing this chapter.

1 Lazare Rivière, *The Practice of Physick* (London, 1655), title page.
2 Ibid., sig. A2v.
3 Ibid., sig. A1v.
4 The English Short Title Catalogue lists editions from 1655, 1658, 1661, 1663, 1664, 1665, 1666, 1668, 1672 and 1678. Until 1666, the work was printed and sold by Peter Cole (sometimes with his brother Edward Cole). From 1668 onwards, the work was printed by John Streater to be sold by George Sawbridge.
5 Rivière, *Practice of Physick* (1655), sig. A1v.
6 For a similar focus on translation, print and text production, see Kinzelbach and Ruisinger, "Trading Information," Chapter 11 of this volume.
7 There is now a growing literature on this topic. Recent work includes Ann Blair, *Too Much to Know: Managing Scholarly Information before the Modern Age* (New Haven, 2010); Lorraine Daston, "The Sciences of the Archive," *Osiris*, 27/1 (2012): 156–87; Volker Hess and J. Andrew Mendelsohn (eds), *Paper Technology: Ein Forschungsinstrument der frühneuzeitlichen Wissenschaft*, special issue of *NTM: Zeitschrift für Geschichte der Wissenschaften, Technik und Medizin*, 21/1 (2013); Richard Yeo, *Notebooks, English Virtuosi and Early Modern Science* (Chicago, 2014).
8 Louis Dulieu, "Lazare Rivière," *Revue d'histoire de la pharmacie*, 190 (1966): 205–11. Dulieu provides a lengthy (yet, alas, incomplete) bibliography of Rivière's works, p. 201.
9 Laurence Brockliss and Colin Jones, *The Medical World of Early Modern France* (Oxford, 1997), p. 153, n. 257.
10 Lester S. King, *The Road to Medical Enlightenment, 1650–1695* (London and New York, 1970), pp. 15–36.
11 Gianna Pomata, "Sharing Cases: The *Observationes* in Early Modern Medicine," *Early Science and Medicine*, 15 (2010): 193–236.
12 Lazare Rivière, *Observationes medicae* (London, 1646), pp. 385–87.
13 These include a number of practitioners described as surgeons working in Montpellier, including Samuel Formio and Denis Pomaret, ibid., p. 403 ff and p. 427 ff. On the significance of place and locality in the *observationes* genre, see Pomata, "A Sense of Place," Chapter 8 of this volume. See Stolberg, "The Many Uses of Writing," Chapter 2 of this volume for a detailed case study of Georg Handsch's letters, the writing of *consilia* and the collation of physicians letters into printed volumes.
14 For a history of the *pratica* genre in the medieval period, see Luke Demaitre, "Theory and Practice in Medical Education at the University of Montpellier in the Thirteenth and Fourteenth Centuries," *Journal of the History of Medicine and Allied Sciences* 30/2 (1975): 103–23; Demaitre, "Scholasticism in Compendia of Practical Medicine, 1250–1450," *Manuscripta*, 20/2 (1976): 81–95.
15 On *practica*, see Joël Coste, "La mèdecine pratique et ses genres littèraires en France à l'èpoque moderne": www.bium.univ-paris5.fr/histmed/medica/medpratique.htm (accessed 12 August 2013); Jerome J. Bylebyl, "Teaching Methodus

Medendi in the Renaissance" in Fridolf Kudlien and Richard J. Durling (eds), *Galen's Method of Healing: Proceedings of the 1982 Galen Symposium* (Leiden, New York, Copenhagen, and Cologne, 1991): 157–89; Andrew Wear, "Explorations in Renaissance Writings on the Practice of Medicine" in Andrew Wear, Roger K. French and Iain M. Ionie (eds), *The Medical Renaissance of the Sixteenth Century* (Cambridge, 1985): 118–45; Chiara Crisciani, "Histories, Stories, *Exempla* and Anecdotes: Michele Savonarola from Latin to Vernacular" in Gianna Pomata and Nancy Siraisi (eds), *Historia: Empiricism and Erudition in Early Modern Europe* (Cambridge, MA, and London, 2005): 297–324.

16 Bylebyl, "Teaching Methodus medendi," p. 166.

17 Paris, 1641 and subsequent editions. For a full list of editions, see Dulieu, "Lazare Rivière," p. 210.

18 Dulieu, "Lazare Rivière," p. 210. The *Methodus curandorum febrium* was published in Paris in 1641, in Lyon in 1649 and the Hague in 1651.

19 See "Index Librorum et capitum Praxeos Medicae," in Rivière, *Praxis medica* (Paris, 1640 and Lyon, 1653).

20 Rivière, *Praxis medica* (Paris, 1640), pp. 126–29.

21 Rivière, *Praxis medica* (Lyon, 1653), vol. 1, pp. 506–17.

22 Ibid., p. 510. This could be a reference to Petrus Salius Diversus, *Liber de affectibus particularibus* (Bologna, 1584).

23 For a discussion of student lecture notes and textbooks, see Ann Blair, "The Rise of Note-Taking in Early Modern Europe," *Intellectual History Review*, 20/3 (2010): 303–16; Blair, "Student Manuscripts and the Textbook" in Emidio Campi et al. (eds), *Scholarly Knowledge: Textbooks in Early Modern Europe* (Geneva, 2008): 39–74.

24 For a discussion of how readers ruminated on medical works, see Jennifer Richards, "Useful Books: Reading Vernacular Regimens in Sixteenth-Century England," *Journal of the History of Ideas*, 73/2 (2012): 247–71.

25 Mary Fissell, "Popular Medical Writing," in Joad Raymond (ed.), *The Oxford History of Popular Print Culture: Cheap Print in Britain and Ireland to 1660* (Oxford, 2011): 417–30; Fissell, "The Marketplace of Print," in Mark Jenner and Patrick Wallis (eds), *Medicine and the Market in England and Its Colonies, c. 1450 – c. 1850* (Basingstoke and New York, 2007): 108–32; Paul Slack, "Mirrors of Health and Treasures of Poor Men: The Uses of the Vernacular Medical Literature of Tudor England," in Charles Webster (ed.), *Health, Medicine and Mortality in the Sixteenth Century* (Cambridge, 1979): 237–73.

26 Rivière, *Practice of Physick* (1655), sigs. B r-v.

27 Studies of early modern translation is a flourishing field. Recent studies include Sara K. Barker and Brenda Hosington (eds), *Renaissance Cultural Crossroads: Translation, Print and Culture in Britain, 1473–1640* (Leiden, 2013); Harold J. Cook and Sven Dupré (eds), *Translating Knowledge in the Early Modern Low Countries* (Vienna, 2013); Peter Burke and R. Po-chia Hsia (eds), *Cultural Translation in Early Modern Europe* (Cambridge, 2007).

28 See, for example, Faye Getz, "Charity, Translation and the Language of Medical Learning in Medieval England," *Bulletin of the History of Medicine*, 64/1 (1990): 1–17; Peter Murray Jones, "Four Middle English Translations of John of Arderne," in Alastair J. Minnis (eds), *Latin and Vernacular: Studies in Late-Medieval Texts and Manuscripts* (Cambridge, 1989): 61–89; Slack, "Mirrors of Health."

29 Charles Webster, *The Great Instauration: Science, Medicine and Reform, 1626–1660* (London, 1975), p. 269.

30 Culpeper, *A Physicall Directory* (London, 1649).

31 Jean Prevost, *Medicaments for the Poor* (London, 1656), Letter to the Reader by Nicholas Culpeper, R4r.

32 See also, for example, Culpeper's diatribe against the physicians in his letter to the reader in *Galen's Art of Physick* (London, 1652), sigs. A4r to B1v (esp. A4v).

33 For detailed discussion, see Webster, *The Great Instauration*, esp. ch. 4; Christopher Hill, "The Medical Profession and Its Radical Critics," in Christopher Hill (ed.), *Change and Continuity in Seventeenth-Century England* (London, 1974): 157–78.

34 Sanderson, "Nicholas Culpeper and the Book Trade," pp. 92–93; Furdell, *Publishing and Medicine*, p. 42.

35 See Adrian Johns, "Streater, John (*c*.1620–1677)," in H. C. G. Matthew and Brian Harrison (eds), *Oxford Dictionary of National Biography* (Oxford, 2004); online edn., Lawrence Goldman (ed.), January 2008, www.oxforddnb.com/view/article/26656 (accessed 25 April 2014); Adrian Johns, *The Nature of the Book* (Chicago, 2000), Ch. 4.

36 This was not the first attempt to bring Rivière's *Praxis medica* to England. A few months earlier, on 26 November 1653, James Flesher registered the title "Lazari Riveri Praxis Medica" in the Stationer's Company's Register under the supervision of a College of Physicians member Francis Prujean. It was common for publishers to register titles as a way of establishing ownership of the text, and it seems that Flesher never followed through in publishing the text. Flesher was responsible for publishing Rivière's *Observationes medicae* in London in 1646. This publication was endorsed by the College of physicians as it was registered under the hands of a college member John Clarke: Sanderson, "Nicholas Culpeper and the Book Trade," pp. 67–70.

37 Sanderson, "Nicholas Culpeper and the Book Trade," p. 108; McCarl, "Publishing the Works of Nicholas Culpeper," p. 238.

38 It is not unusual, in this period, to find vernacular translations of *practica* texts. For example, Arnold de Villanova's *Praxis Medicinalis* was not only printed in Latin in the late sixteenth century, but a German edition also appeared in 1619. As Chiara Crisciani tells us, Michele Savonarola also rewrote parts of his *Practica major* into a series of Italian texts within the *regimina sanitatis* genre. In crafting these treatises, Savonarola made substantial changes to the text in order to adapt it to his new urban and courtly audience: Wear, "Explorations in Renaissance Writings," p. 119; Crisciani, "Histories, Stories."

39 The format and style of the Latin and French editions follows the convention of the learned medical book market in the early modern period; Ian Maclean, *Logic, Signs and Nature in the Renaissance: The Case of Medicine* (Cambridge, 2007), p. 59. For an overview of Latin medical books, see Ian Maclean, "The Diffusion of Learned Medicine in the Sixteenth Century through the Printed Book," in Maclean, *Learning and the Market Place: Essays in the History of the Early Modern Book* (Leiden and Boston, 2009): 59–86.

40 Fissell, "The Marketplace of Print"; Fissell, "Popular Medical Writing."

41 Rivière, *Practice of Physick* (1655), sig. A1v.

42 There is a growing body of literature on household medical practice in early modern England; see, for example, Lucinda Beier, *Sufferers and Healers: The Experience of Illness in Seventeenth-Century England* (London, 1987), ch. 8; Doreen Evenden Nagy, *Popular Medicine in Seventeenth-Century England* (Bowling Green, OH, 1988), ch. 5; Elaine Leong "Making Medicines in the Early Modern Household," *Bulletin of the History of Medicine*, 82/1 (2008): 145–68.

43 For a discussion of the medical notebooks and reading practices of these two women, see Elaine Leong, "Herbals She Peruseth: Reading Medicine in Early Modern England," *Renaissance Studies*, 29 (2014): 556–78.

44 The most successful examples of this genre include: *A Choice Manual of Rare and Select secrets in Physick and Chyrurgery* (London, 1653) and *The Queens Closet Opened* (London, 1655). The first is associated with Elizabeth Grey, Countess of Kent (1581–1651), and the latter is reportedly the recipe book of Queen Henrietta Maria. Both titles are designed and geared towards a female reading audience. See Lynette Hunter, "Women and Domestic Medicine: Lady Experimenters, 1570–1620," in Lynette Hunter and Sarah Hutton (eds), *Women, Science and Medicine, 1500–1700: Mothers and Sisters of the Royal Society* (Stroud, 1997): 89–107.

45 Rivière, *Praxis medica* (1653), sig. **5v; Rivière, *Practice of Physick* (1655), sig. Cv.

46 Rivière, *Practice of Physick* (1655), sig. A2r.

47 Ibid.

48 Ibid., sig. Lllll1r.

49 Ibid., sigs. Lllll2r, Lllll2v, Lllll4v, Mmmm2v, Mmmm3v and Mmmm4r.

50 Thomas Brugis, *The Marrow of Physick* (London, 1640), pp. 87–88.

51 These kinds of crib sheets can also be found in manuscript medical notebooks. For example, the notebook of Valentine Bourne contains a list offering the "interpretation of strange words"; Bodleian Library, Oxford: Tanner MS 397, fols. 6r–8v.

52 Jukko Tyrkkö, "*A Physical Dictionary* (1657): The First English Medical Dictionary," in John Considine (ed.), *Ashgate Critical Essays on Early English Lexicographers, Volume 4: The Seventeenth Century* (Farnham, Surrey, 2012): 323–39.

53 *The Physitian's Library, Containing all the Works of the Most Famous Physitians Following, viz. Dan. Sennertus. Laz. Riverius. Fel. Platerus. Tho. Bartholinus. Joh. Riolanus. Joh. Veslingus. Joh. Johnston. Nich. Culpeper. Mart. Ruland. Zacut. Lusitanus. Wil. Rnd. Joh. Fernelius & Abdiah Cole. All which are of Excellent use for Rational Persons; especially for all Chyrurgeons at sea in his Most Royal Majesties ships; And all others that are on Trading Voyages, for the Advancement of the Wealth and Honor of His Kingdoms* (London, 1663).

54 Mario Biagioli has made this argument with reference to print and scientific instruments: "From Print to Patents: Living on Instruments in Early Modern Europe," *History of Science*, 44 (2006): 139–86.

55 Sanderson, "Nicholas Culpeper and the Book Trade," pp. 98–99.

56 Many of these editions were newly type-set, suggesting that they were not all reissues or unsold stock sold with a new title page.

57 Rivière, *The Practice of Physick* (London, 1672), title page.

58 The history of reading is a rich field, and references are too numerous to cite here. For a recent overview, see Jennifer Richards and Fred Schurink, "Introduction: The Textuality and Materiality of Reading in Early Modern England," *Huntington Library Quarterly*, 73 (2010): 345–61. Key works on reading in early modern Europe include Robert Darnton, "First Steps Towards a History of Reading," *Australian Journal of French Studies*, 23 (1986): 5–30; Roger Chartier, *The Order of Books: Readers, Authors and Libraries in Europe between the Fourteenth and Eighteenth Centuries*, trans. Lydia Cochrane (Cambridge, 1994); Anthony Grafton and Lisa Jardine, "'Studied for Action': How Gabriel Harvey Read His Livy," *Past and Present*, 129 (1990): 30–78. For a focus on early modern England, see among others William Sherman, *Used Books: Marking Readers in Renaissance England* (Philadelphia, 2007); James Raven, Helen Small, and Naomi Tadmor (eds), *The Practice and Representation of Reading in England* (Cambridge, 1996); Kevin Sharpe, *Reading Revolutions: The Politics of Reading in Early Modern England* (New Haven and London, 2000); Jennifer Andersen and Elizabeth Sauer (eds), *Books and*

Readers in Early Modern England: Material Studies (Philadelphia, 2002); Kevin Sharpe and Steven Zwicker (eds), *Reading, Society and Politics in Early Modern England* (Cambridge, 2003).

59 See references in note 7 above.
60 Medical notebooks containing references to Rivière's works include Cambridge University Library MS Dd 2 45 (notebook of Dru Burton with notes and translations from Lazare Rivière and others); Glasgow University Library Hunter MS 485 and MS 487 and Folger Shakespeare Library MS v.a. 452 (medical recipe book of Thomas Sheppey).
61 Although I am studying individual readers' engagements with the "English" Rivière in my larger project, in this chapter I have concentrated on analyzing annotated copies of *The Practice of Physick* in the Wellcome, Folger Shakespeare, and Huntington Libraries. For recent detailed discussions on medical and natural history commonplace books, see Michael Stolberg, "Medizinische Loci communes: Formen und Funktionen einer ärztlichen Aufzeichnungspraxis im 16. und 17. Jahrhundert," *NTM: Zeitschrift für Geschichte der Wissenschaften, Technik und Medizin*, 21/1 (2013): 37–60; Volker Hess and J. Andrew Mendelsohn, "Fallgeschichte, Historia, Klassifikation: François Boissier de Sauvages bei der Schreibarbeit," *NTM: Zeitschrift für Geschichte der Wissenschaften, Technik und Medizin*, 21 (2013): 61–92; Leong, "Herbals She Peruseth."
62 Lazare Rivière, *The Practice of Physick* (London, 1678). Folger Shakespeare Library copy shelfmark R1555.2, back cover, fols. 1r and 2r.
63 University of Illinois at Urbana-Champaign Library IUQ02081; Wellcome Library EPB/44149/C/2 (1668), title page, sigs. Dr and Rr2r.
64 Huntington Library 300900; Wellcome Library EPB/44150/C/2, title page and A2r.
65 Rebecca Laroche, *Medical Authority and Englishwomen's Herbal Texts, 1550–1650* (Farnham, Surrey and Burlington, Vermont, 2009); Leong, "Herbals She Peruseth."
66 Wellcome Library EPB/44149/C/1, verso of final index page; Wellcome Library EPB/44146/C, recto of front flyleaf.
67 Wellcome Library EPB 44151/C/3. In his *Ludus Literarius, or The Grammar Schoole* (1612), John Brinsley recommends using the imprint of the fingernail as a method of annotation. Heidi Brayman Hackel has argued that female readers may have shied away from writing in the open and public space of communal book margins. The anonymous marking of book margins with a fingernail was thus a practice sometimes adopted by women. Hackel presents the case of Anne Boleyn annotating Tyndale's *Obedience of a Christian Man* for the king as an example: Hackel, *Reading Material in Early Modern England: Print, Gender and Literacy* (Cambridge, 2005), pp. 205–06.
68 Wellcome Library EPB 44151/C/2, sig. Fff5r.
69 Ibid., back flyleaves.
70 There is now a rich and large body of literature on household recipe collections in early modern Europe. Most relevant to this point and within the English context, see among others Sara Pennell, "Perfecting Practice? Women, Manuscript Recipes and Knowledge in Early Modern England," in Victoria Burke and Jonathan Gibson (eds), *Early Modern Women's Manuscript Writing: Selected Papers from the Trinity/Trent Colloquium* (Aldershot, 2004): 237–58; Elaine Leong and Sara Pennell, "Recipe Collections and the Currency of Medical Knowledge in the Early Modern 'Medical Marketplace'," in Jenner and Wallis (eds), *Medicine and the Market*: 133–52; Elaine Leong, "Collecting Knowledge for the Family: Recipes, Gender and Practical Knowledge in the Early Modern English Household," *Centaurus*, 55/2 (2013): 81–103.
71 Wellcome Library EPB 44151/C/2, first back flyleaf verso.

11 Trading Information

The City of Nuremberg and the Birth of a Latin Medical Weekly

Annemarie Kinzelbach and Marion Maria Ruisinger

Commercium litterarium was the first weekly medical journal in the German-speaking world. It ran successfully from 1731 to 1745, a remarkably long duration at a time when scholarly periodicals lasted, on average, only four years. Evaluating this journal in the context of medical journalism in the Holy Roman Empire, Tilman Rau pointed out that its "medical" purview included all topics of natural history; he also identified the advantages of the publication's organization as well as flaws that finally led to its being discontinued.[1] In accordance with his aim of characterizing the periodical and analyzing its development in the context of contemporary scholarly discourse, Rau based his study on the whole 15-year run of the *Commercium*, which was dominated by Christoph Jacob Trew, who acted as its director from 1733.[2] Focusing on the printed journal, Rau drew little on the rich source material provided by Trew's letter collection and other relevant manuscripts in the Erlangen University Library. How the journal was launched, funded, and produced and the aims and networks of its initiators have remained somewhat vague.[3] Various research projects have been and still are trying to fill these gaps, such that we are now in a position to analyze more closely the process of founding the journal.[4] In this chapter, we concentrate on the birth and first steps of the *Commercium litterarium*. We aim to determine what was distinctive and significant about this journal in the history of knowledge. Our answer will explain how and why such an enterprise was undertaken by a society of civic medical officers and why this happened in a particular German Imperial city. We will argue that an acceleration of "knowledge in motion" made this journal different from other medical periodicals.[5] Nuremberg made this acceleration possible: as one of Europe's foremost trading cities and as the home of physicians who were not merely competing practitioners but comprised an organized community that understood its mission as a broad public one. As Fritz Dross points out in Chapter 4 of this volume, *all* physicians in Nuremberg held public office and were members of the city's Collegium Medicum, a corporative organization that

DOI: 10.4324/9781315554693-16

provided medical advice for the city council and fulfilled several public tasks and services.[6] The public these doctors strove to create through their enterprise of reading, rewriting and distributing was continuous with this local one, yet much wider: a new kind of medical and scientific republic of letters.

Commercium litterarium

The Erlangen University Library preserves a complete run of the *Commercium litterarium*. Its 15 quarto volumes are uniformly bound in leather and form an impressive row on the library shelf. The front page of the first volume reveals interesting information: the complete title reads *Commercium litterarium / ad / rei medicae et scientiae / naturalis incrementum / institutum / quo / quicquid novissime observatum / agitatum scriptum vel / peractum est / succincte dilucideque exponitur.*[7] The first connotation of *commercium* was trade; however, *commercium litterarium* may be translated as "exchange of letters," which is a clue to the kind of sources that served to constitute the journal.[8] Its full title announced the aim of enhancing medicine and the natural sciences (*ad rei medicae et scientiae naturalis incrementum*) and claimed to spread the very latest (*novissime*) information about observations, experiences, and publications (*quicquid [...] observatum, agitatum, scriptum vel peractum est*) in this field of knowledge. The journal was printed, as the front page also reveals, in Nuremberg (*Norimbergae*) in the office of Johann Ernst Adelbulner (1665–1737). An unnamed society (*sumptibus societatis*) was responsible for the whole project.

The main characteristics of this *Societas* have been elucidated by Rau and others.[9] It was founded in Nuremberg in 1730 with the one and only purpose of establishing and running the *Commercium litterarium*. In this respect, it differed fundamentally from other scholarly societies, such as the Royal Society of London, whose purposes were much wider and more varied.[10] The name *sumptibus societatis* evokes economic features by alluding to business companies and to joint investing or spending.[11] The Nuremberg society was composed of six members belonging to the Collegium medicum: five town physicians and one professor teaching at the faculty of medicine in nearby Altdorf, where Nuremberg ran its university.[12] Their respective roles and interaction are examined below. Here, we give basic information on these men.

Oldest among them, Johann Heinrich Schulze (1687–1744), was 43 when the society began.[13] In 1720, Schulze had moved from Halle to Altdorf as successor to Lorenz Heister (1683–1758) in the professorship of anatomy and surgery. As part of the medical faculty, he automatically joined the Nuremberg Collegium medicum. The next year he was elected Fellow of the Academia Caesareo Leopoldina-Carolina Naturae Curiosorum ("Leopoldina").[14] His wide range of knowledge meant that Schulze was an important member of the society.[15] In 1732, Schulze returned to Halle.

Johann Christoph Götz (1688–1733) was a year younger at 42. In 1713, he had settled as physician in his home town of Nuremberg and was appointed member of the Collegium medicum; in 1726, he became Fellow of the Leopoldina.[16] Götz was the only *Societas* member who already had practical experience in publishing a periodical, albeit not a very successful one. In 1726, he had begun publishing the German weekly journal *Der aufrichtige Medicus* (The Honest Physician).[17] However, the hoped-for dialog with his readership did not evolve as expected, and in the following year, Götz brought the endeavor to a halt. He was eager to make a second attempt, and he had learned his lesson: a weekly journal could not be shouldered by one man alone. He became the driving force behind the *Commercium litterarium*. After his untimely death in 1733, Trew honored him as an "outstanding and enriching father, director and promoter" of their common project.[18]

Next in age was 35-year-old Christoph Jacob Trew (1695–1769).[19] He was born the son of an apothecary in Lauf, a small town in the territory of Nuremberg. In 1721, he moved to Nuremberg, where he became a member of the Collegium medicum, which entrusted him with running its Theatrum anatomicum. From 1727, he was a member of the Leopoldina. In 1733, after Götz's death and Schulze's move to Halle, Trew took over the main responsibility for the *Commercium litterarium* and remained its director for years.

Georg Nicolas Stock (1701–1753), Christoph Wilhelm Preißler (1702–1734) and Johann Christoph Homann (1703–1730) were the younger members of the society. Homann was son of the geographer and publisher Johann Baptist Homann, had traveled extensively during his *peregrinatio academica*, and therefore provided important contacts for the society. Preißler, son of a Nuremberg painter, had an elegant writing style that distinguished him for collaboration in the publishing project.[20]

The language of this weekly journal was exclusively Latin. Vernacular letters received were translated into Latin by the editors. This distinguished their journal from others. In the journal *Sammlung von Natur- und Medicin [...] Geschichten* edited by Johann Kanold in Breslau, for example, or the *Philosophical Transactions* of the Royal Society of London, vernacular and Latin texts were mixed.[21] The Nuremberg society's insistence on Latin resembled the politics of the journal of the Leopoldina, the German scholarly scientific society with Imperial privilege, except that the Leopoldina editors defined Latin style as a means of discriminatory segregation.[22] Another trait shared by the two journals was dependency on correspondence to provide content.[23] A major difference between the *Commercium* and other journals was the insistence on *Neuigkeit* (novelty). Not only was this announced in the journal's title (*novissime*), but it was also discussed among its founders: the timeliness of information delivered immediately to the subscriber was the explicit aim of the *Societas* and the explicit difference in comparison with other published journals.[24] The founding members of the *Commercium* guaranteed this dynamic to their subscribers. Their success depended—as the following sections will show—on specific means of cooperation and production enhanced by the opportunities available in Nuremberg.

The front page of the *Commercium litterarium* (Figure 11.1) provides not only written, but also pictorial information about the society's program. A small copperplate engraving illustrates how the ambitious project was to be realized: the beehive in the center (a reference to the iconography of the journal of the Leopoldina) symbolizes the collective struggle to gather pollen (that is, information) to a central place (Nuremberg), where it is processed into honey (the journal). The figures on each side of the beehive show the attributes of Athena and Mercury, the ancient gods of science and commerce. They epitomize the enterprise: the collecting, reshaping, and distributing of scientific news and information by the means of commerce.

Commercial Infrastructure in Nuremberg

We turn now to argue that the *Commercium* was enabled by Nuremberg's commercial infrastructure. Moreover, a specific commercial model prevailing there—a variant of "putting out" called the *Verlagssystem* (see below)—inspired the members of the *Societas* in their organization of a process that (1) gathered raw material (information) from various locations and sources by means of a complex local and inter-local net of coordinators; (2) evaluated, translated, and structured this material into a tradable form of knowledge and news; and (3) pre-financed the print version and distributed and sold it via an established web of agents making use of the abundant communication infrastructures available in Nuremberg.

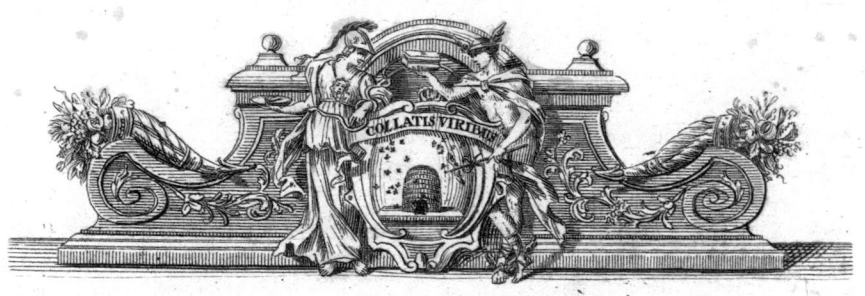

Figure 11.1 Vignette from the front page of eighteenth-century medical weekly *Commercium litterarium*. Courtesy of and © Universitätsbibliothek Erlangen-Nürnberg: Sign. H61/4 TREW.E-II b.

Producing the *Commercium* involved no simple or direct transfer of an economic system into publishing. Rather, the members of the *Societas* borrowed important aspects of the *Verlagssystem* that were widespread in Nuremberg.[25] Since the fourteenth century, the *Verleger* (merchants, rich artisans) had separated production from trade: they pre-financed or bought raw material or equipment that was costly and demanded expertise in its acquisition. This they provided to dependent artisans or homeworkers, who processed the raw material into the end product that was sold by the *Verleger*.[26] It was helpful for the editors to be familiar with this system, as they played the role of *Verleger* in several respects. They pooled their expertise in acquiring the latest scholarly news and made use of their extensive networks to distribute and sell their product. Moreover, they or their printer pre-financed the technical part of production (printing), and they benefited from the local availability of the expensive material (paper) in varying qualities.[27] Without such a model system and resources, the editor of the shorter-lived *Sammlung von Natur- und Medicin* in Breslau, by comparison, had had to establish a *Correspondence Cassa* to which sponsors contributed in order to cover at least part of the expense of producing the journal.[28] Götz, identified by some authors as the first "director" of the *Commercium*, most probably initiated transfer of the *Verlagssystem* into publishing by taking those aspects most relevant to the specific needs of the journal. Götz could rely on experience gained by his upbringing in a family with close ties to the world of merchants and by communicating with friends and family members working as *Verleger* in the gold trade.[29] His great-grandfather, the renowned humanist physician and traveling botanist Leonhard Rauwolf (1535–1596)—from the neighboring center of trade, Augsburg—had already made a good case for a close link between merchants and scholars, a relationship that would combine and enhance economic profit, information-gathering, and the gaining of knowledge.[30]

Producing the *Commercium* differed in several ways from the *Verlagssystem*. Unlike *Verleger*, the editors and not only their providers contributed processed material: news and observations. Here, the economic dependency characteristic of the *Verlagssystem* became instead a win–win situation accelerating the transfer of valued information and condensed knowledge. There were other differences. Unlike *Verleger*, the *Commercium* editors generally did not profit financially. Rather, they increased their social and symbolic capital by their involvement in such an enterprise, which also allowed them to communicate and shape scholarly values.[31] This involvement also enhanced their ability to publish their own observations rapidly and to expand their scholarly networks, as we will show below through the example of a contribution by Götz to the journal and through the dynamic development of the *Commercium*'s supporters.[32]

Since the Middle Ages, Nuremberg had been a communication center fostered not only by its merchants, but also by its councilors. The council, Nuremberg's governing body, gathered information by sending and receiving messengers from all parts of Europe and by interviewing independent individuals. This receiving and spreading of information formed an indispensable element of the domestic and foreign affairs of the Imperial City of Nuremberg, a sovereign "republic" within the Holy Roman Empire.[33] The merchants exchanged letters with partners in most of the important cities of the commercial world. By the eighteenth century, inhabitants could make use of the vigorous traffic of postal and communal messengers, coaches, and transport coming into and going out of the city throughout the day.[34] Consequently, Nuremberg's publishing and bookselling trade was differentiated and well established, if partly limited by censure.[35]

The *Societas* did not choose one of the big publishing houses in Nuremberg to publish its weekly journal. Instead it commissioned the printer Johann Ernst Adelbulner (1665–1737). His son Michael (1702–1779), a mathematician, medical doctor, and printer, participated in his father's business.[36] A topical analysis of Adelbulner publishing reveals interests in religion, in gathering and transforming information from all over the world, and in observing nature. Moreover, direct and indirect personal ties came to the fore. Trew, for example, had already begun publishing with Adelbulner when the journal began. Further links will be discussed below.[37] The closest bonds were with Michael Adelbulner, who in 1735 started a follow-up project, the *Commercium litterarium ad astronomiae incrementum*, whose preface referred to the example set by the medical *Commercium*.[38]

Raw Material: Channeling the Flow of Information Toward Nuremberg

Information was the "raw" material gathered by the agents and members of the *Societas*. Early modern physicians, like other scholars, used direct (oral) as well as indirect (written) communication to gather and transmit information. From the early humanists through the eighteenth century, scholarly sociable networks supported and shaped the exchange of medical and other news.[39] Networks of trade, especially in medicines, a major focus of recent research, did this still more widely and came to include "countless people from all around the world."[40] Here, we shift focus from such networks to how they fed into print. A young scholar's network typically began or intensified through his *peregrinatio academica*, during which he met other learned men, even with leaders in his field of knowledge. Back home, he cultivated these first contacts by regular correspondence, thus turning ephemeral direct conversation into indirect communication materially fixed in writing.[41] When six members of Nuremberg's Collegium Medicum founded the *Societas*, they merged their individual nets of correspondence into one, thus forming a common network of wide reach and dense coverage. This merged correspondence provided the supporting structure for the flow of information to Nuremberg and the spreading of the final product, *Commercium litterarium*, into the world. It was the backbone of the publication project.[42]

Cooperation among the society's members extended so far that, in case of death, they even inherited the correspondents of their late colleague. The imperative of continuing the exchange of letters was felt not only by the society, but also by its correspondents, as the example of Johann Balthasar Ehrhart (1700–1756) shows.[43] Ehrhart, town physician of the Imperial town Memmingen in the Allgäu region, was a correspondent of society member Homann, who died in 1730. When Erhart learned that his contact in the *Societas* had passed away, he sent a letter to Trew, although the two were not acquainted, expressing his wish to continue corresponding with the society.[44] His letter to Nuremberg crossed with a letter from Trew to Memmingen that had the exact same intention.[45] Ehrhart and Trew exchanged letters until 1749, and the Memmingen town physician remained an assistant to the *Commercium*. This indicates that relations among the society's members and its correspondents were characterized by a strong sense of mutual purpose and devotion. It also shows that the enterprise generated exchange and cooperation that transcended the personal relations that characterized much scholarly correspondence.

The "assistants" formed one of the three groups that the editors of the *Commercium* described as vital "promoters" for their enterprise: *assistentes* (assistants), *lectores* (readers), and *collaborantes* (authors, contributors).[46] The assistants can be described as the commercial agency of the *Societas*. They participated in both directions of the *Commercium*'s system of collecting and distributing, serving as relays between the three aforementioned groups and the society in Nuremberg. The assistants recruited new *lectores*, collected money from subscribers, and received letters and materials from the *collaborantes*. They gathered these heterogeneous materials together and sent them in bundles to the *Societas*. Furthermore, they received the printed *Commercium* from Nuremberg and distributed it to subscribers. This indicates that assistants had to be trustworthy persons who were selected from the society's correspondents or on a correspondent's recommendation.[47] Moreover, the assistants were supposed to live in busy and well-connected commercial centers.[48]

In November 1730, the *Societas* published the names of 12 "assistants"—nine in major German cities, one in Strasbourg, and two in Switzerland—and asked urgently for more persons willing to serve in this enterprise for the honor of being named in print at regular intervals and the recompense of receiving a free copy of each issue of the journal, as well as a percentage of the earnings. The appeal's success suggests that the web of this Nuremberg publishing society included enough prominent names (including university teachers as well as town physicians) to attract further promoters. By the first full issue of 1731, the number of assistants had increased to 28, and the geographic reach now included Prague and Vienna to the east, Danzig and Konigsberg to the northeast, and Venice to the south.[49] Soon Paris was included as well.[50] Later, the *Societas* collaborated with about 24 assistants who were spread as far east as St. Petersburg, south to Rome and Pisa, and north to Flensburg.[51]

What kinds of "raw material" did the *Societas* try to channel to and gather in Nuremberg? Trew made this explicit in a letter that he sent early in 1731 to Paris. The recipient was the young Nuremberg physician Georg Leonhard Huth (1705–1761), whose extensive *peregrinatio* led him to Strasbourg, Paris, Amsterdam, and Leiden. Back home, this physician's brother was unhappy about the prolonged travel, and Trew had just put in a good word for the young man.[52] He asked Huth a favor in return: Trew sent "some printed pages" with information about the newly founded *Societas* and asked Huth to communicate them to "some interested physicians and naturalists in Paris."[53] The "*Societas* would be much obliged," Trew continued, "if Huth could procure a person in Paris who would be ready to inform it without delay about new books, inventions, and other relevant news."[54] In his answer, Huth expressed his ready willingness to provide the *Societas* with information himself. Then Trew added a more precise request: Huth should send "the complete title, format and size of the medical and physical *Dissertationes* and publications printed in the last and the current year" in Paris.[55]

The *Societas* needed different kinds of material to produce the periodical. An important part of it was formed by the kind of news Trew requested from Huth: remarks on inventions and in general everything relevant to the periodical's field of interest, which formed the basis for the rubric *nova*. Bibliographic details about recently published dissertations and books were needed for the rubric *libri novi*. By way of information about recent books, these news items also served as a starting point for the rubric *recensiones*, which, however, usually required submission of the work to be reviewed. Furthermore, some personal correspondents sent letters accompanied by elaborated original articles written in German or Latin. These texts provided the material for the fourth and last rubric of the journal, the *observationes*.

Any of these texts could, moreover, be treated as material for an article by an editor. One such by Götz is headed *relatio* (report) and relates his own disease experience.[56] It begins by citing from a letter Götz received from Johann Samuel Carl. This colleague and friend provided advice for the *podagra* (gout of the foot) from which Götz was suffering, and offered to send him a drink to try, which was supposed to help if properly used. The first part of the citation ends with details of adjuvant measures. Götz then gave his own sensory observations on the received fluid and on a residue formed when heated. Citing again from Dr. Carl's letter, he related an appraisal of a remedy recommended by D. D. Dippelius, a prominent Pietist and physician.[57] With the end of citations from the letter, Götz returned to sensory description over time and then focused on the effects this remedy had when he suffered from a seizure of pain. In relating a mixed success in nine steps instead of a single conclusive recommendation or rejection, Götz implied that his readers could judge for themselves.

The members of the *Societas* stressed that their periodical provided "brand new" (*novissime*) information. They therefore faced not only the challenge of procuring news to Nuremberg, but also of procuring it as fast as possible. Organizing the exchange of letters with the least possible delay was crucial for the success of their publication project. The speed of transmission, however, depended to a large extent on the traffic infrastructure provided by their home-town. In this regard, Nuremberg turned out to be exactly the right place.

In the 1730s, the arrival and departure of messengers and coaches in Nu-remberg was dense. Even the *Adresskalender*, which detailed only the official messenger and mail itineraries, shows high frequency for early modern times. Twice a week, for example, people, letters, and parcels could travel to the northern boundaries of the Holy Roman Empire, to the Netherlands, and to England by two outgoing coaches leaving on Wednesday mornings at eight o'clock. One of these headed due north through the most important Saxon towns to the Brandenburg towns, Berlin, and finally Hamburg. Another headed northwest, through Kassel, Paderborn, Munster, the Netherlands, and finally England—returning on Friday. The same route was serviced on Satur-days at eight in the morning. On Saturday at noon, a slightly different route into Saxony led to Leipzig. The same day at three in the afternoon, a coach left for the east via Regensburg to Vienna and then Hungary. Frequent incom-ing coaches and numerous coaches belonging to other territories increased the dynamic of exchange and linked Nuremberg with towns and territories in, for example, Switzerland and Italy. According to the detailed transport tariffs ("post-taxa") for persons, letters, and parcels, routes connected still more towns not mentioned in the route descriptions. This web of communication was strengthened and augmented by ordinary and extraordinary messengers providing opportunities for swift exchanges with major cities and with all towns in the region. Finally, the transport of merchandise, with more than 50 regularly incoming and outgoing carts per week, added further opportunities for sending and receiving information.[58] This remarkable traffic and the infra-structure of its urban hub made the *Commercium* possible. In some cases, we know the exact time a letter took, because Götz and Trew sometimes noted on the received letter the date of its "presentation."[59] This date may not always be the same as the day of its arrival in Nuremberg but gives an idea of the maximum time needed for letters to make the journey: from Coburg, between one and three days; from Halle, seven days; from Weimar, eight days; from Leipzig, three to 13 days; and from Paris 11 days.[60] Slow by our standards, this resulted in a product appreciated by early modern readers as *novissime*—not without much work at the hub.

Production: Processing Letters in a Scholarly Society

The *Societas*, in cooperation with the printer, processed the information into the specific form of news and knowledge required for publication in a weekly journal. The success of this form of production is attested not only by the remarkable duration of the enterprise, but also by the fact that it impressed the printer enough to launch an astronomical *Commercium*.[61] The collaborative processing of letters into a weekly print product needed an appropriate infrastructure. This, too, Nuremberg provided.

Nuremberg's Collegium Medicum comes first to mind in thinking about what institutions the city could offer for sustaining a journal run by doctors. Yet it may have been less important than we would expect. The Collegium hosted communication between Nuremberg medical practitioners and Alt-dorf medical professors, which probably helped establish or deepen contact between Trew and Götz (Nuremberg) and Schulze (Altdorf).[62] Whether issues of interest for the *Commercium* were discussed in Collegium meetings remains an open question because the manuscript volumes of its proceedings for the relevant period have been lost. All in all, the impact of the Collegium as institution of exchange among doctors can be judged relatively low because only a few of its members joined the *Societas*. Other opportunities and forms of communication, however, show profound impact.

Nuremberg's Theatrum anatomicum was situated in the former refectory of the St. Catharine Convent, close to Trew's house and in the same parish as Götz's home (Figure 11.2). Trew regularly gave public anatomy lessons, attended by the printer Michael Adelbulner and younger members of the *Societas*, a regular opportunity for exchanging and testing information concerning anatomy.[63]

Nuremberg also provided opportunities to develop astronomical and meteorological expertise, which were seized by members of the *Societas*. The observatory built by Georg Christoph Eimmart (1638–1705) on the walls of Nuremberg was transferred in 1711 to the roof of the Collegia building in Nuremberg's university town, Altdorf. The observatory was a social hotspot for discussing as well as observing the weather and the sky, attracting medical doctors as well as astronomers.[64] Götz entered meteorological and astronomical observations in one of his medical note-books. He was closely connected to the Rost brothers, who published their observations of the skies in a journal.[65] Homann's father wrote and con-structed an astronomical atlas. Moreover, the society's printer, Michael Adelbulner, had studied mathematics, astronomy, and physics and had published, together with his father, observations by the mathematician and astronomer Johann Leonhard Rost.[66]

Botanical expertise was contributed by Trew and his family.[67] His father had developed such a deep interest in botanical issues that the famous Volk-amer family had established links, despite the fact that Trew's father lived as an apothecary in a small town in the territory of Nuremberg.[68] As Trew wrote to Huth in 1732, he had a "small garden" at his house in Nuremberg, which gave him the opportunity to cultivate "foreign plants for his information."[69] His private garden may have been better attended than the Hortus medicus of the Collegium Medicum, located in the former refectory of the Carthusians. Numerous garden palaces and garden houses outside the

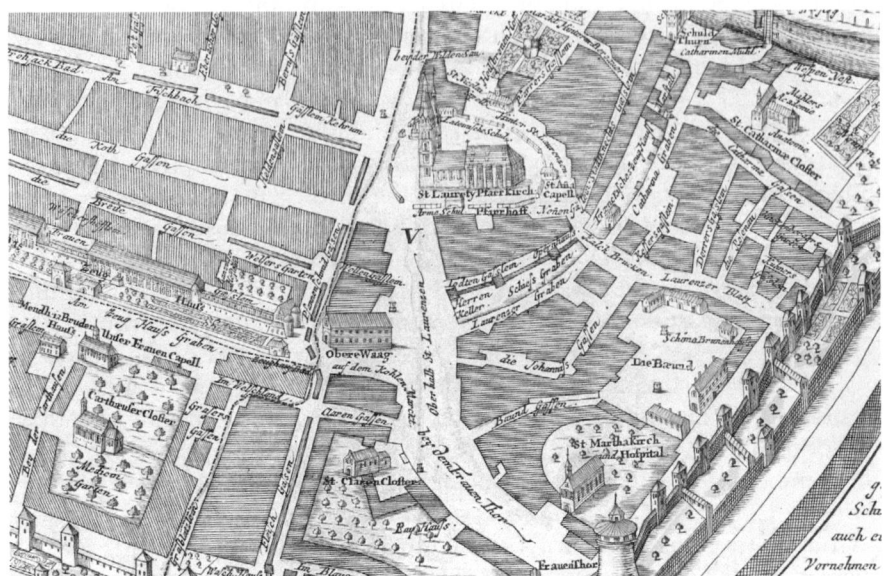

Figure 11.2 The topography of medical scientific Nuremberg in the eighteenth century featured a cluster in the parish of St. Lorenz, with the Collegium Medicum's "Medical Garden" (lower left) and "Anatomy" (upper right), Trew's house with its small garden and extensive library in the "Wespen Nest" behind "Anatomy," and the home of Götz in the "Breite Gasse" (middle left). Courtesy of Germanisches Nationalmuseum Nürnberg: Kupferstichkabinett, Sign. Kapsel 1039b, Sp. 6374.

walls of Nuremberg provided space for botanical experiments—and, as entries in Götz's medical notebook document, for sociable and informational encounters between scholars, patricians, and regional or traveling noblemen.[70] For the *Societas*, these were crucial opportunities for developing bonds with the social elite and future patrons.

Beyond making use of opportunities arising in and around institutions, members of the *Societas* in its early years shared other interests and had developed personal bonds that promised harmonious cooperation. Schulze taught Stock and Huth at Altdorf; Preißler and the printer Michael Adelbulner were friends. Academic valuation and pious association were often shared. By the early decades of the eighteenth century, religion in the form of pietism provided further commitment and deepened interdependence, not least because pietism was no longer sanctioned by the Nuremberg authorities but tolerated in those who did not openly confess. This is illustrated by the example of the well-known pietist preacher Ambrosius Wirth (1656–1723). He lost his office as pastor in a village in the territory of Nuremberg and was transferred to a minor office in the city, where he could be kept under observation by the authorities.[71] Members of the Nuremberg Collegium Medicum would not openly adhere to pietism but could quietly make use of the specific bonds provided by shared religious orientation. Wirth was one among several pietist patients of Götz who had also established family bonds with pietism and whose medical practice showed this religious influence.[72] He obviously shared his esteem for pietism with the printer of the *Commercium*. Adelbulner printed a catechism and a songbook by Wirth, along with many geographic and astrographic books.[73] His press also issued a book on the "exulants," a group exiled from Salzburg, whose cause was often taken up by pietist preachers.[74] The pietist medical professor in Halle and member of the Nuremberg Collegium Medicum, Michael Alberti (1682–1757), shared Götz's appraisal of Stahl's theories and was the academic teacher of Homann.[75] The closest link to pietism in Halle was provided by Schulze: he was raised in a pietistic orphanage by August Hermann Francke (1663–1727). In close connection to the pietist leader, Schulze also studied ancient and Arabic languages and then botany, anatomy, and alchemy.[76] The collaborative effort to produce the weekly journal needs to be viewed against this background of local opportunities and manifold personal bonds.

The weekly rhythm of the *Commercium* structured the workflow of its editorial board, the *Societas*. Members met every Wednesday at Trew's house, with its ever-growing library (Figure 11.3), to prepare and finalize material for that week's issue (always dated a Wednesday) and outline the next.[77] These meetings were open to outsiders, as a letter from Schulze to Trew reveals. In May 1734 Schulze wrote to Trew from Halle, saying that he had provided two medical doctors from Siebenbürgen and Hungary with letters of recommendation to Trew and requesting they be allowed to join the Wednesday meeting.[78] Thus editorial meetings served not only the selecting and shaping of written communication for print, but oral exchange as well, which could in turn be the beginning of fresh written exchange and gain new correspondents for the *Commercium*.[79] The editorial process, with its selecting, translating and perhaps even rewriting of texts submitted by contributors, cannot be fully reconstructed because contributors' letters are only partly preserved in the Trew letter collection. Thus, for example, it is not possible to define precisely the features of the general filter used by the members of the *Societas*. The *observationes* rubric included a broad range of subjects, such as anatomy, chemistry, physics, and pharmacy as well as epidemiology, meteorology, balneology, astronomical observations, and medical case studies. This range of subjects at least shows what the filter let through as *observationes*.[80] In the final section of this chapter, we compare an original letter with its printed version in the *Commercium* as an example of how information was changed by the editing process.

The next step in production of the *Commercium* took place in the printer's shop. The manuscript for the new issue was handed over to

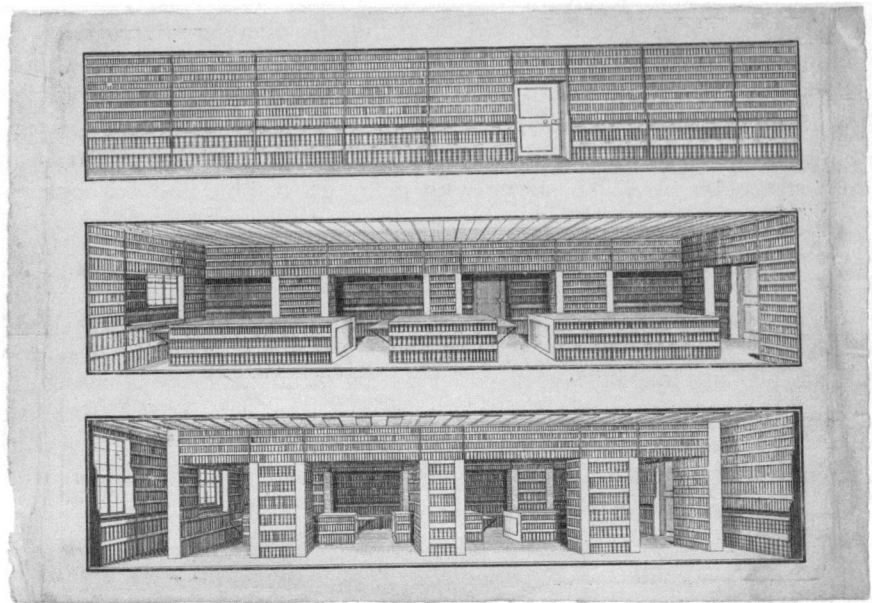

Figure 11.3 Physician Christoph Jacob Trew's private library in his house in Nuremberg in the Wespennest. Copperplate by Johann Michael Stock from an
original by Johann Christoph Keller, Nuremberg, ca. 1760. Courtesy of
Germanisches Nationalmuseum Nürnberg: Kupferstichkabinett, Sign.
Kapsel 1422, Ms. 155. Photograph: Georg Janßen.

Adelbulner's office. As soon as the typesetting was complete, a copy was
printed for proofreading—and presumably for the keen eyes of the censors
as well. Unfortunately, no sources exist on the handling of censorship in the
case of the *Commercium*. In general terms, however, we know that the
magistrate of the Imperial City of Nuremberg had decided in 1701 that journal editors should pay the censor an annual fee of 50 Gulden. Furthermore,
we know that one of the censors responsible for the *Commercium* was the
lawyer Philipp Ludwig Huth (1696–1752), the older brother of *Societas*
member Georg Leonhard. When this young physician returned to Nuremberg from his *peregrinatio academica*, he was appointed a member of the
Societas, thus providing a close familial bond to the Nuremberg censors.[81]

Distribution: Sending the *Commercium litterarium* into the World

Typesetting, proofreading, censoring, printing, and packing of the weekly issue
had to be completed by Saturday. This was the ideal dispatch day. Coaches
left, as described above, in all directions for destinations all the way to England

and Hungary, Vienna and Prague, from which further centers were served. Sundays saw *Commercium* bundles leaving for Imperial cities and places of distribution, such as Augsburg, Frankfurt, Lindau, Memmingen, and Munich. And the *ordinari* messengers could take smaller packages to Hamburg on Sunday and to Breslau and other places with no preset schedule.[82] As Tilman Rau argues, the far reach of the *Commericum*'s system of distribution is still evident today in the existence of complete editions of the journal in the libraries of Paris, Strasbourg, Naples, Florence, Rome, Basel, Neuchatel, Oxford, London, Helsinki, Stockholm, and many German cities.[83]

Every week, one sheet of paper, covered with nicely printed Latin text and neatly folded twice into *quarto* format, was produced for each subscriber of the journal and was directed to its destination. The *Societas* learned from the merchants' *Verlagssystem* how to solve this major logistical problem. The sheets of the *Commercium* did not leave Nuremberg individually to each subscriber. They were packed in bundles and sent to the assistants to be distributed in regional networks. To facilitate this process, the editors offered different frequencies of distribution, as a letter from Trew to a Berlin correspondent reveals: new subscribers were asked if they preferred to receive the *Commercium* in weekly, monthly, or even quarterly dispatches. As this departed from the idea of getting news at its newest, Trew suggested, first, providing the *lectores* in each city with a single weekly copy that could be circulated among them and, second, sending the rest of the copies for subscribers every quarter.[84]

Distributing the *Commercium* to its readers, the society's *assistentes* also dispatched readers' complaints back to Nuremberg. Complaints usually concerned delayed delivery of the annual supplements: *frontispicium, dedicatio, praefatio, recensio synoptica*, and three *indices*.[85] Subscribers needed these before handing over each year's worth of issues to a bookbinder. Binding the stack of loose sheets of weekly information into a solid volume transformed the temporality of the *Commercium* from dynamic carrier of news to reservoir of knowledge for an indefinite future. The bound volume could be handled like a book and thus also became potential merchandise for booksellers. However, subscribers often had to wait long into the following year. In 1733, for example, the supplements for 1732 still had not been distributed as late as May.[86] Pharmacist and naturalist Johann Heinrich Linck (1674–1734), who committed himself to being the society's assistant in Leipzig, wrote angrily to Götz about this. He had not only to appease impatient subscribers, but also to witness how tardiness was damaging the *Societas*. He had just tried to launch the *Commercium* at Leipzig's important Easter fair, without success:

> I would have been able to sell 10 of the *Commercio* 1732 to foreign book merchants if the title[-page] and the *praefatio* had been included. Nobody, however, wanted to buy an incomplete work. [...] You [i.e., the *Societas*] do yourself much harm [by this].[87]

This and many other complaints preserved in the Trew letter collection give the impression that the small *Societas*, which never really recovered from the early loss of Götz, Homann, and Preißler, was working at its limit just to process the weekly edition. Its members had no time to spare for writing the *dedicatio* and *praefatio* and compiling the *recensio synoptica* and the *indices* punctually, which must have been time-consuming tasks. Rau argues that failure to solve the problem of delayed supplements was one of the reasons for the *Commercium*'s abandonment at the close of 1745. The other reason was that Trew had been appointed *Director ephemeridum* of the Leopoldina in summer 1744 and could not manage the double task of editing both the *Commercium* and the Imperial Academy's *Acta physico-medica*.[88]

The Saxon Expedition to Africa: an Example

We close with an example from the *Commercium litterarium*. It illustrates how news was transmitted over a long distance and via different people until it reached the *Societas* in Nuremberg, passed through the editing process and, finally, was widely distributed as part of the printed journal.

Pharmacist and naturalist Linck, whom we just met as the *Commercium*'s assistant in Leipzig, was also a regular correspondent of Götz. Linck reported on his scientific work on starfish and sent Götz items of news, local and not so local. One of his favorite topics was the scientific expedition researching North Africa by order of August II (1670–1733), King of Poland and Elector of Saxony.[89] The head of the enterprise, the physician Johann Ernst Hebenstreit (1703–1757), sent reports of the journey to the Dresden Court. These became the talk of the day in learned circles. In a letter to Götz on 15 January 1733, Linck recounted that Hebenstreit's collection of 50 dried exotic fish skins for the king's cabinet of naturalia had arrived and had been prepared in the manner of a *herbarium vivum*.[90] This letter arrived in Nuremberg on January 26. The society selected the passage about Hebenstreit's fish collection, translated it into Latin for the *nova*, and published it on 4 February 1733 in the fifth weekly issue for that year.[91]

Linck's next letters contain interesting information about the political situation in Leipzig and Dresden after the death of August II of Saxony on 1 February 1733. Linck speculated that the successor to the throne might not be interested in continuing to support scientific enterprises and that Hebenstreit might have to return to Leipzig.[92] These political, speculative, personal, and fragmentary pieces of news, however, were not introduced into the *Commercium litterarium*.

On 27 May 1733, Linck was able to send a more detailed report about the expedition's fate, based on a letter from Hebenstreit written in Tunis on March 24. This letter was so detailed and interesting that Linck copied it as a report ("relation") for the readers of the *Commercium litterarium* and attached it to his letter.[93] This report was translated into Latin and published as a lengthy *nova* in the 24th weekly issue on 17 June 1733.[94] It describes Hebenstreit's departure from Tripoli in December 1732, his sailing via Lampedusa and Malta to Tunis, and the expedition from Tunis to the south, "right to the outermost boundaries of the inhabited lands."[95] Thus, over a period of about three months, news about ancient sites, exotic plants, and animals unknown in Europe traveled from North Africa to Dresden, was discussed in Leipzig, sent to Nuremberg, discussed and translated there by *Societas* members, multiplied in print, and then communicated to the greater part of the *Respublica litteraria*.

The original letters from Linck to Götz are preserved in the Trew letter collection. This makes it possible to compare them with their published versions, thus shedding light on the extent to which information was transformed in passing through the publishing process. Change in language was most obvious: the German text of the letters was translated into Latin, and some long sentences in the vernacular were reshaped into shorter ones. The content of the original text was transferred in its entirety into the Latin version. The editors changed it only by adding (1) an introductory sentence to the news about the dried fish skins, and (2) scientific nomenclature for some of the animals mentioned in the long report.[96] In one instance, Linck had chosen slightly disrespectful language when speaking about Hebenstreit's expedition. The editors put this more courteously in Latin.[97] At least in the case of Linck's letters, the editing process did not change the content of the text but shifted it slightly into a more scientific and respectful language. Praising the activity of Hebenstreit in Africa, the *Societas* signaled their common aim: collecting and distributing scientific data.

In sum, an eighteenth-century society of town physicians sharing interests and values created a novel information enterprise by seizing opportunities provided by the Imperial City of Nuremberg. They translated the economically successful *Verlag* model of production and trade into the world of publishing medical and scientific news. This collaborative effort of continuous, fast-paced production in Nuremberg was made possible not only by the city's institutions and resources, but also by more personal characteristics, such as scholarly interests and religious orientation. It depended on individual physicians' networks of correspondence, yet merged these in a new, less personal, more publicly oriented way. Whereas physician translators and publishers in seventeenth-century London, as Elaine Leong shows in Chapter 10 of this volume, created new medical publics and communities of knowledge by turning a Latin book of university lectures into an English-language household book, the Nuremberg physicians created a more united and up-to-date, novelty-valuing scholarly public by turning sundry vernacular news and individual correspondence into that unique product and medium, a Latin weekly.

Notes

Acknowledgments: The research for this collaborative chapter began in Ingolstadt with the project Ärztliche Praxis im frühen 18. Jahrhundert: Der Nürnberger Arzt Johann Christoph Götz (1688–1733), funded by the DFG (Deutsche Forschungsgemeinschaft), under the direction of Marion Maria Ruisinger, and was continued in the ERC-funded project Ways of Writing: How Physicians Know 1550–1950, under the direction of Volker Hess and Andrew Mendelsohn in Berlin. The chapter benefited greatly from comments and discussions by participants in the three workshops leading up to this volume. We are much indebted to Harun Küçük and Sebastian Kühn for their supportive and critical review as commentators during the final workshop.

1   Tilman T.R. Rau, *Das Commercium litterarium: Die erste medizinische Wochenschrift in Deutschland und die Anfänge des medizinischen Journalismus* (Bremen, 2009); for the remarkable duration of the journal, pp. 29–30.
2   On Trew, see especially Thomas Schnalke, *Medizin im Brief: Der städtische Arzt des 18. Jahrhunderts im Spiegel seiner Korrespondenz* (Stuttgart, 1997).
3   For example, Rau provided little information about the first director of the journal, the medical doctor Johann Christoph (erroneously Christian) Götz; Rau, *Commercium*, pp. 46–47. Götz has now been identified as publisher of a medical journal and author of several thousand pages of medical notebooks.
4   These projects are the above-mentioned DFG-funded project Ärztliche Praxis, as well as a number of dissertations at the Friedrich-Alexander-Universität Erlangen-Nürnberg under the co-direction of Marion Maria Ruisinger.
5   Pamela H. Smith, "Knowledge in Motion: Following Itineraries of Matter in the Early Modern World," in Daniel T. Rodgers, Bhavani Raman, and Helmut Reimitz (eds), *Cultures in Motion* (Princeton, 2014): 109–33.
6   Thomas Schnalke, "Collegium Medicum Norimbergense" in Michael Diefenbacher and Rudolf Endres (eds), *Stadtlexikon Nürnberg* (Nuremberg, 1999), p. 187; Fritz Dross, "Vom zuverlässigen Urteilen: Ärztliche Autorität, reichsstädtische Ordnung und der Verlust 'armer Glieder Christi' in der Nürnberger Sondersiechenschau," *Medizin Gesellschaft und Geschichte*, 29 (2010): 9–46, pp. 9–15.
7   For a German translation of the title, see Rau, *Commercium*, p. 43.
8   Adam Friedrich Kirsch, *Adami Friderici Kirschii Abvndantissimvm Cornvcopiae Lingvae Latinae Et Germanicae Selectvm [...] Editio Qvinta, Prioribus multo correctior & auctior* (Nuremberg, 1731), p. 246.
9   Rau, *Commercium*, pp. 44–49.
10 Lorraine Daston, "The Moral Economy of Science," *Osiris*, 10 (1995): 2–24, pp. 13–14; Steven Shapin, "The House of Experiment in Seventeenth-Century England," *Isis*, 79 (1988): 373–404.
11 For the business connotation of *Societas* in 1730s Nuremberg and for *sumptibus* referring to jointly investing or spending money, see Kirsch, *Cornvcopiae Lingvae Latinae*, pp. 1009, 1050.
12 Georg Andreas Will, *Geschichte und Beschreibung der Nürnbergischen Landstadt Altdorf* (Altdorf, 1796).
13 For a short biography of Schulze and an annotated edition of his correspondence with Trew, see Heidrun Mitzel-Kaoukhov, *Die Briefe Johann Heinrich Schulzes (1687–1744) an Christoph Jacob Trew* (Diss. med. Erlangen, 2011).
14 Mitzel-Kaoukhov, *Schulze*, p. 23.
15 Mitzel-Kaoukhov (*Schulze*, pp. 94–95) stresses the importance of Schulze, whereas Rau (*Commercium*, p. 48) argues against it.

16 Academiae Cesareae Leopoldino-Carolinae, *Acta Physico Medica [...] Ephemerides sive observationes[...]* (Norimbergae, 1727), Catalogus No. 391.

17 Susan Splinter, *"Der aufrichtige Medicus*: Eine Zeitschrift des Nürnberger Arztes Johann Christoph Götz (1688–1733) als Vorläufer des *Commercium Litterarium*," *Jahrbuch für Kommunikationsgeschichte*, 13 (2011): 5–15.

18 "Merito est, quod parentem directoremque et amplificatorem nominemus optimum et locupletem"; quoted in Rau, *Commercium*, p. 47.

19 Marion Mücke and Thomas Schnalke, *Briefnetz Leopoldina: Die Korrespondenz der Deutschen Akademie der Naturforscher um 1750* (Berlin, 2009), pp. 49–60.

20 Rau, *Commercium*, p. 48.

21 Johann Kanold, *Sammlung von Natur- und Medicin: Wie auch hierzu gehörigen Kunst- und Literatur-Geschichten [...]*, 1–38 plus 4 Suppl. (1717–26); Royal Society of London, *Philosophical Transactions [...]* (1665–), consulted using ISTOR Reprint 1963.

22 The editors decided not to publish the *observationes* of Johann Friedrich Glaser, citing their lack of Latin style; Ruth Schilling, *Johann Friedrich Glaser (1707–1789): Scharfrichtersohn und Stadtphysikus in Suhl* (Cologne, 2015), pp. 167–68.

23 Mücke and Schnalke, *Leopoldina*, pp. 21–28.

24 Trew: "... anderen journalisten u[nd] collectoribus, ... das meinste [sic] sehr spat erst communiciret wird und dahero als eine novität, die doch nicht alleine angenehm ist, sondern auch offt ihren besondern Nutzen hat, nicht mehr passiren kan." Trew also emphasized that the group would publish only "the new and special" parts of received "observationes," which later might appear in full in already established journals. Letter of Trew to Caspar Neumann, draft, ca. 1731 (Universitätsbibliothek Erlangen-Nürnberg, Briefsammlung Trew [hereafter: UBE BT], Trew 581).

25 Michael Diefenbacher, "Verlagswesen," in *Stadtlexikon*, p. 1135.

26 Stadtarchiv Nürnberg (hereafter: StadtAN) B12 and E5/1; Herbert Maschat, *Technik, Energie und Verlagswesen: Das Beispiel der spätmittelalterlichen Reichsstadt Nürnberg* (Munich, 1988).

27 Lore Sporhan-Krempel and Wolfgang von Stromer, "Das Handelshaus der Stromer von Nürnberg und die Geschichte der ersten deutschen Papiermühle," *Vierteljahreshefte für Sozial- und Wirtschaftsgeschichte* 47 (1960): 81–104.

28 Kanold, *Sammlung* (1717–18), preface.

29 Landeskirchliches Archiv der Evangelisch-Lutherischen Kirche in Bayern, Nuremberg: St. Lorenz Taufen Sign. L_26, fol. 523 (researched by Susan Splinter); St. Sebald Taufen S_011, 932; Annemarie Kinzelbach, Kay Peter Jankrift, and Marion Maria Ruisinger, "Arztpraxis im frühneuzeitlichen Nürnberg: Johann Christoph Götz (1688–1733)" *Jahrbuch für fränkische Landeskunde*, 72 (2012): 123–49, p. 134.

30 Leopoldina-Archiv MS 359, 1. Mark Häberlein, "Botanisches Wissen, ökonomischer Nutzen und sozialer Aufstieg im 16. Jahrhundert: Der Augsburger Arzt und Orientreisende Leonhard Rauwolf," in Gernot M. Müller (ed.), *Humanismus und Renaissance in Augsburg: Kulturgeschichte einer Stadt zwischen Spätmittelalter und Dreissigjährigem Krieg* (Berlin, 2010): 101–17, pp. 103–04.

31 For social and symbolic capital, see Kay-Peter Jankrift, Annemarie Kinzelbach, and Marion M. Ruisinger, "Ernst von Metternich (1656–1727): Ein patientenzentrierter Einblick in den medizinischen Markt um 1720," *Gesnerus*, 69 (2012): 12–35, pp. 29–32; for scholarly values, see Daston, "Economy," pp. 4–6.

32 For the difficulty of getting published, see Ian Maclean, *Scholarship, Commerce, Religion: The Learned Book in the Age of Confessions, 1560–1630* (Cambridge, MA, 2012), pp. 47–48.

33 For the latter, see Walter Bauernfeind, "Reichsstadt," in *Stadtlexikon*, p. 877.

34 Lore Sporhan-Krempel, *Nürnberg als Nachrichtenzentrum zwischen 1400 und 1700* (Nuremberg, 1968), pp. 21–30; Joseph Paul Nigrino, *Verzeichnus der Republic Nürnberg Regenten, Beamten und Bedienten, sowohl in der Stadt als auf dem Land* (Freyburg, 1732–1733), pp. 137–80; see generally Sheilagh C. Ogilvie, *Institutions and European Trade: Merchant Guilds, 1000–1800* (Cambridge, 2011), pp. 344–90.

35 Michael Diefenbacher, Wiltrud Fischer-Pache, and Manfred H. Grieb (eds), *Das Nürnberger Buchgewerbe: Buch- und Zeitungsdrucker, Verleger und Druckhändler vom 16. bis zum 18. Jahrhundert* (Nuremberg, 2003); the censoring council forced some printers to print anonymously and without giving the place of printing, Sporhan-Krempel, *Nürnberg*, pp. 67–71.

36 Manfred H. Grieb, *Nürnberger Künstlerlexikon* (Munich, 2007); Georg Andreas Will, *Nürnbergisches Gelehrten-Lexicon [...]* (Nuremberg, 1755), vol. 1, pp. 3–6.

37 Survey of the 50 Adelbulner imprints for the period 1701 to 1736 preserved in the Bavarian State Library (BSB); including a bulky, anonymous booklike journal *Das Neueste von der Zeit [...]* (Nuremberg, 1703); Christoph Jacob Trew, *Beschreibung der Grossen Americanischen Aloe [...]* (Nuremberg, 1727).

38 He named the editors and several assistants as supporters; Michael Adelbulner, *Commercium litterarium: ad astronomiae incrementum inter huius scientiae amatores communi consilio institutum* (Norimbergae, 1735), preface.

39 Gábor Almási, *The Uses of Humanism: Johannes Sambucus (1531–1584), Andreas Dudith (1533–1589), and the Republic of Letters in East Central Europe* (Leiden, 2009); Laurence W. B. Brockliss, *Calvet's Web: Enlightenment and the Republic of Letters in Eighteenth-Century France* (Oxford, 2002).

40 See recently the special issue edited by Harold J. Cook and Timothy D. Walker and their introduction, "Circulation of Medicine in the Early Modern Atlantic World," *Social History of Medicine*, 26 (2013): 337–51, quotation on p. 344.

41 Thomas Schnalke, "Sammeln und Vernetzen: Christoph Jacob Trew (1695–1769) in seiner botanischen Matrix," in Regina Dauser et al. (eds), *Wissen im Netz: Botanik und Pflanzentransfer in europäischen Korrespondenznetzen des 18. Jahrhunderts* (Berlin, 2008): 172–200, pp. 175–79; Annemarie Kinzelbach, Susanne Grosser, Kay P. Jankrift, and Marion M. Ruisinger "*Observationes et Curationes Noribergenses*: Die Praxis von Johann Christoph Götz (1688–1733)" in Martin Dinges et al. (eds), *Medical Practice, 1600–1900: Physicians and Their Patients* (Leiden, 2016).

42 Rau, *Commercium*, pp. 58–59.

43 For an annotated edition of the correspondence between Ehrhart and Trew, see Ruth Heinzelmann, *Johann Balthasar Ehrhart (1700–1756) und seine Korrespondenz mit Christoph Jacob Trew (1695–1769)* (Diss. med. Erlangen, 2011).

44 Letter from Ehrhart to Trew, 17 January 1731 (UBE BT, Ehrhart 1); Heinzelmann, *Ehrhart*, pp. 23–24, 73.

45 Trew's letter was written on 18 January 1731 and is not preserved in the UBE BT; Heinzelmann, *Ehrhart*, pp. 23–24, 74.

46 *Commercium litterarium* 1 (1731), *Consultatio* 1730, Nov. 20; see Rau, *Commercium*, pp. 55–56.

47 UBE BT, Trew 379.

48 "Assistentes [...] in magnis vrbibus, vbi commerciis cum vicinis colendis occasio [...] suppetit"; *Commercium litterarium* 1 (1731), *Consultatio* 1730, Nov. 20.

49 *Commercium litterarium* (1731), preface.

50 *Acta physico-medica Academiae Caesareae Leopoldino-Carolinae Naturae Curiosorum [...]*, 50 (1740), IL Catalogus 465; *Commercium litterarium* (1733), preface.

51 Rau, *Commercium*, p. 64.
52 Letter from Trew to Huth, 28 July 1729, draft, UBE BT, Trew 376.
53 Presumably these printed pages were the *Consultatio* and *Ulterior consultatio*; letter of Trew to Huth, before 14 February 1731, draft, UBE BT, Trew 377.
54 UBE BT, Trew 377.
55 Letter from Trew to Huth, 30 January 1733, draft, UBE BT, Trew 379.
56 Johann Christoph Götz, "Relatio de effectu medicinae cuiusdam antipodagricae," *Commercium litterarium* (1731): 172–74. Many thanks to Conrad-Jakob Schiffner for translating this text.
57 Stephan Goldschmidt, *Johann Konrad Dippel (1673–1734)* (Göttingen, 2001); for Carl and Dippel, see Christa Habrich, *Untersuchungen zur pietistischen Medizin und ihrer Ausprägung bei Johann Samuel Carl (1677–1757) und seinem Kreis* (Habil. TU Munich, 1981), pp. 51–54.
58 Nigrino, *Verzeichnus*, pp. 140–80.
59 We thank Anna Hofmann for providing us with her transcription of the Götz-Trew correspondence.
60 UBE BT, Albrecht 1, Fritsch 2, Webel 1, Fritsch 1, Linck 1–7, Huth 4.
61 Adelbulner, *Commercium*.
62 Staatsarchiv Nürnberg Rst N, *Medicinalordnung Nuernberg 1700: Erneuerte Gesetz und Ordnung Eines Hoch Edlen und Hochweissen Raths [...] Dem Collegio Medico, den Apotheckern [...]* (Nuremberg, 1700); Mitzel-Kaoukhov, *Schulze*.
63 Will, *Gelehrten-Lexicon*, vol. 1, pp. 3–4; vol. 2, p. 4; vol. 4, pp. 65–67; Christoph Gottlieb von Murr, *Beschreibung der vornehmsten Merkwürdigkeiten in der Reichsstadt Nürnberg*, 2nd edn. (Nuremberg, 1801), 383–86; Christoph Jacob Trew, *Vertheidigung der Anatomie ... Auf dem Nürnbergischen Theatro Anatomico bey öffentlichen Demonstrationibus eines Männlichen Cörpers den 21. Jan. A. 1728 vorgetragen* (Nuremberg, 1729); Thomas Schnalke, "Anatomie für alle! Trew und sein Projekt eines anatomischen Tafelwerks," in Thomas Schnalke (ed.), *Natur im Bild: Anatomie und Botanik in der Sammlung des Nürnberger Arztes Christoph Jacob Trew* (Erlangen, 1995), 53–73.
64 Will, *Gelehrten-Lexicon*, vol. 1, pp. 333–37; vol. 3, pp. 397–401; vol. 4, pp. 58–60.
65 UBE Ms 1200/1, 15, 17, 20, 24, 28, 31 ff., Ms 1200/2, 256 (last entry). For Nuremberg meteorology, astronomy, and the Rost brothers, see Kanold, *Sammlung*, vol. 8 for 1719 (1720), 381–757, p. 390, and subsequent volumes. The astronomer Rost was Götze's patient; the astronomer's brother, a medical doctor, collaborated with Götz; see Kinzelbach, Grosser, Jankrift, and Ruisinger, *"Observationes et Curationes."*
66 Will, *Gelehrten-Lexicon*, vol. 1, pp. 196–98; Johann Leonhard Rost, *Warhafte, ... Beschreibung desjenigen ... Nordscheines, der sich An. 1721 Sonnabends den 1. Martii ... zu Nürnberg ... hat sehen lassen ...* (Nuremberg, 1721).
67 For botanical themes in the *Commercium*, see Tilman Rau, "Das 'Commercium Litterarium' ein 'Commercium plantarum'? Botanischer Wissensaustausch in der ersten medizinischen Wochenschrift Deutschlands," in: Arbeitskreis Orangerien in Deutschland e.V. (ed.), *Nürnbergische Hesperiden und Orangeriekultur in Franken* (Petersberg, 2011), 117–27.
68 Will, *Gelehrten-Lexicon*, vol. 4, 60–67; Johann Christoph Volkamer, *Nürnbergische Hesperides ...* (Nuremberg, 1708).
69 Letter from Trew to Huth, 17 November 1732, draft, UBE BT, Trew 378; botanical topics also played a major role in Trew's correspondence with Heister; Marion Maria Ruisinger and Thomas Schnalke, "Der Lehrer und sein Schüler: Die Korrespondenz zwischen Lorenz Heister und Christoph Jacob

Trew," *Gesnerus, 61*, special issue on Medical Correspondence in Early Modern Europe (2004): 198–231.

70 Volkamer, *Hesperides*; Kinzelbach, Grosser, Jankrift, and Ruisinger, "*Observationes.*"

71 Horst Weigelt, "Der Pietismus in Bayern," in Martin Brecht and Hartmut Lehmann (eds), *Geschichte des Pietismus: Der Pietismus im achtzehnten Jahrundert* (Göttingen, 1995), vol. 2, 296–318, p. 302.

72 Kinzelbach, Jankrift, and Ruisinger, "Arztpraxis," pp. 130, 137, 142–43.

73 Ambrosius Wirth, *Neu-eingerichtetes und vermehrtes Geistliches Blumen- und Würtz-Gärtlein* ... (Nuremberg, 1725); Ambrosius Wirth, *Einfältige Anweisung Für diejenigen, welche der zarten, und mit dem theuren Blut Christi erkaufften Jugend, den kleinen Catechismum Lutheri beybringen sollen* ... (Nuremberg, 1714).

74 Georg Jeremias Hoffmann, *Abrahams Emigranten-Stab, oder das Erbauliche Exempel Abrahams, für Christliche Emigranten* (Nuremberg, 1732); James Horn van Melton, "Pietism, Print Culture, and Salzburg Protestantism on the Eve of Expulsion," in Jonathan Strom, Hartmut Lehmann, and James Horn van Melton (eds), *Pietism in Germany and North America, 1680–1820* (Farnham, 2009), 229–49, p. 229.

75 Some members of the Collegium Medicum were not resident in Nuremberg: Nigrino, *Verzeichnus*, p. 108; on Alberti, see Jürgen Helm, *Krankheit, Bekehrung und Reform* (Tübingen, 2006), p. 43.

76 Mitzel-Kaoukhov, *Schulze*, pp. 16–21.

77 Schulze refered to this meeting as their "Mittwochs-Konvent": Letter from Schulze to Trew, 15 May 1734 (UBE BT, Schulze 63), cited by Mitzel-Kaoukhov, *Schulze*, pp. 71, 249; UBE BT, Stock 2.

78 UBE BT, Schulze 63.

79 "I do not doubt that both will be very ready for correspondence"; UBE BT, Schulze 63.

80 Rau, *Commercium*, pp. 114–15.

81 Rau, *Commercium*, p. 85.

82 Nigrino, *Verzeichnus*, pp. 139–41, 151–52, 164–65, 172–73.

83 Rau, *Commercium*, p. 69.

84 UBE BT, Trew 581.

85 Rau, *Commercium*, p. 181.

86 Letter from Linck to Götz, 13 May 1733, UBE BT, Linck 5.

87 UBE BT, Linck 5.

88 Rau, *Commercium*, pp. 93–96; Mücke and Schnalke, *Briefnetz*, p. 60.

89 For another perspective on physicians in Saxony-Poland at this time, see Schilling, "Physical City," Chapter 9 of this volume.

90 Letter from Linck to Götz, 15 January 1733 (UBE BT, Linck 1).

91 *Commercium litterarium* 3 (1733), p. 35.

92 UBE BT, Linck 5.

93 Letter from Linck to Götz, 27 May 1733; UBE BT, Linck 6.

94 *Commercium litterarium* 3 (1733), pp. 185–87.

95 UBE BT, Linck 6.

96 For example, *Sechs Antelopen oder Gazellen* (six antelopes or gazelles) was translated into *ex genere caprarum silvestrium, quas Antelopen, seu Gazellen vocant, sex* ("of the species *caprarum silvestrium*, which are called antelopes or gazelles, six"); UBE BT, Linck 6, and *Commercium litterarium* 3 (1733), p. 186.

97 "Er [Hebenstreit] streiche das Land durch" (he is crisscrossing the country) was translated as "terram a se diligentissimo studio perquiri" (the country was searched by him with utmost zeal); UBE BT, Linck 6, and *Commercium litterarium* 3 (1733), p. 185.

Index

Page numbers followed by *f* indicate figures; page numbers followed by *t* indicate tables.